Case Studies in Global Health: Millions Saved

Ruth Levine, PhD
and the What Works Working Group

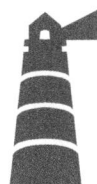

JONES & BARTLETT
LEARNING

World Headquarters
Jones & Bartlett Learning
40 Tall Pine Drive
Sudbury, MA 01776
978-443-5000
info@jblearning.com
www.jblearning.com

Jones & Bartlett Learning books and products are available through most bookstores and online booksellers. To contact Jones & Bartlett Learning directly, call 800-832-0034, fax 978-443-8000, or visit our website www.jblearning.com.

Substantial discounts on bulk quantities of Jones & Bartlett Learning publications are available to corporations, professional associations, and other qualified organizations. For details and specific discount information, contact the special sales department at Jones & Bartlett Learning via the above contact information or send an email to specialsales@jblearning.com.

Production Credits
Publisher: Michael Brown
Production Director: Amy Rose
Associate Production Editor: Rachel Rossi
Associate Editor: Katey Birtcher
Marketing Manager: Sophie H. Fleck
Manufacturing Buyer: Therese Connell
Composition: Shawn Girsberger
Cover Design: Kristin E. Ohlin
Senior Photo Researcher and Photographer: Kimberly Potvin
Associate Photo Researcher and Photographer: Christine McKeen
Illustrations: Louis Ochoa
Printing and Binding: Malloy, Inc.
Cover Printing: John P. Pow Company

Library of Congress Cataloging-in-Publication Data
Levine, Ruth, 1959-
  Case studies in global health : millions saved / Ruth Levine and the What Works Working Group.
    p. ; cm.
  Rev. ed. of: Millions saved. c2004.
  Includes bibliographical references and index.
  ISBN-13: 978-0-7637-4620-9
  ISBN-10: 0-7637-4620-7
  1. World health. 2. Public health--Developing countries. I. Levine, Ruth, 1959- Millions saved. II. What Works Working Group. III. Title.
  [DNLM: 1. World Health. 2. Developing Countries. 3. Public Health Administration. WA 530.1 L665c 2007]
  RA441.L48 2007
  362.1--dc22
                            2006030012

6048
Printed in the United States of America
17 16 15 14 13   10

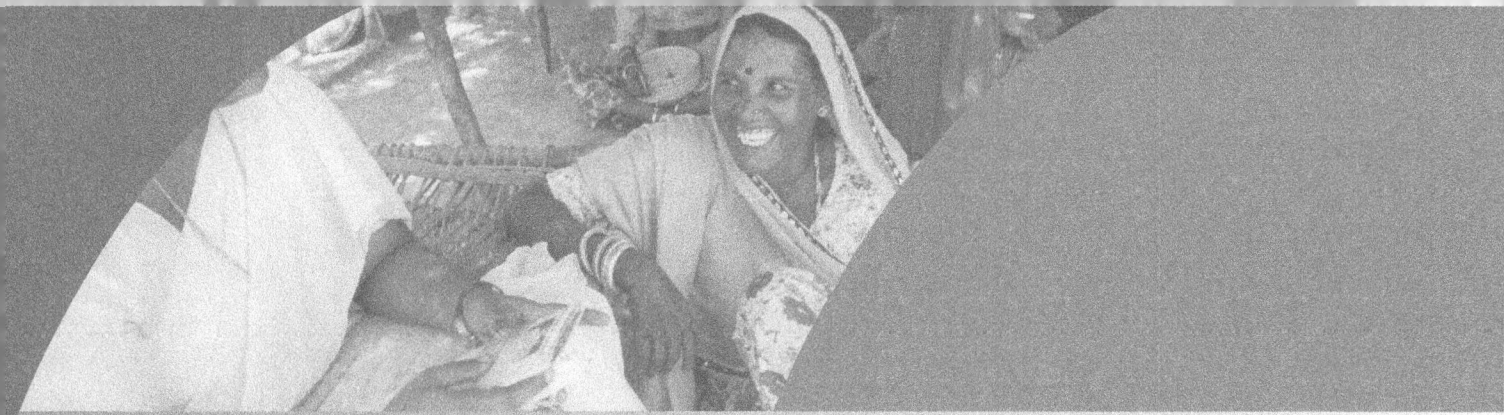

Dedication

Dedicated to
public health workers around the world,
who save lives every day

Table of Contents

Tables

Figures

Boxes

Prologue

The issues of global health have finally arrived in the consciousness of the developed world through a unique union of efforts by former presidents, software pioneers, and rock stars. It is now time that students have a textbook and accompanying casebook that systematically lead them through the issues of global health from basic principles, to the burden of disease, to examples of successful efforts to improve lives and livelihoods.

Ruth Levine's text, *Case Studies in Global Health: Millions Saved,* and Richard Skolnik's *Essentials of Global Health* completely and artfully fulfill this need. Both authors bring to their writing the clarity of thought and organization of scholars, the excitement of storytellers, and the commitment of activists to making a difference. Their casebook/book bundle takes the big picture population health perspective, building upon classic public health principles and extending them to include the impact of the health care system and the relationship of health to social and economic development.

Global health belongs as an integral part of public health education as taught in schools and programs in Public Health. In addition, the global health curriculum needs to reach beyond public health students to the future educated citizens who will make a difference in global health as clinicians, health administrators, lawyers, business executives, academics, politicians, etc., all of whom will shape the world's future from global trade to international migration to environmental sustainability. Levine and Skolnik's casebook and book are, in many ways, designed to ensure that in the future the educated citizenry from Wall Street to Main Street understands public health issues and their impact on all of our lives.

I am proud that Levine's and Skolnik's efforts are part of our **Essential Public Health** series. The materials included in their books have been carefully coordinated with other books in the series to ensure that they utilize the same definitions and terminology. The content of the books has also been coordinated across the series to provide only intended overlap. You will find many of these books key to broadening and deepening your understanding of public health and global health. The full list of materials in the **Essential Public Health** series can be found at http://www.jbpub .com/essentialpublichealth.

I am confident that you will enjoy learning from the work of Levine and Skolnik. They bring to you the world of global health and arrange it before you so it makes sense. The links between health and social and economic development are indisputable and fascinating. You will find an abundance of examples of ways that you can impact global health as part of your career, no matter in which direction you head. The authors take you on an adventurous journey through the world of global health. Enjoy the ride.

Richard Riegelman, MD, MPH, PhD
Series Editor—Essential Public Health

The Essential Public Health Series

Log on to *www.jbpub.com/essentialpublichealth* for the most current information on availability.

CURRENT AND FORTHCOMING TITLES IN THE ESSENTIAL PUBLIC HEALTH SERIES:

ABOUT THE EDITOR:

Richard K. Riegelman, MD, MPH, PhD, is Professor of Epidemiology-Biostatistics, Medicine, and Health Policy, and Founding Dean of The George Washington University School of Public Health and Health Services in Washington, DC. He has taken a lead role in developing the Educated Citizen and Public Health initiative which has brought together arts and sciences and public health education associations to implement the Institute of Medicine of the National Academies' recommendation that "…all undergraduates should have access to education in public health." Dr. Riegelman also led the development of George Washington's undergraduate major and minor and currently teaches "Public Health 101" and "Epidemiology 101" to undergraduates.

Foreword

There is little doubt about the magnitude of the problems: Combined, AIDS, malaria, and tuberculosis kill 6 million people each year in developing countries, and another 7 million children die of infectious diseases that have long been forgotten in the rich world. This represents both the humanitarian tragedy of lives cut short and the loss of productivity that puts a drag on economic growth.

Does anything really work to solve profound health problems that face poor countries? Does development assistance from rich countries make any difference at all?

Under the auspices of the Center for Global Development's Global Health Policy Research Network, we invited 15 experts in international health, development economics, public policy, and other relevant fields to identify and examine experiences of large-scale success in international health—national, regional, or global programs that worked to improve health. To find those cases, we collaborated with the Disease Control Priorities Project of the National Institutes of Health and solicited nominations from many of the world's leading health authorities. The conclusions of the "What's Worked in Global Health" Working Group leave little doubt that some efforts to save lives and livelihoods through health interventions have worked and have done so at remarkably low cost compared with the benefits.

Published in 2004, *Millions Saved: Proven Success in Global Health*, told the stories of 17 of these successes. This casebook serves as an updated edition with three entirely new cases, revised data, and supplementary information. These 20 success stories (or, more formally, the evidence-based cases) show that major public health efforts can and have changed the world for the better—well beyond what would have occurred through income growth alone. The magnitude and profundity of current health challenges facing the developing world—from AIDS to chronic malnutrition to the looming threat of tobacco-related cancers—can seem daunting. But past challenges have been surmounted and serve as object lessons: Even in countries with few financial resources and limited health infrastructure, sensible and systematic efforts to improve health have worked.

Looking toward the future, the stories told here suggest essential elements of success. At a time when the international community is scanning the horizon for hints about how to "scale-up" health programs and systems to accelerate progress toward better health for the world's poorest children and their parents, a close look at these successes can tell us what factors may need to be in place today—individually or in combination—to increase the chances that "scaling-up" will work.

This effort puts to rest the notion that nothing works in global health. But it raises new challenges to tackle: The first is how we make sure there are more and even bigger successes in the future. If the humanitarian impetus isn't enough, surely the knowledge that economic progress is hastened by health improvements should spur scientists, public health workers, government officials, and funders to action. The second is how we make sure that we know what works and what doesn't. Rigorous evaluation should no longer be seen as an optional academic add-on to major programs. It should be required so that both successful and failed experiences yield knowledge for smarter policymaking and program design in the future. Only with high-quality evaluation will we have a credible basis for claiming the effectiveness of foreign assistance. (Those interested in the opportunities to improve evaluation may wish to read *When Will We Ever Learn: Improving Lives through Impact Evaluation*; CGD 2006.)

I invite you to dip into this book—to learn a bit more about how people and institutions have worked together in impressive ways to save lives. This is inspiration for the challenges ahead.

Nancy Birdsall
President
Center for Global Development

Acknowledgments

This casebook, which started as the 2004 volume *Millions Saved: Proven Successes in Global Health* (Center for Global Development), owes both its inception and its completion to the contributions of many. We would first like to offer profound thanks to the members of the What Works Working Group, who took on the challenge of selecting success cases and who scrutinized every word to ensure that both tone and substance were appropriate. Our discussions about the criteria for success, the quality of the evidence base, and the commonalities across cases infused the work with a strong sense of purpose. And, although invisible to readers, the cases excluded and the conclusions discarded for lack of evidence are testimony to how seriously the Working Group members took their charge. Working Group members are profiled in the About the Authors section. We would also like to thank the editors of the Disease Control Priorities Project, whose close collaboration has guided our work since the very early days of the project. Furthermore, we are grateful to the authors of *Disease Control Priorities in Developing Countries*, 2nd edition (2006), who nominated success cases and shared expertise on each of the book's chapters.

Thanks are also due to several writers, who drafted cases, including Gail Vines, Jane Seymour, and Elaine Richman, and in particular to Phyllida Brown. We are also grateful to Ayesha Siddiqui, who devoted a summer internship to this project, and to Morissa Malkin, Steve Fishman, Nancy Hancock, Valerie Norville, Marla Banov, Madona Devasahayam, and Paul Karner, who contributed to the original book.

We thank Bruce Benton for his valuable additions to the onchocerciasis case in this version, and Disha Shah for her contributions to the new text boxes appearing in this edition. We thank Disha and her fellow students at George Washington University, Dawn Pepin, Edward Morgan, and Ami Joglekar, for excellent background research that provided a foundation for drafting new cases.

Many reviewers helped us to accurately represent both the central elements of each case and the nuances. The reviewers include Richard Adegbola, Mercy Ahun, Dariush Akhavan, Robin Biellik, Maureen Birmingham, David Brandling-Bennett, Joel Breman, Tim Brown, Jesse Bump, Donald Bundy, Flavia Bustreo, Sandy Cairncross, Anupong Chitwarakorn, Joseph Cook, Felicity Cutts, Isabel Danel, Lola Dare, Joy de Beyer, David DeFerranti, Ciro de Quadros, Shanta Devarajan, Chris Dye, Saskia Estupinan, Christa Fischer, William Foege, Olivier Fontaine, Kevin Frick, Rae Galloway, Suzanne Gilbert, Renato Gusmao, Ken Gustavsen, Davidson Gwatkin, Ross Hammond, DA Henderson, Eva Hertrampf, Janet Hohnen, Donald Hopkins, Robin Houston, Prabhat Jha, Jacob Kumaresan, Orin Levine, Jerker Liljestrand, Elizabeth Lule, Tom Merrick, Philip Musgrove, Luke Nkinsi, David Olson, Gordon Perkin, Frank Richards, Juan Rivera, Wiwat Rojanapithayakorn, Ebrahim Samba, Gabriel Schmunis, Christopher Schofield, Paul Schultz, Adelaide Shearley, Ram Shrestha, Werasit Sittitrai, Peter Small, Alfredo Jose Solari, Jonathan Struthers, Varachai Thongthai, RD Thulasiraj, Ernesto Ruiz Tiben, Corne van Walbeek, Judith Watt, Diana Weil, Keith West,

Derek Yach, Zaida Yadon, and Witold Zatonski. We also benefited from the published reviews of the original *Millions Saved* text, which were written by Brian Bilchik, Henry Mosley, Robert Northrup, James Phillips, and Robert Trautman. All remaining errors remain the responsibility of the authors.

Our colleagues at the Center for Global Development have been generous with their suggestions, constructive critiques, and moral support. We would particularly like to thank CGD President Nancy Birdsall, as well as Maureen Lewis, Sheila Herrling, Sarah Lucas, Lawrence MacDonald, and Steve Radelet.

Molly Kinder worked on the original *Millions Saved* and devoted the better part of two years to finding the cases, supporting the working group in all phases, and drafting several chapters. Jessica Gottlieb joined the Center for Global Development in 2005 and took on the challenge of updating the material and drafting two new chapters. Their intelligence, professionalism, and spirit infuse each and every page of this book.

Finally, we are grateful to the Bill & Melinda Gates Foundation for financial support and technical feedback—and particularly to Blair Sachs, who showed unflagging enthusiasm for this project, and Raj Shah for setting this in motion when he asked the question, "So, what's worked?"

About the Authors and Contributors

Ruth Levine, PhD, is a Senior Fellow and Director of Programs at the Center for Global Development (CGD) and head of CGD's Global Health Policy Research Network. An expert on health and education, she was previously a Senior Economist at the World Bank and Social Sectors Advisor at the Inter-American Development Bank. She has worked in 14 developing countries and on global programs such as the Global Alliance on Vaccines and Immunization. Levine holds a doctoral degree in economics and public health from Johns Hopkins University and is co-author of *The Health of Women in Latin America and the Caribbean* and *Making Markets for Vaccines: Ideas to Action.*

The What Works Working Group

The CGD's Global Health Policy Research Network convened the What Works Working Group to identify, describe, and analyze proven successes in global health. The Working Group includes 16 prominent experts in international health, development economics, public policy, and other fields. The Working Group collaborated closely with leading authorities on specific diseases and interventions through the Disease Control Priorities in Developing Countries Project of the Fogarty International Center of the US National Institutes of Health.

MEMBER CONTRIBUTORS:

George Alleyne, *Pan American Health Organization (retired)*
Dr. George Alleyne, a national of Barbados, entered academic medicine in the University of the West Indies in 1962, and his career included research in the Tropical Metabolism Research Unit for his doctorate in medicine. Alleyne joined the Pan American Health Organization (PAHO) in 1981 as chief of Research Promotion and Coordination. From 1995 to 2003 he served as director of PAHO. In 1990, Alleyne was made Knight Bachelor by Queen Elizabeth II for his services to medicine, and in 2001 he was awarded the Order of the Caribbean Community. Sir George Alleyne was appointed by the UN Secretary-General in February 2003 to serve as his special envoy for HIV/AIDS in the Caribbean region. In July 2003, the Caribbean Community (Caricom) appointed Alleyne as the head of a new commission to examine health issues confronting the region, including HIV/AIDS, and their impact on national economies. In October 2003, he was appointed Chancellor of the University of the West Indies.

Victor Barbiero, *George Washington University*
In December 2005, Dr. Victor K. Barbiero joined the George Washington University (GWU) School of Public Health and Health Services as a Visiting Associate Professor of Global Health in the Department of Global Health. In addition to his full-time associate professor duties, he also serves as Director of Student Programs. Prior to joining GWU,

Barbiero was a Foreign Service Officer with the United States Agency for International Development (USAID) for 21 years in Washington, East Africa, and India. He served in the USAID East Africa Regional Office in Kenya as the Deputy Director for Population, Health, and Nutrition (PHN) and served as the Director for PHN in Ethiopia and India. He also served as Chief of the Child Survival Division and Chief of the Implementation Support Division for HIV/AIDS in Washington. Dr. Barbiero worked on tropical disease epidemiology in Sudan with Michigan State University and with the World Health Organization in Burkina Faso, and was a Fulbright Scholar in Liberia. Barbiero holds a doctorate in pathobiology and a master of health sciences, both from Johns Hopkins University School of Hygiene and Public Health.

Scott Barrett, *Paul H. Nitze School of Advanced International Studies*
Scott Barrett is professor of international political economy at the Paul H. Nitze School of Advanced International Studies, Johns Hopkins University. A specialist on international environmental policy, Barrett was previously on the faculty of the University of London. He has published widely on the strategy of negotiating international environmental agreements and received the Erik Kempe Prize for his research in this field. His book on this subject, *Environment and Statecraft: The Strategy of Environmental Treaty-Making*, was published by Oxford University Press in 2003. In addition to his many academic contributions, Barrett has advised international and other organizations, including the European Commission, the Global Environment Facility, the OECD, the Intergovernmental Panel on Climate Change, the IUCN Commission on Environmental Law, various agencies of the United Nations, the World Bank, and the World Commission on the Oceans. Among other professional affiliations, he is a member of the board of the Beijer Institute of the Royal Swedish Academy of Sciences, and an International Research Fellow of the Kiel Institute of World Economics. Barrett received his PhD in economics from the London School of Economics.

Mariam Claeson, *World Bank*
Dr. Mariam Claeson is a Program Coordinator for HIV/AIDS in the Human Development Network, South Asia Region, of the World Bank. Previously, she was the Lead Public Health Specialist in the Health, Nutrition and Population (HNP), Human Development Network managing the HNP Millennium Development Goals work program to support accelerated progress in countries. She coauthored the health chapter of the *Poverty Reduction Strategy* source book, and as a coordinator of the public health thematic group, she lead the development of the strategy note *Public Health and World Bank Operations*. Before joining the World Bank, Claeson worked with WHO as program manager for the WHO Global Program for the Control of Diarrheal Diseases. She has several years of field experience working in developing countries, in clinical practice at the rural district level; in national program management on immunization and diarrheal disease control; and in health sector development projects in middle- and low-income countries.

Mushtaque Chowdhury, *Bangladesh Rural Advancement Committee Foundation*
A native of Bangladesh, Dr. Mushtaque Chowdhury is the Deputy Executive Director of the Research and Evaluation Division of BRAC (formerly known as the Bangladesh Rural Advancement Committee) in Bangladesh. BRAC is one of the largest indigenous NGOs in the world, which is particularly concerned with poverty alleviation, education, empowerment of women, environment, and health issues. He has also played a crucial role throughout the expansive introduction of oral rehydration therapy by BRAC in Bangladesh. Chowdhury completed his undergraduate work in Dhaka, and he later obtained his PhD from the London School of Hygiene and Tropical Medicine. Many articles and books in the areas of public health, education, and poverty eradication can be accredited to Chowdhury. He has worked in China, Ethiopia, Nepal, and Thailand and has been a consultant to governments in South Asia and Africa as well as multilateral organizations including UNICEF, the World Bank, and the Red Cross.

William Easterly, *New York University*
William Easterly is Professor of Economics at New York University, joint with Africa House, and codirector of NYU's Development Research Institute. He is also a nonresident Fellow of the Center for Global Development in Washington, DC. Easterly received his PhD in economics at MIT. He spent 16 years as a Research Economist at the World Bank. He is the author of *The White Man's Burden: How the West's Efforts to Aid the Rest Have Done So Much Ill and*

So Little Good (Penguin, 2006), *The Elusive Quest for Growth: Economists' Adventures and Misadventures in the Tropics* (MIT, 2001), three other co-edited books, and 46 articles in refereed economics journals. Easterly's areas of expertise are the determinants of long-run economic growth and the effectiveness of foreign aid. He has worked in most areas of the developing world, most heavily in Africa, Latin America, and Russia. Easterly is an associate editor of the *Quarterly Journal of Economics*, the *Journal of Economic Growth*, and of the *Journal of Development Economics*.

Robert Hecht, *International AIDS Vaccine Initiative*
Robert Hecht is currently Senior Vice President of Public Policy at the International AIDS Vaccine Initiative (IAVI). Before joining IAVI, Mr. Hecht had a 20-year tenure at the World Bank, most recently serving as Manager and Acting Director of the bank's central unit for health, nutrition, and population, responsible for global strategies, knowledge, technical services, and partnerships. His other positions at the bank included chief of operations for the World Bank's Human Development Network, principal economist in the Latin America region, and one of the authors of the 1993 World Development Report, *Investing in Health*. From 1987 to 1996, Hecht was responsible for a number of the bank's studies and projects in health in several countries in Africa and Latin America, most notably in Zimbabwe, South Africa, Brazil, and Argentina. From 1998 to 2001, Hecht served as an Associate Director of the Joint United Nations Programme on HIV/AIDS (UNAIDS). Mr. Hecht has a BA from Yale and a PhD from Cambridge University.

Dean Jamison, *University of California, Los Angeles*
Dean Jamison became Professor of Development Economics at the University of California, San Francisco, in July 2006 and concurrently (for 2006–2008) the T. & G. Angelopoulos Visiting Professor of Health and International Development in the Kennedy School of Government and the School of Public Health, Harvard University. Jamison also serves as an adjunct professor in both the Peking University Guanghua School of Management and in the University of Queensland School of Population Health. Before joining the UCSF and Harvard faculties, Jamison had been at UCLA (1988–2006) and previously at the World Bank where he was a senior economist in the research department, division chief for education policy, and division chief for population, health, and nutrition. In 1992–1993 he temporarily rejoined the World Bank to serve as Director of the World Development Report Office and as lead author for the bank's 1993 World Development Report, *Investing in Health*. More recently Jamison has led the Disease Control Priorities Project, where he was senior editor of *Disease Control Priorities in Developing Countries*, 2nd edition, and an editor of *Global Burden of Disease and Risk Factors*, both published by Oxford University Press in 2006. Jamison studied at Stanford (AB, philosophy; MS, engineering sciences) and at Harvard (PhD, economics, under K.J. Arrow). In 1994, he was elected to membership in the Institute of Medicine of the US National Academy of Sciences.

Carol Medlin, *University of California, San Francisco*
Carol Medlin is a faculty member at the Institute for Global Health at the University of California, San Francisco. Her current work focuses on the evaluation and assessment of a variety of global health initiatives and international health projects, including an evaluation of a Rotary-sponsored malaria control project in Vanuatu. She is a contributing author to the second edition of *Disease Control Priorities in Developing Countries* and is a member of the International Health Policy Reform Network sponsored by the Bertelsmann Foundation. She coauthored the final report of the external review of Roll Back Malaria (RBM), an international partnership dedicated to malaria control. Between 2000 and 2002, she served as the project director of Working Group 2 of the Commission on Macroeconomics and Health, leading an international team of policy practitioners, researchers, and scientists to evaluate multicountry collaborations in topics of special importance to global health. She received her doctoral degree in political science from the University of California, Berkeley, completed a master's degree in public affairs from the Woodrow Wilson School of Public and International Affairs at Princeton University, and has been a consultant to the United Nations in Chile.

Anthony Measham, *World Bank (retired)*
Dr. Anthony Measham has spent more than 30 years working on maternal and child health, family planning, and nutrition in developing countries. After completing a medical degree from Dalhousie University of Halifax, Nova Scotia, Dr. Measham worked at the Population Council in the Latin American region and subsequently at the Ford

Foundation in Dhaka as program officer and project specialist in population, community health, and nutrition. He joined the World Bank in 1982, and during his tenure worked in 25 developing countries. He was Special Professor of International Health at the University of Nottingham Medical School from 1989 to1998 and has published more than 70 monographs, book chapters, and scientific articles. Since his retirement in 1999, Measham has continued to work for the World Bank as a consultant on immunization, nutrition, and public health. He was co-managing editor of *Disease Control Priorities.*

Germano Mwabu, *University of Nairobi*
Germano Mwabu, an associate professor of economics, is chairman of the Economics Department at the University of Nairobi. He was previously a senior research fellow and project director at the World Institute for Development Economics Research in Helsinki. He is a former dean of commerce and chairman of the Economics Department at Kenyatta University. He received his PhD in economics from Boston University.

Blair Sachs, *Bill & Melinda Gates Foundation*
Blair Sachs is a program officer in the Policy and Finance team at the Bill & Melinda Gates Foundation, where she develops the global health policy research portfolio and provides policy and finance guidance and analytics to the foundation global health divisions. Originally, her finance efforts focused on a major grantee in the immunization program, the Vaccine Fund and Global Alliance for Vaccines and Immunizations (GAVI). More recently, she has been concentrating on policy and financial issues related to the HIV and reproductive health programs. Prior to joining the foundation, Sachs operated in the business development team of a microbicide biotechnology firm. She also managed health programs with CARE International in Ecuador and assisted a USAID project, Juhudi Women's Association, to initiate a medical dispensary in a rural ward in Tanzania. Sachs earned her master's in business and public health from Johns Hopkins University School of Professional Business and Education and School of Public Health, respectively.

William Savedoff, *Social Insight*
William D. Savedoff is currently senior partner at Social Insight, an international consulting firm. He has worked extensively on questions related to improving the accessibility and quality of public services in developing countries, first as an Associate Researcher at the Instituto de Pesquisa de Economia Aplicada (Rio de Janeiro) and later as an economist at the Inter-American Development Bank and the World Health Organization. In addition to preparing, coordinating, and advising development projects in Latin America, Africa, and Asia, he has published books and articles on labor markets, health, education, water, and housing, including *Organization Matters: Agency Problems in Health and Education in Latin America* (IDB, 1998), *Spilled Water: Institutional Commitment in the Provision of Water Services* (IDB, 1999), and *Diagnosis Corruption: Fraud in Latin America's Public Hospitals* (IDB, 2001).

Rajiv Shah, *Bill & Melinda Gates Foundation*
Rajiv Shah is the director for Strategic Opportunities at the Bill & Melinda Gates Foundation, where he leads efforts to explore new strategic areas of giving and manages the foundation's special projects portfolio, including grants to extend financial services to the poor; expand access to improved water, sanitation, and hygiene; and improve agricultural productivity to reduce poverty and hunger. Shah previously served as the foundation's deputy director for Policy and Finance for Global Health and as its senior economist. Before joining the foundation, he served as a health care policy advisor on the Gore 2000 presidential campaign. He co-founded Health Systems Analytics and Project IMPACT and currently serves on boards for the Global Development Network, City Year Seattle, and Time to Vote. Shah has coauthored articles, book chapters, and working group reports on topics ranging from the quality of domestic cardiovascular care to the effective financing and implementation of global health and development initiatives. He earned his MD from the University of Pennsylvania Medical School and his MSc in health economics at the Wharton School of Business, where he received a National Institutes of Health Medical Scientist Training Grant.

Holly Wise, *US Agency for International Development (retired)*
Through her consultancy practice, Wise Solutions LLC, Ms. Wise brings international development, corporate social responsibility, public–private alliance, and business development expertise to corporations, foundations, and

nonprofit organizations. She teaches enterprise development at Georgetown University's graduate school of foreign service and sits on the board of GlobalGiving, an online auction site for global development organizations. Wise is also a member of the Council on Foreign Relations. Ms. Wise spent 26 years in the foreign service with the US Agency for International Development (USAID), achieving the diplomatic rank of Minister Counselor. She is the founder and first Secretariat Director of the Global Development Alliance, USAID's business model that forges strategic alliances between public and private partners in addressing international development issues. Under her leadership, 300 alliances were formed with $1.1 billion in USAID funding, which leveraged $3.8 billion in private resources for the world's poor. In addition to overseas tours in Uganda, Kenya, Barbados, the Philippines, and China, Ms. Wise served as USAID chair at the National Defense University where she taught political science, environmental courses, and published research on China. Ms. Wise is a Phi Beta Kappa graduate of Connecticut College and holds advanced degrees from Yale University and the National Defense University.

STAFF

Jessica Gottlieb, *Center for Global Development*
Jessica Gottlieb is a program coordinator with the Center's Global Health Policy Research Network, where she manages the Evaluation Gap initiative, the Working Group on Performance-Based Incentives, and the What Works Working Group. She holds a BA in political science and international studies from Yale University. Before joining the Center, Gottlieb worked at the Academy for Educational Development, where she managed international health projects and participated in health policy and advocacy efforts. She has conducted research on health systems in Mali and France.

Molly Kinder, *Center for Global Development*
Molly Kinder was a program coordinator with the Global Health Policy Research Network, at the Center for Global Development from 2003 to 2005 and coauthored *Millions Saved: Proven Successes in Global Health* (CGD, 2004). Subsequently, Kinder was a consultant with the Bill & Melinda Gates Foundation's policy and finance team. Following the 2005 earthquake in Pakistan, she served as a junior task manager for the World Bank Islamabad office and also worked on a World Bank research study exploring mobility in rural India. Kinder previously worked with Oxfam's trade policy and advocacy team and has conducted research projects and volunteered in Kenya, Mexico, India, and Chile. She graduated from the University of Notre Dame and is pursuing graduate studies at Harvard University.

Introduction

MILLIONS SAVED: PROVEN SUCCESSES IN GLOBAL HEALTH

One of the greatest human accomplishments has been the spectacular improvement in health since 1950, particularly in developing countries. With death rates falling steadily, more progress was made in the health of populations in the past half century than in many earlier millennia.

Average life expectancy—the age to which a newborn baby is expected to survive—was approximately 40 years in developing countries in 1950; 50 years later, life expectancy in these same countries has risen more than 60% to about 65 years today.[1] Each year, nearly four months are added to average life expectancy globally.[2] Most of the improvements in life expectancy are derived from the reduced risks to young children. The death rate among children under 5 has dropped dramatically around the globe, from 148 deaths per 1,000 children in 1955 to fewer than 59 deaths in 2000.

Economic growth only partially explains the overall improvement in health in the past 50 years in developing countries.[3,4] In fact, researchers have estimated that income growth accounts for less than half the health gains between 1952 and 1992.[5] The role of the technological innovation and diffusion, including the spread of health-related knowledge, is seen as a main driver of the improvement of health in recent decades, particularly in low-income countries.[6,7] There is little doubt, in fact, that specific actions within the health sector have contributed to the improvements observed in global health over the past 50 years.

This book is about part of that success: major achievements in public health programs in the developing world. Not all of those achievements are included in this volume, by any stretch of the imagination, and in no way do the examples here represent the only health programs that have worked. By focusing on experiences that embody the deployment of resources within the health sector to achieve measurable improvement in human health, this book provides a sample of the national, regional, and global public health efforts that we know, with confidence, have saved millions of lives and improved millions more (see Box I-1).

These cases meet a set of rigorous selection criteria: being large-scale, having a duration of five years or more, employing a cost-effective intervention, and having a major impact on an important health problem (see Box I-2). Importantly, for these cases, as for a few others, sufficient investment was made in data collection and analysis to attribute changes in health conditions to the large-scale interventions or programs themselves. (The process of case selection, and the mandate, methods, and limitations of this review of success cases, are described in Appendix B.)

On the basis of impact alone, this sampling of major global public health successes is impressive: Mothers throughout Latin America no longer worry about their children contracting polio; huge regions of Africa are now habitable because river blindness is under control; women in Sri Lanka can give birth without fear of dying—in sharp contrast to women in most poor countries; China has made major inroads against tuberculosis; and much more.

But the stories are about more than the impact itself; they are about how that success came about. What are the common threads running through these success cases that provide useful hints about what might be needed to generate future success? How do these success stories arm policy makers and development practitioners to fight for more successes? And how do these stories challenge the assertion that foreign assistance makes little difference in people's lives?

BOX I-1 Success Case Summaries

Eradicating smallpox. A massive global effort spearheaded by the World Health Organization eradicated smallpox in 1977 and inspired the creation of the Expanded Programme on Immunization, which continues today.

Preventing HIV and sexually transmitted infections in Thailand. In Thailand, the government's "100% condom program" targeting commercial sex workers and other high-risk groups helped prevent the spread of HIV relatively early in the course of the epidemic. Thailand had 80% fewer new cases of HIV in 2001 than in 1991 and has averted nearly 200,000 new cases.

Controlling tuberculosis in China. To address the problem of tuberculosis (TB) patients' early dropout from treatment, a national TB program in China implemented the directly observed treatment, short-course (DOTS) approach in which a health worker "watches" patients with TB daily for six months as they take their antibiotic treatment. The program helped reduce TB prevalence by 40% between 1990 and 2000 and dramatically improved the cure rate in half of China's provinces.

Reducing child mortality through vitamin A in Nepal. Capitalizing on the discovery that vitamin A supplementation could save child lives, in 1995 the government of Nepal began the National Vitamin A Program that has averted nearly 200,000 child deaths.

Eliminating polio in Latin America and the Caribbean. Beginning in 1985, a regionwide polio elimination effort led by the Pan American Health Organization immunized almost every young child in Latin America and the Caribbean, eliminating polio as a threat to public health in the Western Hemisphere in 1991.

Saving mothers' lives in Sri Lanka. Despite relatively low national income and health spending, Sri Lanka's commitment to providing a range of "safe motherhood" services led to a decline in maternal mortality from 486 deaths per 100,000 live births to 24 deaths per 100,000 live births over four decades.

Controlling onchocerciasis in sub-Saharan Africa. A multipartner international effort begun in 1974 dramatically reduced the incidence and impact of the blinding parasitic disease and increased the potential for economic development in large areas of rural west, central, and southern Africa. Transmission has been virtually halted in West Africa today, and 22 million children born in the 11-country area are now free of the threat of contracting river blindness.

Preventing diarrheal deaths in Egypt. Using modern communication methods, a national diarrheal control program in Egypt increased the awareness and use of life-saving oral rehydration therapy, helping reduce infant diarrheal deaths by 82% between 1982 and 1987.

Improving the health of the poor in Mexico. Since 1997, Mexico's Progresa (now known as "Oportunidades") has provided a comprehensive package of education, health, and nutrition interventions to rural families through a conditional cash grants program, resulting in lowered rates of illness and malnutrition and increased school enrollment.

Controlling trachoma in Morocco. Since 1997, the incidence in Morocco of trachoma, the leading preventable cause of blindness worldwide, has been cut by more than 99% among children under 10 through a combined strategy of surgery, antibiotics, face washing, and environmental changes.

Reducing guinea worm in Asia and sub-Saharan Africa. A multipartner eradication effort focused on behavior change reduced prevalence of guinea worm by 99% in 20 endemic African and Asian countries. Since the start of the campaign in 1986, the number of cases has fallen from 3.5 million to fewer than 11,000 in 2005.

Controlling Chagas disease in the southern cone of South America. Through surveillance, environmental vector control, and house spraying, a regional initiative launched in 1991 has decreased the incidence of Chagas disease by 94% in seven countries in the southern cone of Latin America. Disease transmission has now been halted in Uruguay, Chile, and large parts of Brazil and Paraguay.

Reducing fertility in Bangladesh. In Bangladesh, strong leadership of the family planning program, a sustained outreach strategy, and a focus on access to services increased contraceptive prevalence from 3% to 54% (and correspondingly decreased fertility from 7 to 3 children per woman) over three decades, more than what would have been predicted based on changes in economic and social conditions alone.

(continues)

BOX I-1 Success Case Summaries   *(continued)*

Curbing tobacco use in Poland. Starting in the early 1990s, the transition to a market economy and a more open society paved the way for health advocates to implement strong tobacco controls in Poland, a country that had the highest rate of tobacco consumption in the world. A combination of health education and stringent tobacco control legislation averted 10,000 deaths a year, led to a 30% reduction in the incidence of lung cancer among men aged 20 to 44, and helped boost the life expectancy of men by four years.

Preventing iodine deficiency disease in China. China's introduction of iodized salt in 1995 reduced the incidence of goiter among children, from 20% to 9%, and created a sustainable system of private provision of fortified salt.

Preventing neural-tube defects in Chile. Through a successful partnership between the flour industry and the national government, Chile began fortifying wheat flour with folic acid in 2002. This intervention has prevented life-threatening neural tube defects in infants and saved the health system millions of dollars in treatment costs.

Eliminating measles in southern Africa. Measles vaccination campaigns in seven African countries nearly eliminated measles as a cause of childhood death in southern Africa and helped reduce the number of measles cases from 60,000 in 1996 to just 117 cases four years later. The number of reported measles deaths fell from 166 to zero.

Preventing dental caries in Jamaica. Between 1987 and 1995, Jamaica's National Salt Fluoridation Program demonstrated up to an 87% decrease in dental caries in schoolchildren and has been regarded as a model for micronutrient interventions.

Treating cataracts in India. An intensified cataract surgery program implemented in seven Indian states from 1994 to 2001, which was catalyzed by technical and operational innovations developed by a nongovernmental organization, saved more than 300,000 people per year from a lifetime of blindness.

Preventing Hib disease in Chile and the Gambia. A national Hib vaccination program in Chile reduced prevalence of Hib disease by 90% in the early 1990s. In 1997, the Gambia introduced Hib vaccines into its national immunization program, virtually eliminating the disease from the country.

BOX I-2 What Is Success?

Each of the cases in this volume adheres to five selection criteria:

Scale. Interventions or programs that were implemented on a national, regional, or global scale. Programs were characterized as "national" if they represented a national-level commitment, even if they were targeted at a problem that affected only a limited geographic area. Programs implemented on a pilot basis, or within only a few districts, were excluded.

Importance. Interventions or programs that addressed a problem of public health significance. In this case, a measure of burden of disease—disability-adjusted life years (DALYs)—was used as an indicator of importance.

Impact. Interventions or programs that demonstrated a clear and measurable impact on a population's health. Demonstration of impact on process indicators—such as immunization rates—was not taken as a proxy for health outcomes. Rather, genuine changes in morbidity and mortality constituted the criteria.

Duration. Interventions or programs that were functioning "at scale" for at least five consecutive years. Sustainability, including financial self-sufficiency, was not used as a selection criterion.

Cost-effectiveness. Interventions or programs that used a cost-effective approach, determined by a threshold of about $100 per DALY saved.

TAKE NOTE

Six "wows" emerge from a close review of the cases presented in this book.

Success Is Possible Even in the Poorest of Settings

These cases show that major health improvement is possible in the face of grinding poverty and weak health systems. Countries of every region in Africa and South Asia—places where the average citizen earns less than $1,000 per year (often far less, closer to $1 or $2 a day)—have seen major public health successes. Several of the programs highlighted, such as the guinea worm and river blindness control efforts and the Vitamin A supplementation program, employed innovative interventions and involved the community to reach people in some of the most remote terrain on the planet. Other programs, such as those in Bangladesh that improved the health of mothers and children, brought needed health commodities and information through house-to-house visits to many low-income women, who, for cultural reasons, could not venture far from home.

Other programs have improved the health of poor people in middle-income countries through targeted incentives and support. For example, Mexico's Programa de Educación, Salud y Alimentación (Progresa)—now known as Oportunidades—uses a tiered targeting strategy to provide income transfers to the most disadvantaged residents if they take their children for well-child services. In short, we found programs that successfully improved the health of people who are the hardest to reach.

Governments in Poor Countries Can Do the Job—and in Some Cases Are the Chief Funders

In almost all of these cases, the public sector does the daily work of reaching affected populations. This contrasts with the view that governments in poor countries are uniformly inefficient at best and hopelessly corrupt at worst. Through at least the narrow frame of these cases, we found that the public sector was integral to the successful delivery of services at scale in most instances, sometimes in collaboration with nongovernmental organizations (NGOs) or the business community. For example, in Sri Lanka, maternal mortality has been halved at least every 12 years since 1935, in large measure because of the services that are designed, delivered, and monitored within the public health system. In the southern cone of South America, it was the ministries of health that collaborated across borders to greatly diminish the threat of Chagas disease. In these and other instances, such as the measles initiative in southern Africa, the financial support depended not on donors but on local resources—another dimension of the public sector's ownership of the success.

Technology, Yes—but Behavior Change, Too

Despite the fact that technological developments in global health are more likely to grab headlines—and in fact, do constitute a major element in many of these cases—very basic behavior change emerges as a prominent feature in a surprising number of instances. In the control of guinea worm in Africa, for example, families learned to filter their water conscientiously; in the fight against deaths from dehydrating diarrheal disease in Bangladesh, mothers learned and now teach their grown daughters how to mix a simple salt-and-sugar solution; and in Poland and South Africa, long-standing patterns of cigarette consumption have been dramatically altered through a combination of legal measures, taxation, and communication efforts. This is good news in light of the health challenges that now confront us, very few of which can be tackled through improved technology alone.

International Coalitions Have Worked

Many of the cases show the ways in which international agencies can break through institutional and bureaucratic walls to work for a common purpose. In no instance was this collaboration easy, and it was often the source of institutional friction and cumbersome processes. But the benefits are evident: Some parties bring funding, others bring technical capabilities in public health, and still others generate the political will to sustain the effort in the face of competing priorities.

Two examples demonstrate such collaboration: The guinea worm eradication campaign benefits from the participation of a large number of partners—the Carter Center, the US Centers for Disease Control and Prevention, the United Nations Children's Fund (UNICEF), the World Health Organization (WHO), the Bill & Melinda Gates Foundation, the World Bank, the UN Development Program (UNDP), NGOs, more than 14 donor countries, private companies (including Du Pont and Precision Fabric Groups, which have donated more than $14 million worth of cloth for water filters), and the governments of 20 countries in Asia and Africa. Through interagency meetings, held three to four times a year, and annual meetings of coordinators of national eradication programs, exemplary coordination has been achieved among implementers and donors.

The international effort to control onchocerciasis (or river blindness) also demonstrates the power of partnership. The African Programme for Onchocerciasis Control has relied on the long-term participation of the World Bank, WHO, UNDP, the Food and Agriculture Organization, the governments of 19 African countries, 21 bilateral and multilateral donors, more than 30 NGOs, the pharmaceutical giant Merck, and more than 80,000 rural African communities. In both cases, a single coordinating body played a critical role, helping to unite the partners and spur momentum within the project.

Attribution Is Possible

It is indeed possible to know whether large-scale health programs are the key drivers of improved health. Although this might not sound surprising at first blush, policy makers in fact rarely have the opportunity to directly connect investments in major health (or other social) programs to outcomes that have as much meaning as lives saved. Typically, large initiatives, such as immunization programs, are judged by intermediate measures—for example, the number of children receiving vaccination services or the number of doses of vaccines procured. The actual health impact is assumed. In contrast, we insisted on finding evidence that the programs led to specific types of health improvements, and we were able to do so—in most cases because special data collection efforts had been made to look at those outcomes (see Box I-3).

A pathbreaking example of connecting investments to impact is the Progresa program in Mexico, which provided a package of education and health interventions to families through conditional cash grants. Progresa's proponents in government saw the value of an external, independent impact evaluation as a way to establish the program's credibility and help ensure its continuation during a political shift. When a rigorous evaluation demonstrated major impacts on health and welfare of the poor, Progresa survived the transition from one Mexican administration to the next and has inspired the creation of similar "conditional cash transfer" programs in Latin America and elsewhere.

BOX I-3 Attributing Success: How Do We Know?

In each of these cases, solid evidence—summarized in the respective case studies—confirms that the impact on health is largely attributable to the specific public health efforts rather than to broad economic and social improvements. In some instances, this confirmation comes through a randomized experimental design, which permits the comparison of the health of people who were included in a particular program with the health of people who have similar baseline characteristics and yet did not participate in the program. Such experimental designs are rare but not unknown: In Mexico, for example, the Progresa program of income transfers was scaled up in a way that was explicitly designed to assess the program's impact.

In other instances, the confirmation comes indirectly from a composite of information about health changes that occurred simultaneously with a program's implementation. In Sri Lanka, for example, the changes in specific causes of maternal mortality, such as hemorrhage, coincided with targeted improvements in health systems, such as the introduction of transfusion services. In the Gambia, the reduction of a disease that causes meningitis in children was so dramatic and so well documented following the nationwide introduction of Hib vaccine that little doubt exists about the cause of the epidemiologic change. And in other cases, such as the Bangladesh family planning program, statistical analyses provide the grounds for claims of success.

Success Comes in All Shapes

It is commonly held that in low-income countries, the only health programs that really work are those that are disease-specific and centrally managed, delivering medicines and services outside of the routine health system. These are the so-called vertical programs—some of which are highlighted in this book. As the experiences chronicled in this volume attest, many other approaches also have worked, including initiatives that strengthen health systems to effect steady improvements in access and quality, such as the use of female community health volunteers to distribute vitamin A capsules and the improvements in eye care services. Also successful have been traditional public health interventions that employ community-wide interventions such as salt iodation, and legal and regulatory reforms such as tobacco control legislation in Poland. Perhaps more important, several of these stories break down the boundary between vertical approaches and efforts to strengthen health systems by showing disease-specific efforts that work together with routine health service delivery. For example, under the right circumstances, a big push to immunize children can provide the much-needed organizational skills, funding, and motivation to improve basic pediatric health services. And virtually all disease-specific programs are made more successful when functioning training, logistics, surveillance, and referral systems are present in a country's health infrastructure.

CONNECTING THE DOTS FOR SUCCESS

Each of the chapters in this volume tells a unique story, specific to time and place. While they all reveal the tremendous improvements in the lives of millions that public health efforts can achieve, they vary vastly in the health conditions addressed and the interventions used. Each also is distinct in the factors that contributed to the accomplishments. They yield no single recipe that, if followed, will result in success.

Though no single recipe emerges, a remarkably consistent list of ingredients does: political leadership and champions, technological innovation, expert consensus around the approach, management that effectively uses information, and sufficient financial resources. In some of the cases, the participation of the affected community and the involvement of NGOs are also central features. Combined in particular ways, these elements appear to be the main contributing factors to success.

No *single* ingredient was enough in any case. By itself, political leadership could create an opportunity for funding and action, in the face of competing demands within and outside the health sector, but such leadership did not provide the road map to effectively deal with a health problem. That came from strong information sources that identified the breadth and nature of the problem and from appropriate technology that effectively addressed the problem. Implementation then depended on effective management, with close monitoring of processes and results. In many instances, success was derived from a type of collaboration across countries and institutions that defied bureaucratic battle lines.

Whether these factors would lead to success in other programs is a question that our methods did not permit us to answer. Because "failures" are not as well documented as successes, we were unable to undertake a comparative analysis, and so it is not possible to say definitively that these factors, if in place, would guarantee success in the future. However, the common elements suggest a working checklist that policy makers and planners could use to provide large-scale global health programs with greater chances of reaching their full potential.

MOBILIZING POLITICAL LEADERSHIP AND CHAMPIONS TAKES A LITTLE LUCK AND A LOT OF PREPARATION

Virtually all of the cases show the importance of visible high-level commitment to a cause. In Mexico, the director general of Social Security at the time, Santiago Levy, championed the design and evaluation of the Progresa program, a demand-side program for helping poor families, and thereby helped the program to survive a key political transition to an opposition government. In Thailand, the government showed strong leadership and vision in its early efforts to curb a growing AIDS epidemic, making a bold commitment that led to one of the very few successes in HIV/AIDS prevention on a national scale. In South Africa, the strong will of the first health minister of the country's new government allowed for the successful passage of one of the most comprehensive and stringent tobacco control policies in the world, despite fierce opposition from the tobacco industry.

Other cases show the potential for champions to rally resources and international resolve. The near eradication of guinea worm from Africa and Asia is due in large measure to the personal involvement and advocacy of former US President Jimmy Carter and former African heads of state, General Amadou Toumani Touré of Mali and General Yakubu Gowon of Nigeria. These leaders visited endemic countries, mobilized the commitment of political and public health communities, and raised both awareness and financial resources. In the case of the control of onchocerciasis in 11 West African countries, then president of the World Bank Robert McNamara personally committed to spearheading a new initiative after witnessing the devastation the blinding disease caused.

In a few of the cases, political commitment was simply the serendipitous result of a leader's particular interest in taking on a cause. In others, however, political commitment came about because technical experts were able to effectively communicate that a "big win" was possible through the development of plans that were technically feasible, economically possible, and socially desirable. So, when US President Lyndon B. Johnson was looking for an initiative to mark "International Cooperation Year" in 1965, technical personnel from the US Communicable Disease Center* took advantage of the opportunity to promote the eradication of smallpox. And when Chile's Minister of Health was under fire after an outbreak of meningitis, public health researchers seized the moment to make the case for the national introduction of the Hib vaccine—even though the vaccine would not prevent the type of meningitis drawing public attention at the time. In these instances, the ability of the technical experts to make the most of a political opening was the seed of the success.

TECHNOLOGICAL INNOVATION WORKS ONLY WHEN THERE IS AN EFFECTIVE SYSTEM TO DELIVER AT AN AFFORDABLE PRICE

Many of the cases turn on the development of a technology—a drug, vaccine, nutritional supplement, or pesticide—that was appropriate for the conditions in the developing world. Commonly, the new technology permitted an existing program to work more effectively, achieving rapid health gains. For example, the regional initiative to eliminate Chagas disease in South America gained great momentum in the 1980s with the development of a synthetic pesticide that was both more effective and more acceptable to the population than the earlier one. The success of Morocco's trachoma program hinged in part on the use of azithromycin, an antibiotic that in the 1990s was found to be as effective in treating the blinding disease with one dose as a 6-week regimen of the predecessor treatment. The control of onchocerciasis in central and east Africa was possible only after the 1978 discovery that ivermectin, the drug originally developed for veterinary use, was an effective one-dose treatment for many of the most debilitating symptoms of the disease.

However, the development of a new health product is in no way a guarantee that the technology will take hold. In many of the cases in this volume, the technological innovation led to better health only because of a concerted and large-scale effort to make it available at a cost affordable to developing countries and donor agencies—often through a public–private partnership in which the private sector provided the product at concessionary prices or through a donation program, and the public sector (both national governments and donor agencies) took responsibility for distribution. These deals have frequently been brokered or facilitated through international NGOs. For example, one of the largest public–private partnerships is a collaborative effort between Merck and a range of nonprofit institutions, led by the Task Force for Child Survival and Development (an affiliate of Emory University), through which the pharmaceutical giant has donated approximately 470 million doses of ivermectin in the fight against onchocerciasis. Similarly, Pfizer has teamed with the Edna McConnell Clark Foundation and the Bill & Melinda Gates Foundation to provide one of the world's largest donations of a patented drug, Zithromax, as part of a global effort to eliminate blinding trachoma. Another successful public–private partnership is demonstrated by the union of the flour industry and the Chilean government to fortify flour with folate, preventing neural-tube defects.

AGREEMENT AMONG TECHNICAL EXPERTS STRENGTHENS THE SIGNAL, REDUCES THE NOISE

In addition to specific technology and improved medicine, many of the health interventions in this book have benefited from the implementation of new strategies to fight disease, based on technical consensus about the strategies'

---

* In 1970, the name was changed to the Center for Disease Control and in 1992 to the Centers for Disease Control and Prevention.

efficacy. For example, the World Bank and WHO helped China revamp its fight against tuberculosis, the leading cause of adult deaths in China, and recommended the introduction of the DOTS strategy—a way to package the elements of successful TB control. Subsequently China launched the world's largest DOTS program in 1991. In the case of trachoma, the government of Morocco joined forces with WHO and an international partnership in the first national test of a comprehensive strategy to both prevent and treat the disease, including low-cost surgery, antibiotics, face washing, and environmental change. In each of these instances, and in nearly all others, the agreement about the right strategy by an expert community both within international technical agencies and in the broader international public health community was a central factor in the appropriate design of the programs. Such expert consensus does not occur magically, but rather through investment in scientific research and ongoing international expert meetings. With such consensus, programs were seen as fully credible and worth the outlays required.

NGOS COMPLEMENT AND KEEP A VIGILANT EYE ON PUBLIC ACTION

Most of the cases represent achievements of the public sector, but some show the special role that NGOs with broad reach and strong management can play, thus complementing the public sector. In Bangladesh, a national NGO carried out the world's largest oral rehydration program, reaching more than 13 million mothers and preventing child deaths. NGOs have played a key role in the distribution throughout sub-Saharan Africa of ivermectin, the antibiotic that treats river blindness. And India's Cataract Blindness Control Program scaled-up services and improved delivery of high-quality, low-cost eye care through nongovernmental collaboration, particularly with the innovative Aravind Eye Hospital.

Beyond service delivery, NGOs have a valuable role as watchdogs and advocates, going beyond what any public agency can do. For example, health-promoting NGOs in Poland and South Africa formed the backbone of advocacy efforts that led to sweeping tobacco control legislation in both countries.

NO TECHNOLOGY, FUNDING, OR CHAMPION TAKES THE PLACE OF GOOD MANAGEMENT ON THE GROUND

Without question, effective management is an essential element of each and every case. Good health service delivery requires that trained and motivated workers are in place and have the supplies, equipment, transportation, and supervision to do their job right. Although this does not happen without adequate funding, it also does not happen without good management—and in some instances strong management partially compensates for budgetary restrictions. For example, in the case of smallpox eradication, a quasi-military organizational structure was able to respond quickly to new information, managing the multiple logistical challenges of reaching every corner of the globe. During the polio campaign in the Americas, management at the country level was strengthened through the establishment of national interagency coordinating committees in each country. The committees worked with ministries of health to develop national plans of action, setting immunization strategies, and optimizing the use of resources. These plans of action now serve as an important management tool for planning other health interventions.

INFORMATION IS POWER

One facet of each and every case is the use and broad sharing of quality information, particularly in four ways:

- First, information *raises awareness* about a health problem, focusing political and technical attention. In China, for example, research showing that iodine deficiency posed a threat to children's mental capacity prompted government action. In Honduras, a rapid method to estimate maternal mortality highlighted regional differentials, which led to a public-sector response. In Poland, research that linked smoking to the heavy disease burden there, particularly to the exploding cancer problem, helped raise awareness among policy makers and the general public and provided the foundation for initiating tobacco control legislation.
- Second, information in the early stages of a program *shapes design*. Through careful monitoring, program designers measure the effectiveness of various ways to address a health problem and discern which approach merits additional resources. In Egypt, for example, information from community trials and "rehearsals" and from market research revealed consumer preferences—essential for the design of a national oral rehydration program that depended in large measure on effective communication with mothers. In South Africa, research on the impact of tobacco excise taxes shaped the stringent taxes implemented in the late 1990s.

- Third, information *motivates*. In the guinea worm eradication campaign, information was disseminated in monthly publications that highlighted the progress of national programs. The information sharing helped keep countries motivated and focused and pressured those lagging behind. The campaign even used information to spark positive competition between rival countries.
- Fourth, information *facilitates midcourse corrections*. In the India cataract case, the collection of information demonstrated that the government's traditional approach of using "eye camps" was not working well, and many patients were obtaining no benefit from the cataract surgery. This led to the introduction of a better surgical approach and effective collaboration with NGOs.

COMMUNITY PARTICIPATION CREATES A TWO-WAY STREET

In some of the cases, the communities whose health is affected play a strong and active role in the success. Among the best examples are the community-directed ivermectin treatment program for river blindness, in which tens of thousands of communities across central and east Africa organize and manage local distribution of the drug, assuming full responsibility and thus increasing the likelihood of the long-term sustainability of the program; the guinea worm campaign across central and east Africa, in which "village volunteers" serve on the front line distributing filters, raising public awareness, and identifying and containing cases; the vitamin A program in Nepal, in which volunteers, often village grandmothers, distribute the nutrition supplements—a measure that proved crucial to the ability of the program to reach remote areas and sustain activity; and a community-based health education campaign to reduce trachoma in Morocco, which uses mosques, lodgings for young women, local associations, and schools as venues to communicate the program's messages of behavior change.

MORE PREDICTABLE FUNDING, AT ADEQUATE LEVELS, PERMITS THE SYSTEM TO WORK

Last but in no way least, each of these cases demonstrates that making public health programs work takes money. Not vast sums—in each of the cases, cost-effective and often low-cost interventions are employed, and the benefits far outweigh the costs—but steady, adequate funding ensures that the programs can be sustained long enough to have a major impact. In many of these cases, a large share of the funding came from donors—donors who can now claim a resounding public health victory: In the onchocerciasis control program, $600 million over 28 years, contributed by many donors, has virtually halted transmission of the blinding disease in 11 countries—at an annual cost of just $1 per person. A $26 million† grant from the US Agency for International Development (USAID) to Egypt in 1981 helped the country prevent 300,000 child deaths from diarrheal disease—at the remarkable cost of just $6 per treated child. In the guinea worm control program, about $88 million from an extensive list of donors and NGOs has helped reduce guinea worm prevalence by more than 99%, cutting the number of people affected by this profoundly debilitating ailment from 3.5 million in 1985 to less than 11,000 in 2005.

The payoffs have been huge. Eradicating smallpox from the globe cost the donor community less than $100 million; the United States, the campaign's largest donor, saves its total contribution every 26 days because it is not spent on treatment or vaccine. In the onchocerciasis control program, the economic rate of return has been estimated to be 17%—a yield that is comparable to investment in the most productive sectors, such as industry, transportation, and agriculture.

Donor investments in health do not always yield such resounding benefits, but these cases show the proven potential for donor dollars to save individuals, communities, and entire nations from the devastation of preventable death and disease. This is the type of impact that taxpayers in wealthy countries want to see from the foreign assistance budget: major improvements in the well-being of the world's poorest citizens.

THE CHALLENGES AHEAD

The need to learn how to succeed is urgent. Ancient problems remain unsolved, such as the differentials in health between the rich and the poor. Newer ones—from the AIDS pandemic to the growing prevalence of chronic disease—threaten future generations.

---

† Throughout, dollar figures are expressed in nominal terms, unless otherwise noted, and are US dollars.

AIDS

The soaring rates of HIV infection have had a devastating impact on life expectancy in many poor countries and have erased decades of steady improvements in sub-Saharan Africa. An estimated 25 million people are believed to be HIV-positive in Africa alone—a figure that represents nearly two thirds of the total global HIV burden, and 9 in 10 children with AIDS.[8] In countries like Swaziland that have exceptionally high rates, it is estimated that more than one third of the population carries the disease. The death toll in the continent is staggering: 2.8 million adults and children died of AIDS in 2005 alone.[8] As a result, life expectancy in southern Africa, the region with the highest prevalence rates in the world, has decreased from 62 years in 1995 to 48 years today, and is projected to fall even further to 43 years in the next 10 years.[9]

High Child Mortality in Africa

Child mortality has declined in low- and middle-income countries, but more than 11 million children under 5 still die each year, most from diseases that can be treated or prevented with known approaches. And the rate of improvement in child health has slowed dramatically in the past 20 years. From 1990 to 2001, for example, the number of deaths of children under 5 declined by 1.1% each year, compared with 2.5% per year during the years from 1960 to 1990. Even more troubling, while improvements have continued in places where child health is relatively good, it has been slowest in the places that historically have had the highest rates of child mortality. Since the early 1970s, sub-Saharan Africa has experienced a slower rate of decline in child mortality than any other region. Currently, 41 percent of the world's child deaths occur in sub-Saharan Africa; another 34 percent occur in South Asia.[10]

Inequality

There is nothing new about rich people being healthier than poor people. Higher income generally translates into better nutrition, better access and ability to effectively use health services, and greater ability to avoid hazards. But the persistence of these differentials—and the growing gap for some health conditions and some populations—must be taken as a caution on claims of success. In this, average success masks an important failure: The gap in mortality, life expectancy, and disease burden between industrialized and developing countries, and between rich and poor children within most countries, is wide. Ninety-nine percent of total childhood deaths in the world occur in poor countries.[11] The poorest 20% of the population within countries often has significantly higher under-5 mortality rates than the richest 20%. In Indonesia, for example, a child born in a poor household is four times more likely to die by her fifth birthday than a child born to a family in the richest population segment.[12] In short, although overall gains have been impressive, the benefits have not been evenly shared.

Cardiovascular and Chronic Diseases

Chronic diseases, and in particular cardiovascular diseases, have emerged as a "hidden epidemic" in developing countries.[13] Estimates suggest that noncommunicable conditions such as depression, diabetes, cancer, obesity, respiratory diseases, and cardiovascular disease will grow from approximately 40% of the health burden in developing countries in 1998 to nearly 75% in 2020.[5] Responding to the looming disease burden requires that the major risk factors (high cholesterol and blood pressure, obesity, smoking, and alcohol) be addressed through changes in diet, physical activity, and tobacco control and through new government policies to support these desired changes in behavior. There is hope: A small window of 10 to 20 years exists for countries to change behavior patterns and prevent the spiraling health crisis.[13]

TOWARD MORE SUCCESSES

Looking at the past is like shining a flashlight into a mirror: the reflection illuminates both what's behind and what's ahead. In almost all of the cases that we now call successes, there were moments when the disease seemed insurmountable, the technology was still on the drawing board (or too expensive or unusable in developing-country conditions), the funding was nowhere in sight, international agencies were squabbling, and no one appeared ready to take up the challenge. In these instances, a combination of science, luck, money, vision, and management talent came together to overcome daunting obstacles and transform the lives of millions of individuals and the prospects of families, communities, and entire nations.

In the end, the experiences documented in this book say three things loudly and clearly:

- *Success is possible—big success, lasting success, world-changing success.* As the cases themselves show, successes have spanned a vast range of diverse programs and interventions and in many instances have been supported by effective donor assistance and international cooperation. This observation competes with the prevailing sense that little can be done to ameliorate large-scale suffering in the poorest countries—particularly in the face of HIV/AIDS and malaria, for which the successes still are few and far between. And it serves as counterweight to the sense that public-sector action in general, and development assistance in particular, systematically fails to make real improvements in real lives.

- *The ingredients of success are within our reach and not dependent solely on the vagaries of chance.* Because we did not look systematically at failures, we cannot say definitively that combining the ingredients found in these cases will ensure success in future ventures. However, policy makers and planners would be well advised to consider using the common elements we identified earlier as a mental checklist: Are these in place when new initiatives are proposed? If not, what would be required to mobilize the predictable and long-term funding, the political support, the information base, the expert consensus, the managerial skills, and the other elements that form a common thread across these experiences?

- *We don't know enough about what's worked because scaled-up programs are rarely evaluated systematically.* We tapped only a small set of public health successes. In large part, this was because solid evidence of the health impact of many international health programs simply does not exist. In general, although very small programs (particularly pilot programs) may be evaluated, little research is done to estimate the health impacts of large-scale efforts. Even for well-known interventions that have received large amounts of donor support over many years, the base of evidence about what has worked (or not worked) in scaled-up programs—in terms of health outcomes, rather than process measures—is quite slim. The gap in evaluation inhibits the documentation of successes and prevents policy makers from being able to tell the difference between a well-told story and a hard fact as they make decisions about which programs to support. The lack of evaluation also reduces the chances for success in the first place. In many of these cases, high-quality evaluations that clearly established the causal link between programs and impact spurred greater investments, broader application, and, ultimately, more success. Efforts to assess whether programs were yielding the desired benefits have been instrumental in securing continued funding. Employing rigorous evaluation methods that link inputs and impact in large-scale programs is far from simple and often requires financial and technical resources that are otherwise absorbed simply in operating a program. But without such evaluation, policy decisions are based on scanty information from small-scale experiences combined with a large dose of opinion and politics.[15]

Each year, about 3 million children in poor countries die of diseases that can be prevented by immunizations; another 2 million die of the dehydrating effects of diarrheal disease. About half a million women in the developing world die in pregnancy or childbirth. Tobacco-related illness cuts short the lives of 4 million people in less developed countries each year, and cardiovascular disease claims the lives of more than 8 million. Last year alone, 3 million people in sub-Saharan Africa contracted HIV. These are the millions of reasons, and millions of chances, to succeed.

REFERENCES

1. McNicoll G. *Population and Development: An Introductory Overview.* New York, NY: Population Council; 2003. Population Council Working Paper 174.

2. World Health Organization. *Health: A Precious Asset.* Geneva, Switzerland: World Health Organization; 2000.

3. Bloom DE, Canning D, Jamison DT. Health, wealth, and welfare. *Finance & Dev.* 2004;41(1):10–15.

4. Fogel RW. Economic growth, population theory, and physiology: the bearing of long-term processes on the making of economic policy. *Am Econ Rev.* 1994;84(3):369–395.

5. World Health Organization. *The World Health Report 1999: Making a Difference.* Geneva, Switzerland: World Health Organization; 1999.

6. Jamison D, Sandbu ME, Wang J. *Why Have Infant Mortality Rates Decreased at Such Different Rates in Different Countries?* Washington, DC: National Institutes of Health, Fogarty International Center; 2004. Disease Control Priorities Project Working Paper 14.

7. Deaton, AS, *Health in an Age of Globalization.* SSRN; July 22, 2004. Princeton University Research Program in Development Studies Working Paper. Available at http://ssrn.com/abstract=567841. Accessed

8. Joint United Nations Programme on HIV/AIDS. *Report on the Global HIV/AIDS Epidemic 2006.* Geneva, Switzerland: Joint United Nations Programme on HIV/AIDS; 2004.

9. UN Population Division. *World Population Prospects: The 2004 Revision.* ESA/P/WP.193. New York, NY: United Nations; 2004.

10. Black RE, Morris SS, Bryce J. Where and why are 10 million children dying every year? *Lancet.* 2003;361(9376):2226–2234.

11. Shann F, Steinhoff MC. Vaccines for children in rich and poor countries. *Lancet.* 1999;354(suppl II):7–11.

12. Victora CG, Wagstaff A, Schellenberg JA, Gwatkin D, Claeson M, Habicht J-P. Applying an equity lens to child health and mortality: more of the same is not enough. *Lancet.* 2003;362(9379):233–241.

13. The hidden epidemic of cardiovascular disease. *Lancet.* 1998;352,(9143):1795.

14. Raymond, SU. Foreign assistance in an aging world. *Foreign Affairs.* 2003;82,(2):91–105.

15. Savedoff WD, Levine R, Birdsall N. *When Will We Ever Learn? Improving Lives Through Impact Evaluation.* CGD Working Group Report. Washington, DC: Center for Global Development; 2006.

Acronyms/Abbreviations

TERM/ACRONYM	DEFINITION
APOC	African Programme for Onchocerciasis Control
CDC	US Centers for Disease Control and Prevention
ComDT	community-directed treatment
DCPP	Disease Control Priorities in Developing Countries Project
DFID	UK Department of International Development
DOTS	directly observed short course strategy
DTP	diphtheria, tetanus, and pertussis vaccine
EPI	Expanded Programme on Immunization (immunization against diphtheria, pertussis, tetanus, poliomyelitis, measles, and tuberculosis)
FAO	Food and Agriculture Organization of the United Nations
GAVI	Global Alliance for Vaccines and Immunization
Hib	*Haemophilus influenzae* type b
HIV/AIDS	human immunodeficiency virus/acquired immune deficiency syndrome
IDB	Inter-American Development Bank
ICC	Inter-Agency Coordinating Committee
IEC	information, education, and communication
IEDC	Infectious and Endemic Disease Control Program (China)
IPV	inactivated polio vaccine
ITI	International Trachoma Initiative
MDG	United Nations Millennium Development Goals
MDR-TB	multidrug-resistant tuberculosis
Mercosur	Mercado Comun del Sur (Southern Cone Common Market)
MMR	maternal mortality ratio
NCDDP	National Control of Diarrheal Disease Project (Egypt)
NTD	neural-tube defect
OCP	Onchocerciasis Control Programme

ODA	official development assistance
OPV	oral polio vaccine
ORS	oral rehydration salts
ORT	oral rehydration therapy
PAHO	Pan American Health Organization
Progresa	Program de Educacion, Salud y Alimentacion (Education, Health, and Food Program)
SAFE	surgery, antibiotics, face washing, and environment
STI	sexually transmitted infection
UNAIDS	Joint United Nations Programme on HIV/AIDS
UNFPA	United Nations Population Fund
UNICEF	United Nations Children's Fund
USAID	United States Agency for International Development
WHA	World Health Assembly
WHO	World Health Organization

Eradicating Smallpox*

* The first draft of this case was prepared by Jane Seymour.

ABSTRACT

Geographic area: Worldwide

Health condition: In 1966, there were approximately 10 million to 15 million cases of smallpox in more than 50 countries, and 1.5 million to 2 million people died from the disease each year.

Global importance of the health condition today: Smallpox has been eradicated from the globe, with no new cases reported since 1978. However, the threat of bioterrorism keeps the danger of smallpox alive, and debate continues over whether strains of the disease should be retained in specified laboratories.

Intervention or program: In 1965, international efforts to eradicate smallpox were revitalized with the establishment of the Smallpox Eradication Unit at the World Health Organization (WHO) and a pledge for more technical and financial support from the campaign's largest donor, the United States. Endemic countries were supplied with vaccines and kits for collecting and sending specimens, and the bifurcated needle made vaccination easier. An intensified effort was led in the five remaining countries in 1973, with concentrated **surveillance** and containment of outbreaks.

Cost and cost-effectiveness: The annual cost of the smallpox campaign between 1967 and 1979 was $23 million. In total, international donors provided $98 million, while $200 million came from the endemic countries. The United States saves the total of all its contributions every 26 days because it does not have to vaccinate or treat the disease.

Impact: By 1977, the last endemic case of smallpox was recorded in Somalia. In May 1980, after two years of surveillance and searching, the World Health Assembly (WHA) declared that smallpox was the first disease in history to have been eradicated.

The eradication of smallpox—the complete extermination of a notorious scourge—has been heralded as one of the greatest achievements of humankind. Inspiring a generation of public health professionals, it gave impetus to subsequent vaccination campaigns and strengthened routine immunization programs in developing countries. It continues to be a touchstone for political commitment to a health goal—particularly pertinent in light of the United Nations' Millennium Development Goals (MDGs).

But the smallpox experience is far from an uncomplicated story of a grand accomplishment that should (or could) be replicated. Although the story shows how great global ambitions can be realized with leadership and resources, it also illustrates the complexities and unpredictable nature of international cooperation.

THE DISEASE

Smallpox was caused by a variola virus and was transmitted between people through the air. It was usually spread by face-to-face contact with an infected person and to a lesser extent through contaminated clothes and bedding.

Once a person contracted the disease, he or she remained apparently healthy and noninfectious for up to 17 days. But the onset of flulike symptoms heralded the infectious stage, leading after two or three days to a reduction in fever but to the appearance of the characteristic rash—first on the face, then on the hands, forearms, and trunk. Ulcerating lesions formed in the nose and mouth, releasing large amounts of virus into the throat.

Nearly one third of those who contracted the major form died from it, and most of those who survived—up to 80 percent—were left with deeply pitted marks, especially on the face. Many were left blind. In 1700s Europe, one third of all cases of blindness were attributed to smallpox.[1]

POSSIBLE ERADICATION?

In 1798, Edward Jenner announced success in vaccinating people against the disease and went on to claim that his vaccine was capable of eradicating it.[2] With the development in the 1920s of an improved vaccine, mass vaccination programs became theoretically viable. Subsequently, national programs—including the Soviet Union's experience in the 1930s—showed that eradication was possible. However, it wasn't until the early 1950s that eradication became a practical goal, with the development of a vaccine that did not require cold storage and could be produced as a consistently potent product in large quantities.

In its earliest form, the idea of a global effort to eradicate smallpox was far from popular. In 1953, the World Health Assembly (WHA)—the highest governing body of the WHO—rejected the notion that smallpox should be selected for eradication. In 1958, however, the deputy health minister of the Soviet Union and delegate to the WHA, Professor Viktor Zhdanov, proposed a 10-year campaign to eradicate the disease worldwide, based on compulsory vaccination and revaccination—and he promised that the Soviet Union would donate 25 million vaccine doses to initiate the program. A year later, a WHO report on the proposal suggested that eradication could be achieved by vaccinating or revaccinating 80 percent of the people in endemic areas within "four to five years." The Russian proposal was passed in 1959.

Smallpox was a suitable candidate for eradication for several reasons. The disease was passed directly between people, without an intervening vector, so there were no res- ervoirs. Its distinctive rash made it relatively straightforward to diagnose, and survivors gained lifetime immunity. The relatively long time between contracting it and becoming infectious meant that an epidemic took a while to take hold—and because sufferers were likely to take to their beds as they became infectious, due to the severity of the symptoms, they tended to infect few others. Good vaccination coverage, it was reasoned, would disrupt transmission entirely; where an outbreak occurred, the natural course of the disease gave health workers time to isolate victims, trace contacts, and vaccinate the local population.

The vaccine itself has characteristics that also gave reason for optimism. The freeze-dried version produced in the early 1950s eliminated reliance on a **cold chain**; if stored properly, the vaccine maintains its strength for many years. A single vaccination can prevent infection from smallpox for at least a decade, and some studies have suggested that some protection is present even 30 years after vaccination. Even where vaccination failed to prevent infection, the resulting disease tended to be milder and have a lower fatality rate.[1]

BURDEN OF SMALLPOX AT THE START OF THE ERADICATION EFFORT

In 1959, 63 countries reported a total of 77,555 cases of smallpox.[2] Acknowledged at the time to be an underestimate, it was revised to closer to 100,000, although it later became clear that as few as 1 in 100 cases was reported. Despite well-developed health systems, some countries only reported cases that surfaced in major urban hospitals, while others failed to report at all. Information was also lacking from countries that were not then WHO members, such as China.

It has subsequently been estimated that in 1959 smallpox remained endemic in 59 countries containing about 60% of the world's population.[3] In the early 1950s, there were probably around 50 million new cases each year.[1] However, several countries were on the verge of disrupting transmission of the disease, including China, Iraq, Thailand, and Algeria.

A SLOW START

In the early stages the WHO plan relied on national campaigns for which prime responsibility in cost and human resources would rest with national governments. The WHO saw itself in the role of providing technical assistance where called for and helping out by ensuring the production of the vaccine.

In fact, in its earliest days, the smallpox eradication program was a minor concern of the WHO. The reliance on national activities and vaccine donations, and pressures of a campaign against malaria (given the go-ahead four years before smallpox), gave the WHO little incentive to allot significant funds to smallpox eradication.

At the start of the campaign, around 977 million people were estimated to live in endemic areas; to vaccinate them was estimated to cost 10 cents per person, a total of about $98 million. However, the actual amount spent in the first half of the 1960s was around $0.5 million a year, 0.2 percent of the WHO's regular budget. For several years, a medical officer and secretary were the only full-time employees working on the program at the WHO's headquarters in Geneva, and until 1966 only five full-time employees were assigned to field programs.

Each year the WHO's director-general told the WHA that eradication wasn't going as well as hoped because of lack of funds for vehicles, supplies, and equipment. And each year the WHA pressed for more funds to be made available. But they were not.

Political and financial support were in short supply in all quarters. The smallpox effort relied heavily on the donation of vaccines, so there was little to be done when supplies ran short. The problems were illustrated in India in 1963, where the WHO's encouragement led to the announcement of a mass vaccination campaign, only to see the campaign run into trouble when it failed to generate sufficient donations of freeze-dried vaccine.

More fundamentally, the WHO approach of relying on national campaigns and providing only limited leadership gave those who doubted the feasibility of eradication every reason to withhold funds and political support. An expert committee set up in 1964 realized that case reporting was running at 5 percent or less of actual cases—indeed, it was later realized to be closer to 1 percent. This discrepancy meant that no one could tell where progress was being made or where there was a problem. Paradoxically, because the successes in some countries were not tracked with good monitoring systems, progress that was made could not be presented as evidence to bolster support.

The campaign mode was showing its limits in some settings. India, for example, saw vaccination programs that concentrated on the easiest targets to achieve 90 percent coverage in some districts. But outbreaks were still occurring in remote villages and slums, among traveling workers, and even in the heavily vaccinated areas, mainly because of bureaucratic reporting systems and quota-driven campaign efforts. For example, schoolchildren were often revaccinated many times to fulfill quotas for numbers of vaccinations performed, while those not attending school were not vaccinated at all. Thus, in 1964, the WHO recommended that the entire population be vaccinated to achieve eradication.

At the same time, the recognition that the malaria campaign was running into difficulties exacerbated the smallpox situation, and the malaria campaign's shortcomings were threatening to undermine the WHO's credibility. Overall, in the first half of the 1960s, the smallpox eradication effort hardly looked like the global success it would eventually prove to be.

MOMENTUM BUILDS

The program's fortunes then took a turn for the better. New appointments to WHO in 1964 revived the conviction that smallpox was beatable and created the impetus to set up a separate Smallpox Eradication Unit, which provided focused leadership for international efforts. This coincided with the development of a better method of delivering the vaccine. And in 1965, the US government, the WHO's largest contributor, promised more technical and material support to the campaign.

The US decision to provide more support—a key factor in the program's development—came about through a combination of serendipitous circumstances, which started with then President Lyndon B. Johnson's search for an initiative to mark International Cooperation Year in 1965. A combined measles control and smallpox eradication program in western and central Africa was the favored candidate. However, some in the US Communicable Disease Center (now the US Centers for Disease Control and Prevention, or CDC), especially Dr. D. A. Henderson, who later led the WHO's intensified smallpox program, doubted the sustainability of such an effort, due to the high cost of the measles vaccine (at that time more than $1 per dose), which made it unaffordable to many developing countries. An alternative smallpox eradication plan for the region was proposed. Although this wasn't immediately accepted, it started discussions that led to smallpox eradication being put on the US agenda for western and central Africa and, finally, US support for the global effort.

Growing political and financial support from the United States, combined with the long-standing campaign from the Soviet Union, compelled the WHO's director-general, Dr. M. G. Candau, to reenergize the eradication plans. In 1965, at the WHA's prompting, Dr. Candau set out the current understanding of the global spread of smallpox and what would be needed to eradicate it. The WHA resolved that smallpox eradication was one of the WHO's "major objectives."

Several elements figured prominently in the director-general's proposals. First, the budget was divided so that one part remained in the main WHO budget and the other in a dedicated fund. This maneuver allowed countries' commitment to smallpox eradication to be gauged, while at the same time safeguarding the WHO's core budget. Second, the general approach was designed to learn from the problems with the malaria program. For example, rather than setting out a strict set of rules, the program articulated "principles" to allow for flexibility. Indeed, the WHO handbook for the program was written as a "draft," leaving headquarters and national staff to infer that it was not the final word and could be updated. Third, the case reporting system was to be developed right at the start of the program to guide its progress; and fourth, research was encouraged. The proposals also made it clear that all WHO member countries would be required to participate, and their efforts would need to be coordinated.

In 1966, the WHA finally agreed to back the objective adopted the previous year for the Intensified Smallpox Eradication Programme, which started on January 1, 1967. The budget allocation was $2.4 million, which, if divided among the roughly 50 countries where programs were needed, amounted to about $50,000 per country.

At that point, there were between 10 million and 15 million cases worldwide. It was estimated that 1.5 million to 2 million people died of smallpox each year, and those who survived were disfigured; some were left blind or with other disabilities. The 31 endemic countries included many in sub-Saharan Africa, six in Asia, and three in South America. And some of those countries remained divided by war and famine.

A FULL EFFORT

The Smallpox Eradication Unit set to work, with minimal staff and Henderson as the chief medical officer. For most of the campaign, the staff consisted of four medical officers, one administrator, a technical officer, and four secretaries. With strong support from the US CDC, the team produced an epidemiological report every two to four weeks, produced training materials, and dealt with the media.

Vaccine jet injectors, kits for collecting and sending specimens, and training aids were stored in Geneva and sent out on request. The effort also supplied a new breakthrough: the bifurcated needle. The needle was a marvel of simple technology that reduced costs (1,000 needles for only $5) and made vaccinating easier. Each needle could be boiled or flamed and reused literally hundreds of times, and one vial provided enough vaccine for four times as many people due to the smaller amount of vaccine required. Plus, they were very easy to use. A villager could be instructed and trained in its use in 15 minutes.

The quality of the international staff was important to the program, but recruitment wasn't easy. In 1967, few

infectious disease control epidemiologists were familiar with smallpox, and the WHO was not organized to provide specialized training for new recruits.

Despite the limits of personnel, progress was noticeable—initially in western and central Africa, where quick detection and containment of outbreaks took effect. Within two years, 17 of the 21 countries in the region were free of smallpox, despite their overall levels of poverty. Brazil also made spectacular progress, enabling the Western Hemisphere to be declared free of endemic smallpox in April 1971. Provision of enough quality freeze-dried vaccine and the introduction of the bifurcated needle started taking effect, especially in eastern and southern Africa.

NEW METHODS

The following year saw major disruption to the program's successful trajectory, as Bangladesh lost its smallpox-free status to the refugees fleeing the civil war that led to independence. Botswana was faced with an epidemic, and it became clear that Iran and Iraq were both endemic again. Thanks to focused campaigns, however, all except Bangladesh were clear of the disease by the end of 1973. In September of that year, intensified campaigns began in the five remaining endemic countries: Bangladesh, India, Nepal, Pakistan, and Ethiopia.

The momentum was regained as new methods and extra resources were mobilized to cope with the large numbers of refugees from both natural and human-made disasters. With the WHO's persuasion, there was a move away from concentrating on general vaccination campaigns to focusing on actively seeking out cases and containing outbreaks with quarantine and vaccination of local people. Using the surveillance and containment strategy, teams were equipped with Jeeps and motorbikes to search villages, markets, and even houses for cases.

The approach appeared increasingly military, as motorized teams sped to an area as soon as an active case was announced. Massive efforts were then made to isolate cases and vaccinate everyone in the area, whether or not they had been vaccinated before. WHO staff on short-term contracts supplemented the ranks of local health workers.

The military-like approach succeeded even in the most difficult of circumstances. By the end of 1976, tens of thousands of health staff in search and containment programs stopped smallpox transmission in Ethiopia, a country embroiled in civil war and suffering with poverty and little infrastructure. In this final stage, large numbers of volunteers and helicopters were used to respond to outbreaks. As smallpox was contained in Ethiopia, war and the resulting refugees took the disease back into Somalia, but campaign coordinators could see there really was an end in sight, and experienced staff and money from many countries were marshaled to contain the outbreak.

In October 1977—10 years, 9 months, and 26 days after the start of the intensified campaign—the last endemic case of smallpox was recorded in Somalia. National staff and WHO officials embarked on an intense program of tracing contacts, quarantine, and vaccination. In May 1980, after two years of surveillance and searching, the WHA declared that smallpox finally had been eradicated.

COSTS OF ERADICATION

The costs of smallpox eradication have been estimated, although the underlying data are limited. In 1967 the main program cost was associated with vaccine, personnel, and transport. For the developing countries, this amounted to about 10 cents per vaccination. Estimating that about a fifth of the 2.5 billion people living in developing countries were vaccinated each year suggests that $50 million a year was spent on vaccination. However, the actual expenditure was much less, approximately $10 million per year by the endemic countries.[2]

India is the only developing country that has estimated the economic loss due to smallpox. In 1976, it was estimated that the cost of caring for someone in India with smallpox was $2.85 a patient, so the annual total cost of patient care for India alone would be $12 million.[3,4] Based on the proportion of the global smallpox cases that India reported, these figures suggest that caring for people with smallpox cost developing countries more than $20 million in 1967. Estimating a person's economic productivity during his or her lifetime, it has also been calculated that India lost about $700 million due to diminished economic performance each year. Assuming 1.5 million deaths due to smallpox occurred in 1967, it is reasonable to estimate that smallpox was costing developing countries as a whole at least $1 billion each year at the start of the intensified eradication campaign.[2]

Industrialized countries, on the other hand, incurred the cost of vaccination programs to prevent the reintroduction of the disease. In the United States, the bill for 5.6 million primary vaccinations and 8.6 million revaccinations in 1968 alone was $92.8 million, about $6.50 a vaccination. Of those vaccinated, 8,024 people had complications requiring medical attention, 238 were hospitalized, 9 died, and 4 were permanently disabled. With other indirect costs of the vaccination program, such as absences from work, the cost for 1968 was 75 cents per person. Even assuming that other developed countries had lower costs, this puts the annual cost for these countries around $350 million, based on their total population. Overall, the suggested global cost, both direct and indirect, of smallpox in the late 1960s was more than $1.35 billion.[2]

The ultimate expenditures of the intensified eradication program were around $23 million per year between 1967 and 1979, including $98 million from international contributions and $200 million from the endemic countries.[2] It has since been calculated that the largest donor, the United States, saves the total of all its contributions every 26 days, making smallpox prevention through vaccination one of the most cost-beneficial health interventions of the time.[5]

LESSONS LEARNED

Observers attribute much of the program's success to political commitment and leadership, in this case from WHO and its partner the CDC, along with specific funds, staff, and a unit with overall accountability and responsibility for the program. The initial dismal phase of the eradication program in the first half of the 1960s showed how lack of that commitment and organization undermined the efforts.

For national programs, it is generally agreed that success hinged on having someone who was responsible, preferably solely, for smallpox eradication. This individual was the main contact in the country and could be held accountable. Best results were obtained where WHO staff, or supervisory people, went into the field frequently to review activities and resolve problems. Their work showed that relatively few highly committed and knowledgeable people could motivate large numbers of staff successfully, even in unstable areas and the poorest of countries.

No two national campaigns were alike, which points to one of the significant lessons that can be learned from smallpox eradication: the need for a flexible approach. Vaccination programs had to be adapted to different administrative, sociocultural, and geographical situations, and ways of assessing the work had to be devised. Indeed, it was important that funds raised did not come with conditions that prevented their use for different activities in different areas.

Using existing health care systems for the program both took advantage of established ways of working in some countries and forced other countries to bring their services up to standard. This helped develop immunization services more generally—health staff helping with the campaign received training in vaccination and search and containment. This training was especially important for hospital-based health systems that had no experience in setting up preventive campaigns. The knowledge gained this way then went into other campaigns, offsetting the cost of the initial campaign. This work outside hospitals also reinforced how important it was to seek the support of community leaders and thus the participation of their communities. These lessons have provided a strategy for many community-based projects, including the trachoma control program (Case 10) and the guinea worm campaign (Case 11).

It was also discovered during the campaign that more than one vaccination could be given at a time, an idea now taken for granted. In 1970, the Smallpox Eradication Unit proposed an Expanded Programme on Immunization to increase the number of vaccinations administered during a single patient interaction. The proposal sought to add diphtheria, tetanus, pertussis, polio, and measles vaccines to the routine smallpox and BCG (to prevent tuberculosis) vaccines. In 1974, the WHA agreed, and the United Nations Children's Fund (UNICEF) became a major supporter of the Expanded Programme on Immunization in the 1980s.

Routine immunization in the developing world under the program may prove in the end to be the smallpox eradication effort's greatest contribution: By 1990, 80% of the children throughout the developing world were receiving vaccines against six childhood killers, compared with only 5% when the program started.

The importance of monitoring results is another transferable lesson. In the early 1960s, several countries relied on measuring activity as an indicator of success—and duly reported that they had vaccinated a large number of people. Yet the number of new cases remained high. Clearly, there was a problem with the surveillance and program evaluation, but because the monitoring indicator was within an acceptable range, nothing changed. From 1974, standards were established for surveillance and containment as well as for vaccination coverage.

Good reporting ensures that success can be measured, but publicity of that success is essential. The message that the smallpox eradication campaign was working really spread among donors only in 1974, when just five endemic countries remained, thus triggering large donations and more funds.

Impact of Eradication

The eradication of smallpox continues to inspire and highlights the importance of cooperation, national commitment, leadership, reliable epidemiologic information, and appropriate technology. The particular features of smallpox, both in terms of the disease and the vaccine, which made the disease a prime candidate for eradication, may not be found in other diseases. And recent events have highlighted the potential of an eradicated disease becoming a bioweapon (see Box 1-1).

However, the lessons learned from the campaign can be adapted to other circumstances. The lasting legacy to public health of the smallpox eradication campaign is the demonstration of how the combination of good science, outstanding organization, focused monitoring, and international commitment can make a substantial difference to global health, saving generations from disability and premature death.

BOX 1-1 The Eradication Debate

Smallpox was one of only a handful of diseases considered good candidates for **elimination** or **eradication**. (*Elimination* refers to reducing the number of new infections to zero in a defined geographical area, with continued interventions required to prevent reestablishment of transmission. *Eradication* means permanently reducing the number of new infections worldwide to zero, with interventions no longer needed.) Few human ailments meet the six preconditions for disease eradication:[6]

1. No animal reservoir for the virus is known or suspected.
2. Sensitive and specific tools are available for diagnosis and surveillance.
3. Transmission from one individual to another can be interrupted.
4. Nonlethal infection or vaccination confers lifelong immunity.
5. The **burden of disease** is important to international public health.
6. Political commitment to eradication efforts exists.

During the 1900s, global efforts were made to eradicate seven diseases: hookworm, yellow fever, malaria, yaws, smallpox, guinea worm, and polio.[7] Smallpox was eradicated in 1977. Today, worldwide campaigns against polio continue, with the hope that it will become the second disease to be eradicated. Interventions against guinea worm continue in sub-Saharan Africa, the only remaining endemic area.

BENEFITS OF ELIMINATION AND ERADICATION

The most obvious benefits of disease eradication are that no illness or death from that disease will ever occur again.[8] Control programs are no longer needed, and this allows resources, both monetary and otherwise, to be redirected. These benefits result from the two basic objectives of eradication programs: to eradicate the disease and to strengthen and further develop the health system.[9]

The monetary benefits of elimination and eradication can be substantial. One study estimated that if measles were eradicated by 2010, and vaccination could be discontinued, the United States could save $500 million to $4.5 billion.[10] Another study estimated that seven industrialized countries (Canada, Denmark, Finland, the Netherlands, Spain, Sweden, and the United Kingdom) would save between $10 million and $623 million if measles were eradicated, even assuming that measles vaccination would continue.[11]

Other benefits of elimination and eradication relate to the campaigns themselves. Surveillance, logistics, and administrative support are invigorated to achieve a higher standard of performance. If designed with system strengthening in mind, elimination and eradication programs that benefit from high political visibility and financial support can improve the quantity and quality of health workers, bolster health infrastructure, foster coordination among donors, and contribute to other improvements in the backbone of public health.

Potential Pitfalls of Elimination and Eradication Campaigns

Efforts to eliminate or eradicate disease also can inadvertently cause major problems. The near-term risk is that the focused efforts to deal with one ailment detract from a health system's ability to deal with many other causes of human suffering. Particularly in global eradication programs, where large outlays may be required to reach populations in which the disease in question is of relatively small importance (compared with other illnesses), the diversion of resources can be detrimental; local political commitment can waver in the face of pressures to address higher-priority health concerns. This risk can be—but is not always—countered by explicit attention to how the eradication campaigns can strengthen the basic functions of the health system, such as surveillance, human resource development, management, and others.

The longer-term risk is that it may be impossible to obtain all the promised benefits because vaccination (or other preventive actions) must continue, even if the program is successful in reducing to zero the incidence of a disease. As the US Institute of Medicine's Forum on Emerging Infections put it, even in developed countries where infections have been eradicated or nearly eradicated, mass vaccinations will probably have to be maintained at very high levels for an extended time in order to protect against reintroduction from areas where poverty, civil unrest, or lack of political will impede high vaccination coverage and sustain endemicity.[6] In fact, without continued preventive measures, eradication can put the world's population at risk if there are changes

(continues)

BOX 1-1 The Eradication Debate   (continued)

in the natural history of the disease, if the scientific community is wrong about the effectiveness of immunization or other preventive measures, or if bioterrorism is a threat.

Being prepared for outbreaks of long-gone diseases comes at a price. In 1997, for example, the US Department of Defense contracted with BioReliance to deliver 300,000 doses of an improved smallpox vaccine for $22.4 million (about $70 per dose), and in 2000, the CDC contracted OraVax to manufacture 40 million doses of smallpox vaccine beginning in 2004 and continuing through 2020 at a cost of $8 per dose, though this schedule was altered after the 2002 anthrax outbreak. By the end of 2002, the Bush administration had set aside $500 million to procure 300 million doses of smallpox vaccine.[12] As of January 31, 2003, some 291,000 doses were released by the CDC to vaccinate first responders in the United States against smallpox, and $42 million was appropriated to establish the Smallpox Vaccine Injury Compensation Program, even though smallpox was eradicated almost 30 years ago.[13]

REFERENCES

1. World Health Organization (WHO). WHO fact sheet on smallpox. Available at: http://www.who.int/mediacentre/factsheets/smallpox/en/. Accessed January 12, 2007.

2. Fenner F, Henderson DA, Arita I, Jezek Z, Ladnyi ID. Smallpox and its eradication. Available at: http://whqlibdoc.who.int/smallpox/9241561106.pdf. Accessed January 12, 2007.

3. Ramaiah TJ. Cost-benefit analysis of the intensified campaign against smallpox in India. *Natl Inst Health Adm Educ Bull*. 1976;9:169–203.

4. Ramaiah TJ. Cost-effectiveness analysis of the intensified campaign against smallpox in India. *Natl Inst Health Adm Educ Bull*. 1976;9:205–219.

5. Brilliant LB. *The Management of Smallpox Eradication in India: A Case Study and Analysis*. Ann Arbor, MI: University of Michigan Press; 1985.

6. Institute of Medicine, Forum on Emerging Infections. *Considerations for Viral Disease Eradication: Lessons Learned and Future Struggles*. Washington, DC: National Academies Press; 2002.

7. Henderson DA. Lessons from the eradication campaigns. *Vaccine*. 1999;17(suppl 3):S53–S55.

8. Dowdle WR. The principles of disease elimination and eradication. *MMWR*. 1999;48(SU01):2307.

9. Goodvan RA, Foster KL, Trowbridge FL, Figueroa JR. Summary. *Bull WHO*. 1998;76(suppl 2):9–11.

10. Miller MA, Redd S, Hadler S, Hinman A. A model to estimate the potential economic benefits of measles eradication for the United States. *Vaccine*. 1998;20:1917–1922.

11. Carabin H, Edmunds J. Future savings from measles eradication in industrialized countries. *J Infect Dis*. 2003;187(suppl 1):S29–S35.

12. Koplow DA. *Smallpox: The Right to Eradicate a Global Scourge*. Berkeley, CA: University of California Press; 2003.

13. Centers for Disease Control and Prevention (CDC). Smallpox vaccination program: vaccine doses shipped and released for use. Available at: http://www.cdc.gov/od/oc/media/pressrel/smallpox/smallpox.htm. Accessed January 12, 2007.

Preventing HIV/AIDS and Sexually Transmitted Infections in Thailand*

* The first draft of this case was prepared by Phyllida Brown.

ABSTRACT

Geographic area: Thailand

Health condition: Between 1989 and 1990, the proportion of direct sex workers in Thailand infected with HIV tripled, from 3.5% to 9.3% and a year later reached 21.6%. Over the same period, the proportion of male conscripts already infected with HIV when tested on entry to the army at age 21 rose sixfold, from 0.5% in 1989 to 3% in 1991.

Global importance of the health condition today: HIV/AIDS is one of the greatest threats to human health worldwide, with an estimated 38.6 million people infected with the virus in 2005. The vast majority of people with HIV are in sub-Saharan Africa, where **life expectancy** today is just 47 years; without AIDS, it is estimated that life expectancy would be 15 years longer. The number of children who have lost a parent to AIDS is now estimated at 20 million.

Intervention or program: In 1991, the National AIDS Committee led by Thailand's prime minister implemented the "100% condom program," in which all sex workers in sex establishments were required to use condoms with clients. Health officials provided boxes of condoms free of charge, and local police held meetings with sex establishment owners and sex workers, despite the illegality of prostitution. Men seeking treatment for sexually transmitted infections (STIs) were asked to name the sex establishment they had used, and health officials would then visit the establishment to provide more information.

Cost and cost-effectiveness: Total government expenditure on the national AIDS program remained steady at approximately $375 million from 1998 to 2001, with the majority spent on treatment and care (65%); this investment represents 1.9% of the nation's overall health budget.

Impact: Condom use in sex work nationwide increased from 14% in early 1989 to more than 90% by June 1992. An estimated 200,000 new infections were averted between 1993 and 2000. The number of new STI cases fell from 200,000 in 1989 to 15,000 in 2001; the rate of new HIV infections fell fivefold between 1991 and 1995.

Acquired immunodeficiency syndrome (AIDS), caused by the human immunodeficiency virus (HIV), is among the greatest threats to health worldwide. In 2005, an estimated 38.6 million people were living with HIV. During 2005 alone, about 4.1 million people became infected and another 2.8 million lost their lives.[1] Although the vast majority of people with HIV are in sub-Saharan Africa, the epidemic is becoming increasingly serious in Asian countries. Of an estimated 8.3 million infected persons in Asia, more than two thirds are in India.[1] Approximately 572,500 people in Thailand are infected with the virus, with national prevalence rates the second highest of all countries in the Asia and Pacific region.[2]

The negative social and economic impacts of HIV/AIDS are profound. In Africa, the average life expectancy at birth is 47 years; without AIDS it would be 62 years. Household incomes in societies that lack social support mechanisms are declining dramatically, and the number of children orphaned by AIDS is now estimated at 20 million, with 75,000 of those orphans living in Thailand.[2,3]

Well-documented stories of large-scale success in HIV prevention are few and far between, although many small programs have been shown to be effective among specific populations. Changing the behaviors associated with increased risk of HIV, including sexual practices and intravenous drug use, has proven to be a formidable challenge, and technological advances such as a vaccine against HIV or microbicides that can kill the virus are years, maybe decades, away. As the Thai experience illustrates, creating more prevention successes will take sustained and high-level leadership and the development of programs appropriate to local circumstances.

THAILAND'S AWAKENING TO HIV/AIDS

Thai authorities initially recognized the severity of the situation in 1988, when the first wave of HIV infections spread among injecting drug users. A National Advisory Committee on AIDS was established, which developed an initial plan that included surveillance of "sentinel" groups, such as sex workers, male patients with sexually transmitted infections (STIs), and blood donors. This surveillance revealed that the virus was now also spreading swiftly through sex. Between 1989 and 1990, the proportion of direct sex workers infected with the virus tripled, from 3.5% to 9.3%, and a year later it had reached 21.6%.[4] Over the same period, the proportion of male conscripts already infected with HIV when tested on entry to the army at age 21 rose sixfold—from 0.5% in 1989 to 3% in 1991.[5] Researchers found that visits to sex establishments were common among these young men.[6]

Some health officials had already begun to take action on their own. Dr. Wiwat Rojanapithayakorn, an epidemiologist and expert in STI control, who was then director of the Regional Office in Communicable Disease Control in Thailand's Ratchaburi province, argued for a pragmatic approach. As he explains it, "It is not possible to stop people from having sex with sex workers, so the most important thing is to make sure that sex is safe." However, Rojanapithayakorn knew that such an approach would require political leadership. Prostitution is illegal in Thailand, and the government's intervention could imply that it tolerated or even condoned it. Fortunately, the provincial governor agreed that preventing HIV from spreading further was the priority.

NO CONDOM, NO SEX: THE 100% CONDOM PROGRAM

In 1989, the Ratchaburi province pioneered a program whose aim was to reduce the vulnerability of individual sex workers by creating a "monopoly environment" across the province's sex establishments with one straightforward rule: no condom, no sex. Until this pilot study, sex establishment owners and individual sex workers had been reluctant to insist that their clients use condoms because most clients preferred unprotected sex and would just go elsewhere to find it. But by requiring universal condom use in all sex establishments, the provincial government removed the competitive disincentive to individual workers or sex establishments.

Health officials held meetings with sex establishment owners and sex workers, provided them with information about HIV and proper condom use, and convinced them of the plan's benefits. The police helped organize the early meetings, which pressured sex establishment owners to cooperate. Boxes of 100 condoms were supplied, free of charge, directly to sex workers at their regular health checks in government-run clinics, and health officials distributed boxes of condoms to sex establishments.

Tracing contacts supplemented this strategy. Men seeking treatment in government clinics for any STI were asked to name the commercial sex establishment they had used. The presence of infection was regarded as evidence of failure to use a condom. Similarly, infection in a sex worker was taken as evidence that she had engaged in unprotected sex. Provincial health officers would then visit the establishment and provide more information and advice to owners and workers about condom use. In principle, the police could shut down any sex establishment that failed to adopt the policy. While this sanction was used a few times early on, authorities generally preferred to cooperate with the sex establishments rather than alienate them.[5]

The results were rapid. The incidence of STIs such as gonorrhea in sex workers and their clients in Ratchaburi fell steeply within just months.[5] "Sexually transmitted infections became rare diseases in sex workers: that was very convincing," says Rojanapithayakorn. Through meetings and lectures, the health officials in Ratchaburi persuaded 13 other provinces to adopt the program in 1989 and 1990.

GOING NATIONAL AFTER EARLY SUCCESS

The Thai government first implemented its National AIDS Programme and Centre for Prevention and Control of AIDS in 1987, with the goals of raising awareness about the dangers of the disease, reducing risky behavior, and providing care to people suffering from it. The major strategy behind the campaign was to encourage men to use condoms with sex workers.[6] The government strategy included mass advertising and education campaigns. Television and radio advertisements aimed at men explicitly warned them of the dangers of not using condoms when visiting a sex worker. Health workers in government clinics and community workers from nongovernmental organizations (NGOs) trained sex workers in the proper use of condoms and in negotiating their use with clients.[5] In some cases, experienced sex workers were trained to educate their less experienced colleagues.[7]

It was not until August 1991 that the National AIDS Committee, chaired by Prime Minister Anand Panyarachun, resolved to implement the 100% condom program as part of the national campaign.[5] Health officials had initially feared that the committee would reject the idea, but a series of preparatory meetings with members of the National AIDS Committee and others achieved the necessary support. The resolution stated:

> The governor, the provincial chief of police, and the provincial health officer of each province will work together to enforce a condom-use-only policy that requires all sex workers to use condoms with every customer. All concerned ministries will issue directives that comply with this policy.

By mid-1992, all provinces had implemented the program because of the decisive leadership at the highest level. With this increased support, the overall budget for HIV control rose from $2.63 million in 1991 to $82 million by 1996, 96% of which was financed by the Thai government,[8] and some 60 million condoms were distributed annually.[9]

DRAMATIC RESULTS IN BEHAVIOR CHANGE AND HEALTH OUTCOME

Condom use in sex establishments nationwide increased from 14% in early 1989 to more than 90% by June 1992.[6] These data are based on surveys with sex workers and young men conducted by the epidemiology division of the Ministry of Public Health. According to estimates by the Thai Working Group on HIV/AIDS Projection for the Ministry of Public Health, the number of new HIV cases decreased by more than 80% from 1991 to 2001.[9] The incidence of reported STIs (gonorrhea, nongonococcal infection, chlamydia, syphilis, and others) fell even more steeply. In total, for men, the annual number of new cases of STIs fell from almost 200,000 in 1989 to 27,597 in 1994.[6] By 2001 the total number of new cases of STIs in both men and women

was around 15,000 (see Figure 2-1). The decline in new cases of infection closely tracked the increase in rates of reported condom use.[5]

Similarly, HIV surveillance of sentinel groups showed dramatic changes. In 1993, up to 4% of military conscripts were HIV positive. By December 1994, the figure was 2.7%,[6] and by 2001, only 0.5% of new conscripts were infected. The prevalence of HIV in people attending STI clinics almost halved between the mid-1990s and 2002.[9] See Figure 2-2.

Rigorous prospective studies in the northern areas of the country, which are most severely affected by HIV/AIDS, support these national data. Researchers followed successive cohorts of army conscripts, totaling some 4,000 men, and checked their HIV and STI status every six months. The rate of new HIV infections fell fivefold between 1991 and 1995, while the rate of new STIs fell tenfold.[10]

EVALUATING THE PROGRAM: LESSONS, QUESTIONS, ANSWERS—AND MORE QUESTIONS

The data are so dramatic that skeptics might question their accuracy or ask whether the declining infections can truly be attributed to a government program. Independent studies, however, suggest that the strategy was genuinely effective. The Institute for Population and Social Research at Mahidol University in Thailand, supported by the Joint United Nations Programme on HIV/AIDS (UNAIDS) and the Thai Ministry of Public Health, conducted a study to assess the program's effectiveness. The study concluded that the 100% condom program had contributed significantly to large-scale reduction of HIV transmission throughout the country.[5,11] Meanwhile a separate World Bank review concluded that Thailand's success is "an accomplishment that few other countries, if any, have been able to replicate." The review suggests that the program may have prevented some 200,000 HIV infections during the 1990s alone.[12]

Because the program was implemented in a real-life setting rather than in the artificially controlled conditions of a clinical trial, it is difficult to tease out exactly which components of the program were most effective: the 100% condom program, the education that went with it, the media warnings, or other factors. Notably, the public information campaigns may simply have scared many men away from sex establishments in the early 1990s. STI incidence began to fall rapidly in 1990, before all provinces had implemented the 100% condom program.[6] Between 1990 and 1993, the proportion of men visiting commercial sex workers halved, from 22% to 10%.[13] Some researchers believe, therefore, that mass advertising played an important role. However, as Rojanapithayakorn points out, countries that have simply

FIGURE 2-1 STI cases reported compared with condom use rates in Thailand, 1988–2001.

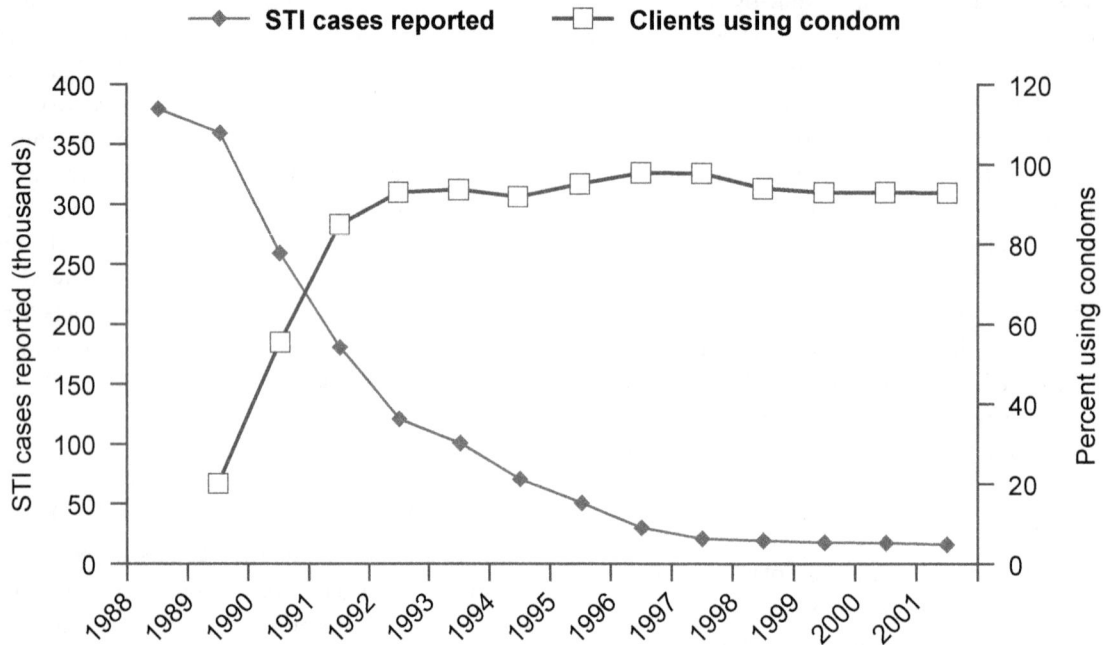

Source: From Dr. Wiwat Rojanapithayakorn. Compiled with data from STI Section, Bureau of AIDS, TB and STI, Department of Disease Control, Ministry of Public Health, Thailand.

provided education about condoms, without also insisting on 100% condom use in the sex industry, have not been so successful in limiting the spread of HIV. He and others argue that the 100% condom program and the information campaign should be seen as complementary components of the same strategy: Neither would have been wholly effective without the other.

Several questions have been asked about the findings. First, was the reported decline in STI incidence genuine, or did some people simply shift away from government clinics to private clinics? In interviews with sex workers, Mahidol University researchers found that the proportion receiving their treatment from government clinics had not changed since the program was implemented. In addition, the researchers interviewed pharmacists. More than 80% reported a 5-year decline in the sale of antibiotics used to treat STIs, casting doubt on any suggestion that patients had simply switched to the private sector.[5]

Another question is whether the reported rates of condom use are inflated. Mahidol University researchers interviewed more than 2,000 sex workers and more than 4,000 clients. There was some regional variation, but overall reported rates of condom use were strikingly high. When sex workers were asked if they would have sex without a condom for more money, only 3.5% said they would, although almost three quarters told the researchers that clients had repeatedly asked them to do so.[5] Among sex workers, 97% reported that they always used condoms with one-time clients, and 93% reported that they did so with regular clients.[6] Other studies indicated that condom use among sex workers may be declining: A 2003 study found a 51% overall condom utilization rate among female sex workers in three Thai cities, and a 2003 cross-sectional survey found that less than half of participants who reported having sex with commercial partners in the past year used condoms consistently.[14,15]

There is also separate evidence that most sex workers have become extremely resistant to demands for condom-free sex. For example, in small studies, male volunteers posing as clients approached sex workers to assess the effectiveness of peer training by sex workers to help each other with the skills needed to insist on condom use. The volunteers asked for sex without a condom, and if they were refused, offered to pay more. In one small study, 72 of 78 sex workers refused sex without a condom even when offered three times the usual fee.[7]

FIGURE 2-2 Prevalence of HIV among direct and indirect sex workers and men attending public STI clinics in Thailand, 1989–2001.

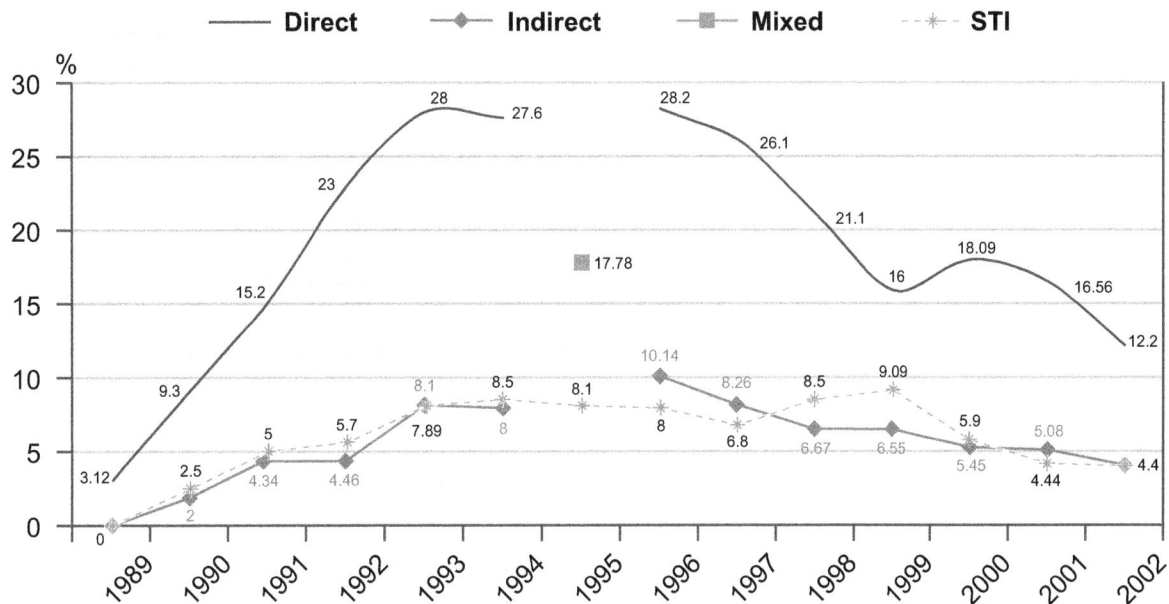

Source: From Dr. Wiwat Rojanapithayakorn. Compiled with data from Bureau of Epidemiology, Ministry of Public Health, Thailand.

A related question is how effectively the program could reach "indirect" sex workers, whom clients would typically find in bars or restaurants. Such establishments often deny that they offer sex, and some have refused to cooperate with the program or distribute condoms to their workers. The relative inaccessibility of these establishments also made them difficult to study in independent evaluations, so estimates of the program's success may be biased if this group is under-represented. This is important, particularly as clients appear to have been shifting from direct sex establishments to indirect workers during the 1990s.[16] However, some studies suggested that most indirect sex workers, like their counterparts in direct sex establishments, insist on condoms with clients. The lowest rates of condom use were reported in hotels, at around 85%; in bars and restaurants the proportion was around 90%, and in massage parlors it was 98%.[5]

WHAT THE PROGRAM DID NOT ACHIEVE

The success of the strategy in slowing HIV transmission is due, at least in part, to the sheer scale and level of organization of the sex industry in Thailand, and the popularity of commercial sex among a wide cross-section of Thai men in

the early years of the epidemic. (See Box 2-1 for a discussion of Cambodia's success in a similar setting.) However, Thailand's public health officials acknowledge that the program has done little to encourage men and women in Thailand to use condoms in casual but noncommercial sex.[9] Among the population as a whole, casual sex without condoms is widespread, particularly among young people, who do not remember the height of the crises in the early 1990s.[12] This suggests that there is still a substantial risk that HIV will continue to spread through heterosexual sex in Thailand. In addition, because the program has focused mainly on sexually transmitted HIV, the most common transmission route, **interventions** among injecting drug users, such as methadone treatment and needle and syringe exchange programs, have not expanded to reach the national scale. In this group, the prevalence of HIV continues to rise and is now as high as 50%.[9]

WHAT MADE IT WORK?

Several important factors enabled the program. First, the sex industry is relatively structured. There are few "freelance" workers; most operate from an establishment. Since the late

BOX 2-1 Replicating Thailand's Success in Cambodia

With its large commercial sex industry and the highest HIV rates in Asia, neighboring Cambodia offers a strikingly similar setting for replicating Thailand's successful 100% condom program. As in Thailand, Cambodia's 100,000 commercial sex workers constitute a particularly high-risk group for transmitting HIV; reported infection rates of sex workers range from 15% to 29%, the highest of any group in the country.[17,18]

Inspired by Thailand's successful experience, Cambodia implemented a pilot 100% condom campaign in 1998 targeting sex establishment-based workers in the high prevalence Sihanoukville province. A survey of sex workers in the region found an increase of consistent condom use from 43% before the program to 93% after the program was fully implemented.[19] This is due in part to the establishment of an effective monitoring system that was able to identify uncooperative establishments through the use of "mystery clients," regular STI checkups, and monitoring of condom stock. The system relied crucially on owners of sex establishments, who actively collaborated with the program to maintain and report condom sale records. The owners also supported **outreach** activities to popular clientele, such as military police.[19]

With the financial support of external donors, Cambodia's National AIDS Authority and National Center for HIV/AIDS, Dermatology and STI scaled up the pilot 100% condom use program nationally in 1999. In 2004 alone, more than 20 million condoms were distributed, largely through social marketing channels. The program has delivered impressive results: According to a recent study, consistent condom use among formal sex workers nearly doubled between 1997 and 2003, from 53% to an estimated 96%.[20] Overall, Cambodia's 2005 adult national HIV prevalence rate of 1.6% was 30% lower than prevalence in the late 1990s.[1]

Source: Adapted and reprinted from ATSDR. 2003 CERCLA Priority List of Hazardous Substances. Available at: http://www.atsdr.cdc.gov/cercla. Accessed January 12, 2007; and ATSDR. Top 20 Hazardous Substances from the CERCLA Priority List of Hazardous Substances for 2003. Available at: http://www.atsdr.cdc.gov/cxcx3.html. Accessed January 12, 2007.

1960s, the Thai government has maintained lists of both "direct" and "indirect" sex establishments, which enabled officials to reach the owners of the establishments and seek their cooperation. Second, the nation already had a good network of STI services, both for treatment and surveillance, within a well-functioning health system. As well as providing essential treatment and advice to sex workers and their clients, the health system supplied decision makers with crucial data both at the baseline and when the program took effect. This could not have happened without an adequate number of trained health workers, epidemiologists, and statisticians. Third, different sectors—health authorities, provincial governors, and police—collaborated well. This multisectoral approach by the national government raised the profile of HIV/AIDS and engaged a variety of stakeholders and others in the policy dialogue to set national priorities.[8] Fourth, strong leadership from the prime minister, backed with significant financial resources, made it possible to act swiftly.

GUESSING THE COST

Surprisingly, given the widespread interest in the Thai government's program, no estimates appear to have been made on the **cost-effectiveness** of the 100% condom program. Rojanapithayakorn points out that most of the program's

cost is human resources: It relies on trained staff in STI clinics and epidemiologists. Because this infrastructure already existed, the costs of implementing the program were very small. Expenditure on the condoms themselves has usually been around $1.2 million per year and has never risen above $2.2 million per year.[9] In addition, the government invested in education and information campaigns. However, the private sector offered financial and in-kind assistance, including an estimated $48 million in donated commercial airtime for HIV/AIDS messages.[21] Total government expenditure on the national HIV/AIDS program has remained steady at approximately $375 million from 1998 to 2001, with the majority of the money spent on treatment and care (65%); this investment represents 1.9% of the government's overall health budget. In return, some 200,000 individuals avoided HIV infection between 1993 and 2000, enabling them to remain productive members of society.

PROGRAM UNDER THREAT

The cost of treating AIDS with antiretroviral drugs—as well as less costly drugs to treat opportunistic infections—has posed a major challenge to Thailand in recent years. Some are concerned that these costs may threaten HIV prevention activities. Between 1997 and 2004, the HIV prevention budget declined by two thirds.[22] Although condom use reportedly remains high among sex workers, there are also concerns about new sex workers, trafficked into Thailand from nearby countries. For these women, access to health care, information, training, and even condoms may be limited. Thailand's success in slowing its HIV/AIDS epidemic to date will continue to require vigorous support.

The Thai experience in preventing the spread of HIV provides no blueprint for other countries, particularly those where the starting conditions may be very different. But it does suggest that major changes in deeply entrenched behaviors can be effected through targeted strategies, and it highlights the courage of political leaders who take risks to improve the public's health.

REFERENCES

1. UNAIDS (United Nations Joint Programme on HIV/AIDS). *Report on the Global AIDS Epidemic*. Geneva, Switzerland: United Nations Joint Programme on HIV/AIDS; 2006.

2. CDC (US Centers for Disease Control and Prevention). *Global AIDS Program, Country Profiles: Thailand*. Atlanta, GA: Centers for Disease Control and Prevention. Available at: http://www.cdc.gov/nchstp/od/gap/countries/docs/04profiles/FY04%20Thailand.Final.pdf. Accessed January 12, 2007.

3. United Nations Joint Programme on HIV/AIDS. *AIDS Epidemic Update* (December). Geneva, Switzerland: United Nations Joint Programme on HIV/AIDS; 2002.

4. Thailand Ministry of Public Health. Results of HIV Sero-surveillance, Thailand 1989–2004 (round 1–22). Available at: http://epid.moph.go.th/Aids/Round6month/R6Mtab1.html. Accessed January 12, 2007.

5. United Nations Joint Programme on HIV/AIDS. *Evaluation of the 100% Condom Programme in Thailand*. Document 00.18E. Geneva, Switzerland: United Nations Joint Programme on HIV/AIDS; AIDS Division, Ministry of Public Health, Thailand.

6. Rojanapithayakorn W, Hanenberg R. The 100% Condom Programme in Thailand. Editorial Review. *AIDS*. 1996;10(1):1–7.

7. Visrutaratna S, Lindan CP, Sirhorachai A, Mandel JS. Superstar and model brothel: developing and evaluating a condom promotion program for sex establishments in Chiang Mai, Thailand. *AIDS*. 1995;9(suppl 1):S69–S75.

8. Ainsworth M, Beyrer C, Soucat A. AIDS and public policy: the lessons and challenges of "success" in Thailand. *Health Policy*. 2003;64(1):13–37.

9. Chitwarakorn A. HIV/AIDS and sexually transmitted infections in Thailand: lessons learned and future challenges. In Narain JP, ed. *AIDS in Asia: The Challenge Ahead*. New Delhi, India: Sage Publications; 2004.

10. Celentano D, Nelson K, Lyles C, et al. Decreasing incidence of HIV and sexually transmitted diseases among young Thai men: evidence for success of the HIV/AIDS control and prevention program. *AIDS*. 1998;12(5):F29–F36.

11. Chamratrithirong A, Thongthai V, Boonchalaksi W, Guest P, Kanchanachitra C, Varangrat A. *The Success of the 100% Condom Programme in Thailand: Survey Results of the Evaluation of the 100% Condom Promotion Programme*. IPSR Publication 238. Mahidol University, Thailand: Institute for Population and Social Research; 1999.

12. World Bank. Thailand's response to AIDS: building on success, confronting the future. *Thailand Social Monitor V*. Available at: http://www.worldbank.orgth. Accessed January 12, 2007.

13. Phoolcharoen W, Ungchusak K, Sittitrai W, Brown T. *Thailand: Lessons Learned from a Strong National Response to HIV/AIDS*. Bangkok, Thailand: AIDS Division, Communicable Disease Control Department, Ministry of Public Health; 1998.

14. Buckingham RW, et al. Factors associated with condom use among brothel-based female sex workers in Thailand. *AIDS Care*. 2005;17(5):640–647.

15. Lertpiriyasuwat C, Plipat T, Jenkins RA. A survey of sexual risk behavior for HIV infection in Nakhonsawan, Thailand, 2001. *AIDS*. 2003;17(13):1969-76.

16. Hanenberg R, Rojanapithayakorn W. Changes in prostitution and the AIDS epidemic in Thailand. *AIDS Care*. 1998;10(1):69–79.

17. Mills E, Singh S, Orbinksi J, Burrows D. The HIV/AIDS epidemic in Cambodia. *Lancet Infectious Diseases*. 2005;5:596–597.

18. UNAIDS/WHO. Epidemiological fact sheets on HIV/AIDS and sexually transmitted diseases: Cambodia. Available at: http://www.who.int/globalatlas/predefinedreports/EFS2004/index.asp. Accessed January 12, 2007.

19. World Health Organization. *100% Condom Use Programme in Entertainment Establishments*. Geneva, Switzerland: World Health Organization Regional Office for the Western Pacific; 2000:20–21.

20. Gorbach PM, Sopheab H, Chhorvann C, Weiss RE, Vun MC. Changing behaviors and patterns among Cambodian sex workers: 1997–2003. *JAIDS*. 2006;42(2):242–247.

21. Viravaidya M, Obremskey SA, Myers C. The economic impact of AIDS on Thailand. In: Bloom DE, Lyons JW, eds. *Economic Implications of AIDS in Asia*. New Delhi, India: United Nations Development Program; 1993.

22. United Nations Joint Programme on HIV/AIDS. *Report on the Global AIDS Epidemic*. Geneva, Switzerland: United Nations Joint Programme on HIV/AIDS; 2004.

Controlling Tuberculosis in China[*]

* The first draft of this case was prepared by Jane Seymour.

ABSTRACT

Geographic area: China

Health condition: Tuberculosis (TB) is the leading cause of death from infectious disease among adults in China. Every year, 1.4 million people develop active TB. In 1990, 360,000 people in China died from the disease.

Global importance of the health condition today: TB currently ranks as the third leading cause of death and disability among adults in the world, and nearly one third of the world's population is infected with the tuberculosis bacillus. Of these cases, more than 9 million people become sick with TB when their immune system is weakened, and 1.76 million die each year.

Intervention or program: In 1991, China revitalized its ineffective tuberculosis program and launched the 10-year Infectious and Endemic Disease Control project to curb its TB epidemic in 13 of its 31 mainland provinces. The program adopted the WHO-recommended TB control strategy, directly observed treatment shortcourse (DOTS), through which trained health workers watched patients take their treatment at local TB county dispensaries. Information on each treatment was sent to the county TB dispensary, and treatment outcomes were sent in quarterly reports to the National Tuberculosis Project Office.

Cost and cost-effectiveness: The program cost $130 million in total. The World Bank and the WHO estimated that successful treatment was achieved at less than $100 per person. One healthy life was saved for an estimated $15 to $20, with an economic rate of return of $60 for each dollar invested. The World Bank ranks DOTS as one of the most cost-effective of all health interventions.

Impact: China achieved a 95% cure rate for new cases within two years of adopting DOTS, and a cure rate of 90% for those who had previously undergone unsuccessful treatment. The number of people with TB declined by over 37% in project areas between 1990 and 2000, and 30,000 TB deaths have been prevented each year. More than 1.5 million patients have been treated, leading to the elimination of 836,000 cases of pulmonary TB.

At any given time, nearly one third of the world's population is infected with tuberculosis bacillus, and every second a new person becomes infected. Of those ill in 2004, an estimated 9 million people became sick with TB disease. Although Asia accounts for over half of all TB patients, the highest rates of TB occur in sub-Saharan Africa.[1] TB kills an estimated 1.7 million people each year and ranks as the third leading cause of death and disease burden among adults aged 15 to 59.[1,2] And there are few signs that the epidemic is subsiding: The global incidence of TB is growing at approximately 0.6% per year and at much faster rates in sub-Saharan Africa, where as much as 4% growth in incidence has followed rising HIV rates.[1]

Over the last decade, China, one of the countries most profoundly affected by TB, has demonstrated the potential for large-scale deployment of DOTS, the WHO-recommended TB control strategy. DOTS is a public health approach focused on the early detection of TB patients via smear microscopy and with a standardized directly observed 6-month treatment in dispensaries or in the community until cure.[†] This strategy was developed primarily to prevent the early dropout from treatment, which can result in the development of bacteria that are resistant to available drugs. China has shown how a combination of adequate funding, leadership, and a sound technical approach, delivered through a relatively strong health system, can dramatically reduce TB over a short period. In the process, China has averted hundreds of thousands of deaths and paved the way for future wins in the battle against TB.

HOW TB KILLS

TB is caused by the bacteria *Mycobacterium tuberculosis* and is contracted by inhaling infected air droplets spread by active TB carriers when they cough, sneeze, or talk. The majority of the people who come into contact with the bacteria can fight the progression of the disease, and the bacteria then lie dormant in the body without the development of any symptoms. Carriers of latent TB cannot spread the infection to others but are still at risk of developing the disease at some point in their lives if their immune system becomes depressed.

Between 5% and 10% of those infected with TB will fall ill.[3] TB occurs when a weakened immune system allows the bacteria to multiply and active disease to develop. TB in the lungs, or pulmonary TB, is the most common form, although the bacilli can cause the disease in any part of the body. The main symptom of pulmonary TB is a persistent worsening cough. If left untreated, night sweats, malaise, weight loss, blood in sputum, and shortness of breath take hold as the lungs are slowly destroyed.

HIV/AIDS and TB are a particularly deadly combination. Because HIV weakens the immune system, it raises the likelihood of latent TB becoming active. Consequently, TB is the leading cause of death among HIV-infected persons and accounts for approximately 11% of all AIDS deaths worldwide. As the number of people infected with HIV has increased so has the number of active TB cases.[3] Unfortunately, the diagnostic tools, which were developed

some 100 years ago, often fail to accurately detect TB in HIV-positive individuals.

The spread of HIV has fueled the TB epidemic, but it is not the only reason TB persists as a major global health problem. TB is both a cause and consequence of poverty. Untreated TB spreads quickly in dense populations, and urbanization and migration accelerate its transmission. Refugees and displaced persons are at an especially high risk because they are usually in crowded refugee camps or shelters and frequently relocate, making compliance with a 6-month treatment regimen extremely difficult. The TB epidemic also is closely associated with the breakdown of financing and infrastructure for public health systems, particularly in the former Soviet Union and in Africa, where access to effective detection and treatment services is limited.

TREATMENT AND THE AGE OF DOTS

For more than half a century, antibiotics have been available to cure standard cases of TB, but their effectiveness depends on strict patient adherence. The drugs must be taken for at least six months, but many patients discontinue use once their coughing subsides, when they suffer from side effects such as vomiting, jaundice, and confusion, or can no longer afford or access treatment. Patients who are only "half-cured" can still transmit TB, which poses a serious public health problem by enabling multi-drug-resistant TB (MDR-TB)[‡] to develop, rendering first-line drugs ineffective in MDR-TB patients.

In the 1970s, Dr. Karel Styblo of the International Union Against Tuberculosis and Lung Disease pioneered a new approach to TB treatment with the ministries of health of Tanzania, Malawi, and Mozambique. The new strategy promoted the integration of TB diagnosis, treatment, and follow-up with an existing health unit. This approach eventually evolved into the DOTS strategy, through which health workers or lay people encourage compliance by watching patients take their medicine. The essential elements of DOTS include the following:

- Government commitment to sustaining TB control activities
- Case detection by microscopic examination of a sputum sample among symptomatic patients who seek health services
- Standardized treatment regimen of six to eight months for at least all patients with positive sputum exams, using DOTS for at least the initial two months

---

† In 2006, WHO launched the Stop TB Strategy, a new strategy for TB control. In addition to the expansion and enhancement of DOTS, the strategy recommends the adoption of TB/HIV collaborative activities as well as MDR-TB treatment as key elements to an integrated approach to TB control.

‡ MDR-TB refers to TB infection that is resistant to at least two of the primary drugs used to treat TB. MDR-TB is the result of improper treatment and is caused most often when patients stop taking TB medicines too early.

- A regular, uninterrupted supply of all essential anti-TB drugs
- A standardized recording and reporting system that allows assessment of treatment results for each patient and of the TB control program as a whole

In the absence of HIV/AIDS or multidrug resistance, DOTS cure rates reach near or over the 2005 target of 85%, even in the poorest countries. DOTS has been ranked as one of the most cost-effective of all health interventions.[4] In some countries, the drugs used in DOTS cost as little as $16 per patient for a 6-month supply.[1]

The WHO first endorsed and recommended DOTS in 1993 when it also declared TB a global health emergency. As of 2004, 183 countries had adopted the strategy, representing 83% of the global population.[1] An estimated 22 million infectious patients were successfully treated under the DOTS programs since 1995, with a reported average cure rate of approximately 82%.[5] In 2004, some 53% of new smear-positive cases were detected under DOTS, and this figure was closer to 60% in 2005.[5] The WHO aims to detect 70% of new infectious TB cases and to cure 85% of those detected.

TACKLING TB IN CHINA

In China, where 400 million people are infected with TB, the burden is especially heavy. TB ranks as the leading cause of death from infectious disease, with 1.4 million people developing active TB each year. A national tuberculosis program was first established in 1981 to reform control efforts, and to expand the reporting system and treatment. Inadequate financial support, however, hampered the program's human resource and technical capacity in many areas, particularly in poorer provinces with the weakest primary health care infrastructure.

Although some important progress was achieved during the 1980s, the program was plagued by poor treatment compliance, a deficient network of diagnostic laboratories, and an inadequate system of reporting and evaluating cases. Furthermore, the treatment offered at urban hospitals was too expensive for many victims of the disease, and patients often abstained from treatment altogether or abandoned the drug regimen early.

As a result, a third nationwide TB random sample survey in 1990 revealed only a slight improvement in TB prevalence compared with rates in 1979 and 1985. In 1990, according to vital registration data, 360,000 people died from TB, making it the leading cause of death among adults. As is typical with TB, the poorest communities were most acutely affected.

Recognizing that the widespread incidence of the disease served as an obstacle to its ambitious social and economic goals, the government of China decided to formally evaluate its TB control program with assistance from the World Bank and the WHO. The analysis highlighted the need for a more effective and efficient method of TB surveillance and treatment of infected patients.

In 1991, with $58 million in financial support from the World Bank, China embarked on a 10-year Infectious and Endemic Disease Control (IEDC) project to help curb its TB epidemic in 13 of its 31 mainland provinces.[6] The project adopted the DOTS strategy and short-course chemotherapy. It set out to improve findings of new smear-positive cases from 35% to 70% and increase the cure rate from less than 50% to more than 90% of these cases by 2005. Accomplishing these goals would avoid an estimated 100,000 deaths each year and slash TB prevalence in half by 2015 in provinces covered by the program.

A RAPID ROLLOUT OF DOTS

The IEDC program was the largest natural experiment in TB control in history. Starting with a pilot project in five counties in Hebei province in April 1991, the program was quickly expanded first to 65 counties and then to approximately half of China's counties. By 1994, the IEDC project in China involved 1,208 counties in 12 provinces and a population of 573 million people. With this expansion of services, China's health system bolstered its TB control support and management services with logistic systems, provincial and township supervision, and monitoring and reporting systems.

Individuals demonstrating symptoms such as a persistent cough for at least three weeks, productive sputum in cough, shortness of breath, night sweats, and fatigue were referred to TB county dispensaries—local TB clinics that are part of the public health system. Free diagnosis was offered, and patients' lungs were examined with chest fluoroscopy. If results gave cause for concern, three sputum samples were taken and a chest X-ray was ordered if appropriate. Patients with positive-testing sputum have the most active and thus infectious TB and are the main targets for observed treatment. In suspect cases, where bacilli do not show up under the microscope, culturing the sputum or a subsequent X-ray may later reveal TB.

From 1991 to 2000, the DOTS program in China evaluated nearly 8 million people in the TB dispensaries, with 3.53 million having sputum smear tests carried out. Of those, 1.3 million had smear-positive results, and more than a half million more people with smear-negative results were later diagnosed with TB. At the start of the project, just over 70% of the smear-positive cases were new cases; this figure increased to a plateau of around 80% after seven years as case-finding improved and fully cured cases did not return for retreatment.

New patients with smear-positive pulmonary TB were started on a course of directly observed treatment of antibiotics, every other day for at least two months and up to six months. Treatment was free, an important feature of the program because fewer than 20% of patients had health insurance and 80% to 90% paid medical expenses out of pocket.[7] Health care workers watched patients every day, or three times a week, depending on the drug regimen, as the patients swallowed their prescribed drugs—the direct observation element.

Smear-positive patients continued to receive free treatment for up to an additional six months, while smear-negative patients were required to pay for their treatment. Sputum specimens were collected after two months of treatment and at regular intervals thereafter to document sputum conversion and cure.[6,8]

DOWN TO THE VILLAGE

The success of the IEDC project depended largely on the involvement of village doctors with basic health training, who played an essential role in patient diagnosis, treatment, and surveillance. In the 1980s, most Chinese doctors had become private practitioners because they were not receiving a salary from the local government. The reliance on payments from patients for services and drugs made free TB care problematic, even with free drugs from the government. To engage doctors in the program and to increase the number of TB patients diagnosed and treated, an incentive scheme was created. Village doctors received $1 for each patient enrolled in the treatment program, an additional $2 for each smear examination carried out at two months in the county TB dispensary, and $4 for each patient who completed his or her treatment.[6]

To monitor the TB epidemic, all infectious TB patients were registered with the county TB dispensary and issued a TB treatment and identity card. A copy of the treatment card was sent to the village doctor to record each dose of treatment. If a patient did not return for treatment, a village doctor visited the patient at home and then reported back to the county TB dispensary.

Furthermore, efforts were made to strengthen the institutions involved. A National Tuberculosis Project Office and a Tuberculosis Control Centre were established. The program worked to strengthen the management and finance of local TB dispensaries and bring them in line with the new DOTS framework. Operational research on management, economic, social, and epidemiological factors was encour-

aged to improve TB control and establish a basis for future health programs.

Quarterly reports summarizing the case findings, treatment outcomes, and other program activities were submitted from each county to the province, the central government, and the newly formed National Tuberculosis Project Office, allowing for consistent monitoring of the project. Involvement of all levels of the government also helped maintain the program's quality.[9]

Careful attention was paid to the implementation of necessary administrative, managerial, and financial changes. Training and supervision was extensive; more than 60 demonstration and training centers were established, which trained tens of thousands of staff from TB dispensaries. Quality was checked through random visits by TB staff to patients' homes, through review of the registry system, and through random examination of smear slides.

IMPRESSIVE AND FAST RESULTS

The DOTS strategy proved powerful (Figure 3-1). The global target of curing 85% of identified patients was quickly achieved—overall, the cure rate was 95% for new cases. This 95% cure rate is the highest for any country undertaking a large-scale TB control program and compares with a rate of just 52% before DOTS was launched in 1991. About two thirds of that improvement happened within the first two years of DOTS implementation.

The IEDC program demonstrated extraordinary cure rates of not only new cases but also of relapsed and retreatment cases. The cure rate for people treated with DOTS who had previously undergone unsuccessful treatment for TB was 90%. These successes have contributed to an MDR-TB rate three times lower in the 12 provinces covered by DOTS than in non-DOTS provinces.[10] Considering China's status as the country with the highest MDR-TB cases in the world—approximately 30%—the success of the IEDC program in reducing MDR-TB cases provides hope to the rest of the world.[11]

From 1990 to 2000, the number of people with TB in the DOTS area declined by 36.1%, about 4.1% each year, compared with a decline of 3.1% in non-DOTS areas. In western China, for example, where five provinces implemented DOTS and seven provinces did not, the prevalence in the DOTS area decreased by 33.3% while the prevalence in the non-DOTS area decreased by just 11.7%.[8] The magnitude of this difference in TB prevalence between DOTS and non-DOTS provinces may also have been influenced by factors other than the DOTS program, such as socioeconomic differences.[12]

FIGURE 3-1 Rates of new and previously treated smear-positive cases among all smear-positive cases by number of years of DOTS implementation.

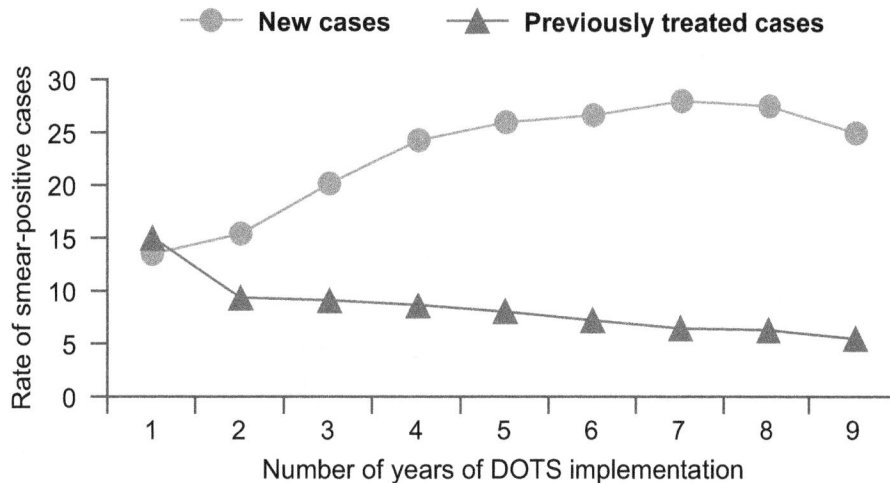

Note: DOTS = directly observed treatment, short-course strategy.
Source: Chen et al. (2002). *Bulletin of the World Health Organization.*

Since DOTS was introduced in China, more than 1.5 million patients have been treated, and approximately 30,000 TB deaths have been prevented each year. DOTS is now available to 96% of the population with a 94% treatment success rate.[1] A national TB prevalence survey carried out in 2000 estimated that the program eliminated 836,000 cases of pulmonary TB disease, 382,000 cases of culture-positive disease, and 280,000 cases of smear-positive disease.[13]

THE PRICE TAG

Funding for China's IEDC project came from the Chinese government at both national and local levels and was supplemented by a World Bank loan. Originally budgeted at $102.5 million, the total cost amounted to nearly $130 million in the end. Most of the resources were devoted to improving case detection and management. Savings were made on the cost of drugs because China bought in bulk and utilized other procurement schemes.

A study conducted by the Ministry of Health and the Shanghai Medical University found that each case detected cost approximately $83 and that the cost per new smear-positive cured was $537. The World Bank and WHO estimated that successful treatment was achieved at less than $100 per person. One life-year was saved for an estimated $15 to $20, with an economic rate of return of $60 for each dollar.[14]

THE PROJECT'S LIMITATIONS

Despite China's success in curing TB, the project achieved lower than hoped for rates of case detection. The case detection rate is the number of notified cases divided by the estimated number of TB cases in the population. The estimated case detection rate in 1998 of 53.5% fell short of the 2005 target rate of 70%.[9] The WHO estimated a much lower case detection rate of 30% for the same year.[7]

One of the main contributing factors to the low case detection rate was inadequate referral of suspected TB cases from hospitals to the TB dispensaries.[9] The 2000 National TB Prevalence Survey reported that just 12% of TB patients received their diagnosis from a TB dispensary. Because hospitals can charge for TB treatment and diagnosis, they have little economic incentive to direct patients to the dispensaries. As a result, despite the existence of regulations requiring referrals to dispensaries, most TB patients are diagnosed in hospitals, where treatment is often abandoned prematurely.

LESSONS FOR THE FUTURE

Several lessons can be drawn from both the outstanding success and the limitations of the Chinese national TB program.

- **DOTS can be rapidly scaled up, while simultaneously achieving high coverage rates**—In less than five years, DOTS coverage increased from 0% to 90% in the program areas.[9] Under rapid expansion, such programs face the risk of sacrificing treatment quality and case management unless adequate levels of training, supervision, and quality control are maintained. In such a scenario, drug resistance could increase. China's experience, however, demonstrated that it is possible to increase the cure rate and lower the treatment failure rate under rapid scale-up and expansion.

- **Political commitment is essential.** Strong political commitment at various levels of government in China contributed to the program's success. Project-leading groups led by the vice-governor or vice-mayor were established at each government level to supervise the program.
- **Creative incentives work.** The provision of incentives to both patients and providers proved essential to the success of the IEDC project. Free diagnosis and treatment for TB patients helped dramatically increase treatment rates over the previous program, and incentives provided to doctors to diagnose and treat patients also contributed to the program's suc-

cess. The resistance from hospitals to refer patients to TB dispensaries exposed a weakness of the program and created the need for further innovative incentives to address this shortcoming.

MAINTAINING AND EXPANDING THE SUCCESS

Despite the success of the IEDC project, which concluded in 2001, TB remains a deadly threat in China (see Box 3-1). More than 300 million people are infected, and 10% of these people will develop TB during their lifetime.[15] The government of China now faces the dual challenge of maintaining high cure rates in the provinces covered by the IEDC project and scaling up the DOTS program to the remaining half of the population. The latter endeavor carries a number of challenges, particularly the need to marshal political support at the local level, increase the numbers of trained staff at the central and provincial levels, increase access to TB dispensaries in the 20% of counties where no dispensary exists, and address increasing drug resistance and TB–HIV coinfection issues.[1,7]

Important progress has been made in recent years. To continue and increase the success of the IEDC project, the State Council of China released a 10-year National Plan for

BOX 3-1 Stop TB: The Quest to Curb MDR-TB

Despite the successes achieved by DOTS programs in China and elsewhere, multi-drug-resistant tuberculosis (MDR-TB) is on the rise. MDR-TB is a more dangerous and difficult to treat form of TB that is resistant to two or more of the most powerful anti-TB drugs currently available. It can arise when patients fail to complete the standard TB treatment regimen for economic or health reasons, or receive improper treatment. Other people they infect will have the same drug-resistant strain.

More than 400,000 MDR-TB cases emerge each year globally, with hotspots in parts of China, India, and the Russian Federation.[1] First-line drugs typically used to control TB are ineffective against MDR-TB, and although new second-line TB drugs for MDR-TB exist, they are particularly toxic and can cost local purchasers 1,000 to 3,000 times as much as first-line drugs, making them largely inaccessible to most MDR-TB patients.

For a long time, these were major barriers in the treatment and control of the highly pernicious MDR-TB, but after a long and hard-won battle, WHO created DOTS-Plus. This new program was initiated in 1999 to curb MDR-TB by preventing the development of new cases through the introduction of second-line drugs, and preventing the spread of resistant strains through adequate laboratory support. The program benefited from the previous work of a joint global program for anti-TB drug resistance surveillance that had been in place since the mid-1990s.

Another critical tool in combating MDR-TB is the Green Light Committee, established in 2000 by the international Stop TB Partnership to promote access to second-line drugs at reduced prices. By defining the market, consolidating various sources of demand, and negotiating prices with pharmaceutical companies, the Green Light Committee and the Stop TB Working Group on MDR-TB were able to reduce the price of high-quality MDR-TB medicines by up to 90%.[16] Thanks in large part to their efforts, MDR-TB detection and treatment can be feasible and cost-effective, even in resource-limited settings. With the expansion of MDR-TB treatment projects, it is estimated that 142,000 deaths from MDR-TB will be prevented between 2006 and 2015.[17]

the Prevention and Control of TB (2001–2010), and the Ministry of Health completed a 4-year implementation plan (2002–2005) and a work plan (2002). While keeping the same high level of treatment success, these projects have been successful in expanding DOTS coverage to 90% of the country and reaching a case detection rate of more than 70%. In line with the new Stop TB Strategy, China is also beginning to tackle MDR-TB.[18]

The World Bank; the Department for International Development of the United Kingdom; the government of Japan through the Japan International Cooperation Agency;

the Damien Foundation Belgium; the Global Fund to Fight AIDS, TB, and Malaria; and other organizations have all contributed funds to the projects, and the central government of China continues to financially support the fight against TB. The WHO, the International Union Against TB and Lung Disease, the Royal Netherlands TB Association, and others are providing expertise to identify new ways for hospitals to work with TB dispensaries to increase case detection rates.[7] With this international financial commitment and technical cooperation, China can achieve its goals and significantly reduce the health burden due to TB.

REFERENCES

1. World Health Organization. *Global Tuberculosis Control Report: Surveillance, Planning, and Financing.* WHO/HTM/TB/2006.362. Geneva, Switzerland: World Health Organization; 2006.

2. World Health Organization. The world health report 2003: shaping the future. Available at: http://www.pso.int/whr/en/. Accessed January 12, 2007.

3. World Health Organization. Tuberculosis fact sheet 104. Available at: http://www.who.int/mediacentre/factsheets/who104/en/. Accessed January 12, 2007.

4. Dye C, Floyd K. Tuberculosis. In: Jamison DT, Breman JG, Measham AR, et al, eds. *Disease Control Priorities in Developing Countries.* New York, NY: Oxford University Press; 2006:289°309.

5. World Health Organization. Global tuberculosis control report 2004: surveillance, planning, and financing. Available at: http://www.who.int/tb/publications/global_report/2004/en/. Accessed January 12, 2007.

6. China Tuberculosis Control Collaboration. Results of directly observed short-course chemotherapy in 112,842 Chinese patients with smear-positive tuberculosis. *Lancet.* 1996;347:358–362.

7. World Health Organization. *Global Tuberculosis Control Report 2003: Surveillance, Planning, and Financing.* Geneva, Switzerland: World Health Organization; 2003.

8. Zhao F, Zhao Y, Liu X. Tuberculosis control in China. *Tuberculosis.* 2003;83:15–20.

9. Chen X, Zhao F, Duanmu H, et al. The DOTS strategy in China: results and lessons after 10 years. *Bull WHO.* 2002;80(6):430–436.

10. World Health Organization Regional Office for the Western Pacific. *DOTS for All: Country Reports.* Geneva, Switzerland: World Health Organization; 2002.

11. Zignol M, Hosseini SM, Wright A, et al. Global incidence of multidrug-resistant tuberculosis. *J Infect Dis.* 2006;194:479–485.

12. Squire SB, Tang S. How much of China's success in tuberculosis control is really due to DOTS? *Lancet.* 2004;364(9432): 391–2.

13. Dye C, Espinal MA, Watt CJ, Mbiaga C, Williams BG. Worldwide incidence of multidrug resistant tuberculosis. *J Infect Dis.* 2002;185:1197–1202.

14. World Bank. *Implementation Completion Report No. 25238.* Washington, DC: World Bank; 2002.

15. World Health Organization Regional Office for the Western Pacific. *DOTS for All: Country Reports.* Geneva, Switzerland: World Health Organization; 2004.

16. Stop TB Partnership. *The Green Light Committee: Leading the Fight Against MDR-TB.* Geneva, Switzerland: World Health Organization; 2006.

17. Stop TB Partnership. *The Global Plan to Stop TB, 2006–2015: Actions for Life.* Geneva, Switzerland: World Health Organization; 2006.

18. World Health Organization Regional Office for the Western Pacific. *Tuberculosis Control in the Western Pacific Region.* Geneva, Switzerland: World Health Organization; 2006.

Reducing Child Mortality With Vitamin A in Nepal*

* Case drafted by Jessica Gottlieb.

ABSTRACT

Geographic area: Nepal

Health condition: In the 1990s, 2–8% of preschool-aged Nepali children experienced severe vitamin A deficiency, or xerophthalmia, associated with blindness and risk of child death.

Global importance of the health condition today: Vitamin A deficiency affects approximately 21% of the developing world's preschool-aged children and leads to the deaths of over 800,000 women and children each year. Because it compromises the immune system, vitamin A deficiency is estimated to be responsible for nearly one fourth of global **child mortality** from measles, diarrhea, and malaria and for a fifth of all-cause **maternal mortality**.

Intervention or program: In 1993, the government of Nepal initiated the National Vitamin A Programme (NVAP) with the support of UNICEF, USAID, and local researchers and nongovernmental organizations (NGOs). The NVAP aimed to reduce child mortality and morbidity related to vitamin A deficiency by providing twice-yearly supplements of vitamin A capsules to children in priority districts; treating xerophthalmia, severe malnutrition, prolonged diarrhea and measles; and encouraging dietary intake of vitamin A and breast-feeding. A large cadre of women who served as community-based volunteers was integral to the rapid expansion of the program to Nepal's 75 districts.

Cost and cost-effectiveness: The cost of delivering two rounds of vitamin A per year was approximately $1.25 per child covered. With an estimated cost of $327–$397 per death averted and $11–$12 per **disability-adjusted life-year (DALY)** gained, the NVAP is considered highly cost-effective.

Impact: The NVAP prevents blindness in approximately 2,000 children each year and was found to reduce by about half the mortality rate for children under 5 years of age in Nepal between 1995 and 2000.

Enveloped in poverty and burdened by its onerous topography, Nepal is hardly an obvious birthplace for a public health success story. And yet, the marriage of scientific and operational innovations provided the foundation for a national program that saves hundreds of thousands of children's lives.

In the early 1980s, a series of studies demonstrated that vitamin A supplementation could reduce child mortality; two of them were carried out in Nepal.[1,2] Following this discovery, Nepal conceived of the National Vitamin A

Program to distribute small, red vitamin A capsules to millions of children each year. Its creative design overcame the country's economic and geographic hurdles by harnessing local capacity and relying on new channels of public health delivery—bridging the once insurmountable gap between where the formal health sector ended and the needs of the poor began. The reduction in child mortality demonstrated by this program and the sustained high levels of coverage would make this innovation in service delivery a model for future attempts to combat vitamin A deficiency and other childhood illnesses.

CARROTS FOR THE EYES

Improved eyesight is perhaps the most familiar benefit of vitamin A. Without sufficient intake of this micronutrient, a condition called xerophthalmia or a dryness of the eyes ensues. Manifesting first as night blindness, severe vitamin A deficiency will eventually cause softening of the corneas and total blindness. Vitamin A deficiency is, however, not only associated with eye problems; it is also an underlying determinant of child mortality. Because of vitamin A's role in epithelial defenses and the immune system, deficiency puts children at greater risk of respiratory, measles, and diarrheal morbidity.[3]

Vitamin A deficiency affects approximately 21% of the developing world's preschool-aged children[4] and leads to the deaths of over 800,000 women and children each year. Furthermore, vitamin A deficiency is responsible for 20% to 24% of global child mortality from measles, diarrhea, and malaria and for 20% of all-cause maternal mortality.[5] It also increases the severity and fatality of measles.[3]

Carrots, spinach, and other green leafy vegetables; ripe yellow fruit; and animal products such as eggs, milk, and liver contain vitamin A. Regularly eating recommended amounts of these foods prevent vitamin A deficiency. In their absence, vitamin A deficiency can also be prevented by consuming dietary supplements. Where vitamin A deficiency is a public health problem, children under five years of age are recommended to periodically take preventive vitamin A in high doses. More specifically, children 6–11 months of age are recommended to receive an oral dose of 100,000 International Units (IU), and children 12–59 months of age should receive a 200,000 IU dose every four to six months.[6] For adults in the United States, the daily recommended dose of vitamin A is 4,000–5,000 IU.

Another target group for vitamin A interventions is pregnant and breast-feeding women. Night blindness, an early symptom of clinical vitamin A deficiency, can be highly prevalent during pregnancy, affecting 10% to 20% of expecting mothers in rural South Asia. Night blind mothers have their own health risks[7] and are more likely to have vitamin A deficient children.[8] Night blindness can be avoided by eating a nutritious diet that is plentiful in foods rich in vitamin A, and it can be treated by taking low doses of vitamin A on a weekly basis. Also, while high doses of vitamin A should be generally avoided in pregnancy due to concerns about risks of birth defects, a high dose of vitamin A can be given to mothers within six weeks after delivery to prevent maternal health problems from vitamin A deficiency and to increase breast milk vitamin A content for breast-feeding infants.[6]

Evidence of the positive health impact of vitamin A supplementation is clear. In a meta-analysis of multiple trials, vitamin A supplementation was shown to be an important way to reduce child mortality.[9] By aggregating similar findings of individual studies, the meta-analysis helped motivate the decision to pursue a sustained national program of vitamin A supplementation in Nepal and elsewhere.

VITAMIN A DEFICIENCY IN NEPAL

In the years before the national program, vitamin A deficiency was an important health problem in Nepal with 2%–8% of preschool-aged children experiencing xerophthalmia or severe vitamin A deficiency.[2,10] Several contextual factors can help to explain this high prevalence rate. Difficult terrain makes it hard to grow or access the types of food that supply vitamin A naturally. Beyond geography, 28% of Nepal's 23 million inhabitants live in absolute poverty, and nutritious foods are more difficult to come by.[11] Even when proper foods may be available, unequal access to them within families can lead to young children and pregnant mothers not getting their fair share.[12] These are the root problems of malnutrition, including vitamin A deficiency, and will take many years to solve. However, in the shorter run, national vitamin A supplementation programs can stave off deficiency and prevent blindness and mortality.

FROM COMMUNITY TRIAL TO NATIONAL PROGRAM

Before the 1980s, the role that vitamin A deficiency played in placing children at risk of death was not widely appreciated. By the early 1980s, however, medical researcher Dr. Alfred Sommer had observed in Indonesia that an exceptional number of children with mild eye signs of xerophthalmia, such as night blindness and Bitot's spots, were dying.[13] Such findings were in line with observations of nutritionists and health scientists in the early part of the 1900s who associated severe xerophalthmia with blindness and risk of child death. However, Sommer's attempt to link vitamin A and child mortality was not immediately accepted by critics.[14]

Sommer, his colleague Dr. Keith West, and their Indonesian colleagues carried out a 30,000-child trial in northern Sumatra in the early 1980s (see Box 4-1). The trial supported Sommer's theory that vitamin A deficiency lead to child deaths and that when given to children vitamin A prevented deaths. Their second trial, among 30,000 children

BOX 4-1 Changing Minds, Saving Lives

In 1983, when Al Sommer published his findings in *The Lancet* showing mild vitamin A deficiency was associated with an increased risk of child death,[13] he was largely ignored. Three years later, he and colleague Dr. Keith West met skepticism when they reported that mortality of young children could be reduced by one third just by giving them a dose of vitamin A every six months, based on data from a community trial in Indonesia.[15] Critics thought such a simple solution to a major global health problem "too good to be true." Finding fault with the fact that the Indonesian study had not used a placebo group, they claimed that chance could have explained the findings.

Sommer decided to challenge the skeptics by "burying them in data." He and his colleagues, as well as other research groups, repeatedly carried out vitamin A supplementation trials using a range of designs in different countries and in populations of varying nutritional and mortality risks to all establish a clear causal link between vitamin A supplementation and reduced child mortality. The trials confirmed the results of Sommer's initial observation and showed reductions in mortality as high as 55%. Through persistent research and spreading the word in scientific papers and meetings, commentaries, and media exposure, the potential of vitamin A supplementation was eventually recognized and brought into the mainstream of child survival activities.[16]

in the southern Nepal plains district of Sarlahi in the early 1990s echoed the results from Indonesia: Periodic vitamin A delivery could reduce mortality in children aged 6–60 months by about 30%.[1] Around the same time, another field trial in Jumla, in the western hills of Nepal, further strengthened the case by reporting an approximate 30% difference in child mortality of children who took vitamin A compared to those who did not.[2]

Aware of these new and dramatic findings and cognizant of the nation's high child mortality rate, the Nepalese Ministry of Health began planning a national vitamin A program with the help of the research community, other ministries, the National Planning Commission, NGOs, and the international agencies United Nations Fund for Children (UNICEF), WHO, and the United State Agency for Internation Development (USAID). In February 1992, the government of Nepal, along with national and international agencies, discussed the data generated during the vitamin A trials and developed an implementation strategy and objectives for a national program. Vitamin A supplementation was made part of His Majesty's Government's Eighth Five-Year Development Plan (1992–1997) with a 10-year goal to reduce the prevalence of xerophthalmia from 1.9% to 0.1% by the year 2001.[17]

With financial and technical assistance from USAID and UNICEF, Nepal's National Vitamin A Programme (NVAP) began in 1993 with the following objectives:

- Reduce child mortality and morbidity through prophylactic supplementation of children 6–60 months with high-dose (200,000 IU) vitamin A capsules twice yearly in 32 priority districts.

- Treat xerophthalmia, severe malnutrition, prolonged diarrhea, and measles in all 75 districts.
- Bring about behavior change to increase dietary intake of vitamin A and improve breast-feeding in the 32 priority districts.

The Nepali Technical Assistance Group (TAG) was an NGO created specifically to assist the health ministry in implementing the program, especially with training, monitoring, motivation, mobilization, and supervision. Since 1999, the Micronutrient Initiative through support from the Canadian International Development Agency (CIDA) has provided vitamin A capsules for the NVAP, and the Australian international aid agency (AusAID) has financially contributed to the training component.

THE CAMPAIGN

As in many poor countries, Nepal's public health system was faced with severe problems from low utilization rates of local health posts (less than 20% for treatment of child illnesses), to absenteeism among health workers, to poor quality healthcare. This was not a setting in which the large-scale NVAP could be successfully launched. Rather than undertake the mammoth task of vastly extending the reach of health post workers, a semiannual campaign approach was adopted to enable vitamin A to reach Nepalese children in a nationally visible, coordinated, focused way. Mass distribution of vitamin A would be carried out in April before the beginning of the high-risk season of xerophthalmia, and in October to boost vitamin A stores to support accelerated child growth that often follows fall harvest season. To achieve high coverage rates, each distribution date would be preceded by training, promotion, and ensuring the availability of vitamin A capsules in each district.[18]

HARNESSING LOCAL RESOURCES TO SAVE LIVES

Based on an existing network of unpaid female community health volunteers (FCHVs) who helped to deliver primary healthcare and family planning to villages, NVAP decided to engage this underutilized and underresourced workforce in vitamin A delivery. In 1993, there were 36,000 FCHVs in 75 Nepalese districts. These mostly illiterate women were not always given respect by their communities, and their credibility was further challenged by oft-lacking medical supplies. With the help of NVAP, this network of volunteers was transformed into 49,000 public health agents who were able to reach 3.7 million children with vitamin A capsules twice per year (Ram Shrestha, Nepal Technical Assistance Group, personal communication, July 2006).

This transformation would have been impossible without the insight and dedication of TAG's leader, Mr. Ram Shrestha. Shrestha noticed that the network of FCHVs, nominated from women's organizations to promote health messages, fell into disuse after the first year of existence. The reason: money. During year one, all FCHVs were given a monthly stipend of 100 rupees (about US$2) as an incentive.[†] After one year, the Nepalese government realized that it was impossible to continue to offer a monthly stipend of 100 rupees; when the incentive ceased, so did the work of the volunteers. Shrestha realized that to motivate community volunteers, he would have to come up with a renewable incentive that would adapt over time to reflect the changing needs of the volunteers. Through a profound knowledge of the community and a wealth of creativity, Shrestha achieved this aim. He relied on a few basic principles—opportunity, respect, recognition, and ownership—knowing that the FCHVs could be motivated without monetary incentives.

Through tactics such as inviting volunteers to speak at meetings, allowing them to pass to the front of the line when awaiting social services, and giving them preference in participating in other government programs, NVAP brought FCHVs newfound respect in their communities and motivated them to carry out public health activities. As one FCHV said, "This [vitamin A] program has made us more active. We undergo training every six months and people come to visit so often for advice."[17] In a culture where women are not often given prominence in society, this program had the added effect of challenging deeply rooted gender biases, giving women responsibilities valued by their families and communities.

The FCHVs did not function in isolation; rather they served as a critical bridge between the public health sector and the community. Although they were engaged in the most direct contact with beneficiaries, the public health system still played a major role. The newly expanded cadre of 49,000 FCHVs was made possible by a method of training the trainers, adopted to enable staff at the district health office to train the chief of the health post in a village, who would then train village health workers, FCHVs, and others. The government supported other key activities such as the provision of supplies and monitoring. Sectors outside of health, such as agriculture and education, also pitched in by integrating messages about the importance of vitamin A into their programs.

The NVAP helped communities take the health of their children into their own hands. The prominence of FCHVs raised the profile of public health, and their integration within the communities they served greatly increased accessibility. The existence of a retrained and invigorated cadre of FCHVs produced a new awareness of and demand for healthcare, as did the public outreach and health education undertaken by them and other NGO partners. This demand is evidenced by the families that brought their children each distribution day to a central village site or health post— sometimes a long walk from home. While FCHVs did not often go door to door, children missed during the first day of distribution were usually traced the next day.

Promoting community ownership over the care of children created a natural constituency that helped to ensure the sustainability and success. When supplies weren't delivered or when FCHVs didn't receive training, beneficiaries in the communities noticed and held the government accountable.

EXPANDING TO A NATIONAL STRATEGY

A critical factor in the success of the national vitamin A program was its phased expansion. In a predetermined sequence, Nepal's 32 priority districts were incrementally phased in to the program at a rate of 8 to 10 districts per year to allow the government time to build local capacity and ownership, and to apply lessons from earlier experience.

By 1997, vitamin A capsule supplementation had been introduced into all 32 districts as mandated in the Eighth Plan. Based upon the high coverage and initial success of the program, the government of Nepal decided to extend vitamin A supplementation to all its 75 districts. Expansion into new districts was facilitated through National Immunization Day activities whereby children would receive one capsule of

---

† Initially, FCHVs were also given a small amount of supplies that were intended to be sold for a small profit, the funds from which could be used to buy more. This did not work well and was eventually stopped.

vitamin A as a temporary measure until NVAP reached those districts with its twice-yearly supplementation.

Skeptics of the program asserted that supplementation was unnecessary because vitamin A deficiency could be averted simply through changing dietary practices.[17] Although one cannot dispute this claim and long-term goal, advocates of the NVAP were able to show by projection the numbers of child lives saved each round; this motivated and moved the program forward. Along with supplementation, education and outreach activities in the villages were introduced to emphasize the importance of healthy dietary practices. Though it took nearly eight years to achieve nationwide distribution, coverage in ongoing program areas remained above 80% to 90%.

COST AND COST-EFFECTIVENESS OF A NATIONAL PROGRAM

In 1997 and again in 2000, cost analyses of the NVAP were undertaken—in part to guide the decision about whether or not to expand the program. Using TAG coverage estimates, the cost of the program per child covered was approximately US$1.25 to deliver two rounds of vitamin A per year (not including volunteer time of the female community health workers).[19] This appears very low-cost, compared with other child survival and nutrition interventions such as breast-feeding promotion, growth monitoring, and micronutrient supplementation, which can cost up to four times as much per child.[20]

The NVAP was found to be highly cost-effective with an estimated cost of US$327–US$397 per death averted and $11–$12 per disability-adjusted life-year (DALY) gained. The NVAP also was estimated to produce cost savings for the Ministry of Health by averting severe episodes of diarrheal disease and measles.[19]

PROGRAM IMPACT

According to a national coverage estimate of 81% of all children 6 to 59 months of age, the NVAP currently prevents approximately 2,000 children from going blind each year.[21] A quasi-experimental evaluation of the program in Nepal demonstrated significant impact on child mortality as well. The study was facilitated by the fact that districts were incorporated into the program at 6-month intervals so the impacts on health in program areas could be compared to the health indicators in nonprogram areas. A demographic and health survey in 2001 provided the child mortality estimates in Nepal necessary to determine the impacts of the Nepal vitamin A program. After controlling for potentially confounding factors such as poverty, disease prevalence, and mother's

education, the effect of 100% community-level vitamin A coverage between 1995 and 2000, relative to no coverage, was found to reduce the mortality of children under 5 years old by about half.[22]

CURRENT CHALLENGES

Can the national vitamin A delivery program be sustained, especially under resource-scarce conditions and amid civil conflict like the one that currently grips Nepal? Now that the nation is covered by the NVAP, a new challenge is to facilitate a longer-term solution to vitamin A deficiency. Such strategies, including strengthening home gardening, small animal husbandry, food markets, and dietary changes, within households can complement supplementation efforts until children receive ample vitamin A through their diet.

In the meantime, attention must also be paid to the sustainability of the NVAP. As occurred with monetary incentives at the outset, the effects of the personal incentives to the FCHVs appear to be waning. A new incentive called the FCHV Endowment Fund is being developed and tested. The Endowment Fund is established by Village Development Committees (VDCs), which place the equivalent of a little more than $1,000 in local currency into an account. The capital remains untouched, and the interest is placed into another savings account controlled by local FCHVs; the earned interest can be used for their welfare. Twenty% of VDCs currently have this sustainable fund at their disposal and early evidence suggests it helps to increase the job satisfaction of the volunteers, according to Ram Shrestha. In VDCs that cannot afford to put aside funds for this purpose, the NVAP is working to involve local industry to contribute to the endowment funds.

LEARNING FROM NEPAL'S SUCCESS

Innovative technical and operational planning can result in a major population impact. Well-designed, nonmonetary incentives to community volunteers have been an efficient and cost-effective way of reaching poor families with primary health care services. The use of FCHVs has been so successful in combating vitamin A deficiency that they are now helping to address deworming, treat pneumonia, and distribute iron supplements to pregnant women. Attention to communities by local health workers and NGOs engendered local ownership of the program and spurred demand for health services, adding to program sustainability.

The success of NVAP reinforces lessons common to other health successes: the importance of local leadership, evidenced by Ram Shrestha's key role in the design and implementation; monitoring of quality, which allowed for the program to make midcourse corrections to improve service delivery; and of partnership, demonstrated by the support system among the district health workers, the NGOs, and the health volunteers.

According to Keith West:

> This case is an exceptional example of how a poor country undertook the required research to demonstrate impact (not in one but two sites in different corners of the country, both of which showed a 30% reduction [in child mortality]), garnered the required political constituencies and funding partners, initiated and learned from mistakes along the way as it scaled up to a national program, undertook periodic and independent evaluations of impact and cost, and has managed to sustain its achievement over time. All of this in the midst of a Maoist insurgency that has otherwise stripped parts of the country of its rural infrastructure; but the vitamin A program continues perhaps because of its known impact by the populace (instilled by its designer, Ram Shrestha) and maybe also by the realization that children need to survive, no matter who rules a country.

REFERENCES

1. West KP Jr. Efficacy of vitamin A in reducing preschool child mortality in Nepal. *Lancet.* 1991;338(8759):67–71.

2. Daulaire N, Starbuck ES, Houston RM, et al. Childhood mortality after a high dose of vitamin A in a high-risk population. *BMJ.* 1992;304:207–210.

3. Sommer A, West KP Jr. *Vitamin A Deficiency: Health, Survival and Vision.* New York, NY: Oxford University Press; 1996.

4. West KP Jr. Extent of vitamin A deficiency among preschool children and women of reproductive age. *J Nutr.* 2002;132:2857S–2866S.

5. Rice AL, West KP, Black RE. Vitamin A deficiency. In: Ezzati M, Lopez AD, Rodgers A, Murray C, eds. *Comparative Quantification of Health Risks: Global and Regional Burden of Disease Attributable to Selected Major Risk Factors.* Vol. 1. Geneva, Switzerland: World Health Organization; 2004:211–256.

6. Ross DA. Recommendations for Vitamin A supplementation. *J Nutr.* 2002;132(9 suppl):2902S–2906S.

7. Christian P, West KP, Khatry SK, et al. Night blindness of pregnancy in rural Nepal—nutritional and health risks. *Int J Epidemiol.* 1998;27:231–237.

8. Semba RD, de Pee S, Panagides D, Poly O, Bloem MW. Risk factors for xerophthalmia among mothers and their children and for mother-child pairs with xerophthalmia in Cambodia. *Arch Ophthalmol.* 2004;122:517–523.

9. Fawzi WW, Chalmers TC, Herrera MG, Mosteller F. Vitamin A supplementation and child mortality: a meta-analysis. *JAMA.* 1993;269(7):898–903.

10. Upadhyay M. Xerophthalmia among Nepalese children. *Am J Epidemiol.* 1985;121(1):71–77.

11. Khatry SK, West KP, Katz J, et al. Epidemiology of xerophthalmia in Nepal: a pattern of household poverty, childhood illness, and mortality. *Arch Ophthalmol.* 1995;113(4):425–429.

12. Shankar AV, West Jr KP, Gittelsohn J, Katz J, Pradhan R. Chronic low intakes of vitamin A–rich foods in households with xerophthalmic children: a case-control study in Nepal. *Am J Clin Nutr.* 1996;64:242–248.

13. Sommer A, et al. Increased mortality in children with mild vitamin A deficiency. *Lancet.* 1983;2(8350):585–588.

14. Hilts PJ. *Rx for Survival: Why We Must Rise to the Global Health Challenge.* New York, NY: Penguin Press; 2005.

15. Sommer A, Tarwotjo I, Djunaedi E, et al. Impact of vitamin A supplementation on childhood mortality. A randomized controlled community trial. *Lancet.* 1986;1(8491):1169–1173.

16. McCarthy M. Alfred Sommer: a life in the field and in the data. *Lancet.* 2005;365(9460):649.

17. United Nations Children's Fund, Regional Office for South Asia. *Getting to the Roots: Mobilizing Community Volunteers to Combat Vitamin A Deficiency Disorders in Nepal.* Kathmandu, Nepal: United Nations Children's Fund; 2003.

18. Houston R. *Elements of Success: National Vitamin A Program—Nepal.* Ministry of Health, HMG/Nepal, JSI, USAID, NTAG, and UNICEF; 1999.

19. Fiedler JL. The Nepal national vitamin A program: prototype to emulate or donor enclave? *Health Policy Plann.* 2000;15(2):145–156.

20. Caulfield LE, Richard SA, Rivera JA, Musgrove P, Black RE. Stunting, wasting, and micronutrient deficiency disorders. In: Jamison DT, Breman JG, Measham AR, et al. *Disease Control Priorities in Developing Countries.* 2nd ed. Washington, DC: World Bank; 2006.

21. Fiedler JL. *The Nepal National Vitamin A Program: Cost Estimates for 2000 and Alternative Configurations of a Nationwide Program.* Special Initiatives Report No. 41. Bethesda, MD: The Partners for Health Reformplus Project, Abt Associates Inc; 2001.

22. Thapa S, Choe MK, Retherford RD. Effects of vitamin A supplementation on child mortality: evidence from Nepal's 2001 Demographic and Health Survey. *Trop Med Int Health.* 2005;10(8):782–789.

CASE 5

Eliminating Polio in Latin America and the Caribbean*

* Case drafted by Molly Kinder

ABSTRACT

Geographic area: Latin America and the Caribbean

Health condition: In the 1970s, Latin America had an estimated 15,000 paralysis cases and 1,750 deaths each year due to polio. The oral polio vaccine was introduced in the region in 1977.

Global importance of the health condition today: Today, polio is on the verge of being erased from the globe. As recently as 1988, 125 countries were endemic for polio, with an estimated 350,000 cases. Through the first half of 2006, just four countries were reported endemic for polio, and fewer than 700 cases were reported worldwide. This dramatic reduction is the result of massive oral polio vaccine (OPV) immunizations through a global eradication campaign.

Intervention or program: In 1985, the Pan American Health Organization began a polio eradication campaign in Latin America and the Caribbean, to complement the routine immunization efforts of the newly formed Expanded Programme on Immunization. To increase immunization coverage in areas with weak routine health services, all endemic countries in the region implemented national vaccine days twice a year to immunize every child under 5, regardless of vaccination status. In the final stages of the campaign, "Operation Mop-Up" was launched to aggressively tackle the disease with house-to-house vaccinations in communities reporting polio cases and with low coverage. An extensive surveillance system helped track outbreaks.

Cost and cost-effectiveness: The first five years of the polio campaign cost $120 million: $74 million from national sources and $46 million from international donors. Taking into consideration the savings from treatment, these donor contributions would pay for themselves in just 15 years. The administration of the vaccine is highly cost-effective, at just $20 for a healthy year of life in a high-mortality environment.

Impact: In 1991, the last case of polio was reported in Latin America and the Caribbean. The disease reemerged briefly in 2000 when 20 vaccine-associated cases were reported in Haiti and the Dominican Republic, but no other cases have been reported since 1991. Today, polio has been eliminated from Latin America and the Caribbean.

As the world struggles to wipe out the last traces of polio, one region has been polio free for more than a decade. The experience of polio elimination† in Latin America and the Caribbean shines a light on what can be done when regional cooperation and support are strong, funding is sufficient, and the strategy covers all the bases. As a result of these factors, polio—which used to cripple thousands in the region each year—is now becoming a distant memory.

† Whereas *eradication* refers to the reduction of worldwide incidence of a disease to zero, *elimination* refers to zero transmission in a specific geographic area or region.

A MIGHTY DISEASE

Polio, short for *poliomyelitis*, is one of history's most feared infectious diseases. It is caused by the intestinal poliovirus, which enters its victim through the mouth or nose and multiplies in the lymph nodes. Polio's most distinguishing symptom, paralysis, develops in less than 1% of all victims and is caused when the virus invades the central nervous system and irrevocably kills the nerve cells responsible for muscle movement. If enough nerve cells are destroyed, the victim is left with lifeless limbs (primarily the legs) in what is called acute flaccid paralysis. In as few as four days, a previously healthy person can become stricken with paralysis and condemned to a lifetime of crutches and wheelchairs. Quadriplegia occurs when extensive paralysis develops in the trunk and muscles of the thorax and abdomen.

The most serious form of the disease, called bulbar polio, occurs when the virus invades the motor neurons of the brain stem and paralyzes the relevant muscles so that the victim loses the ability to swallow, breathe, and speak. Respiratory support is needed to keep bulbar polio victims alive, and fatality runs as high as 40%.[1]

During the virus's incubation period, ranging from 4 to 35 days, infected individuals are extremely contagious and can spread the virus to others through their contaminated feces. The virus can live for as long as two months outside the body and resides in swimming pools, drinking water, food, and clothing. Transmission is silent; 90% of the carriers show no sign of the disease at all, thanks to their development of protective antibodies. Of the 9% of victims who develop nonparalyzing symptoms, their fever, fatigue, headache, vomiting, or stiff neck rarely point conclusively to polio. As a result, for each case of distinctive polio paralysis reported in an area, the community is further threatened by another 2,000 to 3,000 contagious carriers, who may show no further sign than a fever—rendering even a single documented case indicative of an epidemic.[2]

Today, polio is on the verge of being erased from the globe. As recently as 1988, 125 countries around the world were endemic for polio, with an estimated 350,000 polio cases. Through the first half of 2006, only four were endemic, and there were fewer than 700 reported cases.[3] This is due to the coordinated efforts of regional and international polio eradication campaigns that have immunized hundreds of millions of children against the deadly scourge. The regional polio campaign in Latin America and the Caribbean, in particular, is an outstanding success and eliminated polio from the region in just six years.

ROAD TO A VACCINE

In the first half of the 1900s, polio was most prominent in industrialized countries in Europe and North America. Tens of thousands of children became infected with the disease each year in the United States, and thousands more died. Each summer the disease would cause widespread panic when its indiscriminate path left a trail of paralysis and death. Public pools, movie theaters, and beaches were shut down out of fear of the disease, and crippled children supported by crutches and breathing through imposing iron lung machines were common sights.

In the 1930s and 1940s, following a series of prominent outbreaks, the American public rallied behind the drive for a vaccine. The mobilization effort was led by polio's most famous victim, US President Franklin D. Roosevelt, who was left permanently paralyzed after suffering a bout of polio in 1921. In 1938, President Roosevelt created the National Foundation for Infantile Paralysis, later renamed the March of Dimes, to support healthcare for sufferers and to raise funds "a dime at a time" for the urgent quest for a vaccine.

Fourteen years later, in 1952, the millions of nickels and dimes collected through the grassroots March of Dimes campaigns finally paid off. Dr. Jonas Salk made history that year with his discovery of an inactivated polio vaccine (IPV), made from a deactivated ("killed") version of the poliovirus. Administered through an injection, the IPV is capable of protecting against the ravages of polio. The successful results from large community trials were printed in exuberant headlines around the world, and mass immunization led to a rapid and dramatic reduction in disease incidence over the next few years. Between 1955 and 1961, more than 300 million doses were administered in the United States, resulting in a 90% drop in the incidence of polio.[4]

In 1961, a second scientific breakthrough presented the world with a new form of the vaccine, which would later prove ideally suited for widespread use in developing countries. Dr. Albert Sabin's oral polio vaccine (OPV) is made from a live attenuated (weakened) virus and is administered orally. Just three doses of OPV, properly spaced, can confer lifetime immunity to both the user and his or her close contacts. The vaccine works like the IPV by producing antibodies that stop the spread of the poliovirus to the nervous system, thus preventing paralysis. OPV goes a step further, however, by reducing the multiplication of the virus in the intestine, thereby helping to halt person-to-person transmission. At approximately 5 cents per dose, OPV is considerably cheaper than its predecessor.[5] Because no needles are required, administration of OPV is also easier, and volunteers can do it on a wide scale.

The power of the new oral vaccine was first demonstrated during a trial in Chiapas, Mexico, which suffered a polio outbreak in 1961. In as few as four days, Sabin's team reached 80% of children under 11 with the new oral vaccine.[2] After polio was successfully wiped out from the city a few weeks later, Sabin believed he had discovered not only an improved vaccine but also a successful strategy for large-scale immunization. It would take another two decades, however, for Sabin's model of intensive, widespread vaccine campaigns to be deployed.

POLIO IN LATIN AMERICA

Polio was not recognized as a major public health threat to developing countries until the middle of the 1900s, at the same time that the disease was being erased from North America and Europe. In the 1980s, the incidence of paralysis in developing countries rivaled the level in developed countries before the introduction of a vaccine.[6] Estimates suggest that there were more than 250,000 cases of paralytic polio worldwide in 1987.[7]

In Latin America in the 1970s, there were an estimated 15,000 paralysis cases and 1,750 deaths each year due to polio.[8] Countries in the region first added the OPV to regular immunization in 1977 as part of the new Expanded Programme on Immunization (EPI). At the program's outset, immunization in Latin America for the six targeted diseases in the EPI—diphtheria, tetanus, pertussis (which are collectively known as *DTP*), plus polio, measles, and tuberculosis—was quite low at 25%, with OPV coverage among children less than 1 year of age higher, at 38%. With the support of a broad coalition of both international and national partners, EPI promoted the delivery of immunization services for polio and the five other principal diseases through the routine basic health services of Latin American countries. By 1984, coverage with OPV grew to an impressive 80%, the highest of all EPI vaccines. Between 1975 and 1981, the incidence of polio in the region was cut almost in half, and the number of countries reporting cases of polio dropped from 19 to 11.1. See Box 5-1.

The success of EPI in reducing polio in Latin America during the 1970s and 1980s inspired Dr. Carlyle Guerra de Macedo, then director of the Pan American Health Organization (PAHO), to propose the eradication of indigenous wild poliovirus in Latin America and the Caribbean by 1990 through a coordinated regional effort. A polio eradication campaign was seen as a stepping stone to strengthening the entire EPI, to improving health infrastructure throughout the region, and to establishing a greatly needed surveillance system to monitor the impact of interventions on the reduction of polio and other diseases. Encouraged by the success of the smallpox eradication campaign 14 years earlier, the PAHO directing council passed a resolution in 1985 launching the program to eliminate polio from Latin America and the Caribbean.

BOX 5-1 The Expanded Programme on Immunization

In May 1974, the World Health Assembly created the Expanded Programme on Immunization (EPI). The initiative brought together a diverse coalition of both national and international partners to achieve the goal of immunizing by 1990 all children under 5 years of age against six vaccine-preventable diseases: diphtheria, tetanus, pertussis (or DTP), plus measles, tuberculosis, and polio. The second expressed goal of EPI, to "promote the countries' self-reliance on the delivery of immunization service within the context of their comprehensive services," set in motion the strengthening of the overall health infrastructure.

Immunization was integrated into regular maternal and child health services and made a fixture in primary healthcare. Program managers were trained, a comprehensive cold chain established, and a vaccine procurement fund put in place. To decrease the number of visits that mothers with small children would have to make, the program synchronized administration of several vaccines.

The success of EPI has been extraordinary: At the outset of the program in 1974, the average immunization coverage rate in developing countries was just 5%. By 1991, 83% of children in developing countries received three doses of DTP vaccines, and 85% received the polio vaccine.[9]

EPI has succeeded in decreasing the share of the six diseases in the total burden of disease among children under 5 from about 23% in the mid-1970s to less than 10% in 2000. At a cost of just $20, fully immunizing a child against the six diseases is one of the most affordable interventions in existence.

PUTTING TOGETHER THE PIECES: POLITICAL, FINANCIAL, AND MANAGERIAL

The polio campaign was immediately charged with two crucial objectives: mobilizing the necessary political, financial, and social commitment for the intense regional effort; and organizing the managerial oversight to carry out immunization in each country.

To marshal political and financial support, an Interagency Coordinating Committee (ICC) for Latin America and the Caribbean was established. The committee, comprising representatives from PAHO, the United Nations Children's Fund (UNICEF), the US Agency for International Development (USAID), the Inter-American Development Bank (IDB), Rotary International, and the Canadian Public Health Association, contributed more than $110 million between 1987 and 1991. The structure was an innovative model with a level of coordination never before attained in the region. "Prior to the formation of the ICC, many of these agencies had been working independently and sometimes in competition with each other, even duplicating efforts at the country level," explained Dr. Ciro de Quadros, the leader of the regional eradication initiative. "It was the first time that such a mechanism was established in the Americas and it proved to be a fundamental means of securing permanent coordination and continuous support for the program. Its advocacy has been key for the sustained political and social will generated by the initiative." The success of the ICC, according to de Quadros, demonstrated that "diverse organizations can work together to achieve an important health objective."

Because national-level leadership, funding, and management were paramount to the initiative, the ICC model was duplicated at the country level. Each national ICC worked under the coordination of the country's ministry of health to develop a 5-year national plan of action to set immunization program strategies and streamline national resources. The plans delineated objectives, targets, strategies, activities, expected outputs, and time frames. Furthermore, because the cost and expected source of funding (either internal or external) were identified for each activity, the national plans provided a vehicle for systematically analyzing the financing of immunization activities.[5] National commitment in the region was extremely strong and was demonstrated in the financial support from Latin American governments. In the first 5-year plans from 1987 to 1991, 80% of the $544.8 million budget for EPI was derived from national resources. This figure climbed to 90% in the second 5-year plan.

To address managerial needs, PAHO created an EPI technical advisory group of five international health experts to review the initiative's progress and set priorities. Thousands of health workers, managers, and technicians were subsequently trained in tasks ranging from cold chain management to surveillance. Furthermore, "Resources were decentralized to strengthen the response capabilities of the local health systems," added de Quadros.

EXTREME VIGILANCE

Even one confirmed case of polio could threaten an entire community, so the initiative immediately recognized that a well-developed surveillance system capable of detecting even low levels of infection was essential to the program's success and to ensuring immediate investigation of each case. At the outset of the program in 1985, however, such a system was lacking.

The campaign set out to establish uniform indicators throughout the region. *Suspected* cases were cases of acute paralytic illness that a doctor strongly suspected to be polio. Epidemiologists were to investigate each suspected case within 48 hours. For *probable* cases, or instances of acute flaccid paralysis, two stool specimens would be sent for examination to one of the diagnostic laboratories established in the network. A probable case would be dubbed a *confirmed* case if the laboratories found evidence of the wild poliovirus in the sample within 10 weeks, if the patient died within 60 days, or if the patient could not be traced later. To encourage community involvement in case identification at the end of the campaign, PAHO offered a reward of $100 for the reporting of suspected cases.[10]

A *Field Guide for Surveillance and Polio Eradication* was widely disseminated, and hundreds of health workers were trained in surveillance. Surveillance indicators to track program performance were established, and the overall system was computerized by 1989. A reporting network of 22,000 health institutions was established, through which local clinics were required to report weekly on either the presence or absence of suspected cases. Furthermore, eight diagnostic laboratories were equipped to detect wild poliovirus in stool specimens.[11]

IMMUNIZATION STRATEGIES

The immunization strategy of the polio campaign centered around three primary components: achieving and maintaining high immunization coverage, prompt identification of new cases, and aggressive control of outbreaks. Each country in the Latin American and Caribbean region was grouped into one of two categories: (1) "polio-free" countries where no case of polio was reported in the previous three years, and (2) "polio-endemic" countries that had at least one identified case. Countries in the former category were encouraged to maintain their polio-free status through routine immunization—a central pillar of the eradication campaign—and through effective surveillance.

The approach implemented to increase polio immunization coverage in polio-endemic countries was based on Brazil's OPV experience. Beginning in 1980, after disappointing coverage rates in the previous decade exposed that routine health services alone would not accomplish the EPI goals, Brazil embarked on a new strategy of national vaccine days. Held twice a year, one to two months apart, each national vaccine day administered OPV to 20 million children, accounting for nearly all of those in the under-5 age group.[10] The national vaccine days were designed to vaccinate as many children as possible, regardless of their vaccination status, to instantly deprive the virus of its lifeline and halt its transmission.

Brazil's strategy was not new; in fact, it was the very approach that Sabin tested in Chiapas and subsequently recommended. In the 1960s, Cuba used the strategy to interrupt the disease with the help of more than 80,000 local committees that were mobilized to conduct a series of week-long house-to-house campaigns.[2] In fact, every country that had halted polio transmission employed some sort of mass vaccination campaign. Brazil's experience, however, was a powerful example of how poor countries in the region with less developed health infrastructures could bolster coverage and interrupt polio transmission.

By 1987, all 14 countries in the polio-endemic category had incorporated national vaccine days to complement, but not replace, regular immunization, and immunization coverage quickly rose. DTP and measles vaccines were likewise incorporated into the national vaccine days to help boost the overall EPI goals.

"OPERATION MOP-UP" AND THE FINAL CASE

Although the national vaccine days helped slow polio's transmission in most of Latin America by 1989, the disease still lingered in 1,000 of the 14,000 districts. "Operation Mop-Up" was launched that year to aggressively tackle the virus in its final bastions. The initiative targeted the communities where polio cases had been reported; where coverage was low; or where overcrowding, poor sanitation, weak health care infrastructure, and/or heavy migration prevailed. In these communities, two house-to-house vaccination campaigns were conducted to finally wipe out the disease.

In 1991, just seven cases of polio were confirmed: six in Colombia and one in Peru. An aggressive mop-up campaign was launched in Colombia to vanquish the disease. House-to-house vaccination campaigns reached almost a million

households, and nearly a million children under 5 were immunized.

In August 1991, 2-year-old Luis Fermin Tenorio of Pichinaki, Peru, made history as the last polio victim in Latin America. By the end of 1993, two years later, 9,000 stool specimens had been examined, and no poliovirus was found. In 1994, vaccine coverage rates through routine immunization services peaked at 86% in the region, meeting the high surveillance standards set by the International Commission for Certification of the Eradication of Poliomyelitis in the Americas.[1] Polio was then declared eliminated from Latin America and the Caribbean (see Figure 5-1).

IMPACT OF ELIMINATION

In addition to the tangible benefits to the health and welfare of residents in Latin America following the eradication of polio, the program's success has left an indelible mark on the region's health infrastructure and its capacity to control other infectious diseases. Thousands of trained epidemiologists and health workers with experience in surveillance, disease control, cold chain management, and operational research currently are addressing new health challenges. The program's surveillance system is considered to be the "most comprehensive surveillance system for human health that has ever existed in the Western Hemisphere," and the network of diagnostic laboratories now detects and controls additional public health threats, such as measles, cholera, and tetanus.[10]

The health planning capacity of national governments also has improved considerably. The annual national plans of action continue to serve as an important program management tool and have expanded to cover broader mother and child health services. Finally, the polio campaign succeeded in advancing the overall goals of the EPI. By the end of 1990, coverage for the six EPI vaccines reached a historic high: Coverage for every vaccine was above 70% and in many regions exceeded 80%.[10]

ECONOMICALLY JUSTIFIED?

Administration of an oral polio vaccine is both an inexpensive and an extremely cost-effective intervention. It is estimated that the cost of immunizing a child with three doses of the polio vaccine (along with the DTP vaccine) is about $14. The cost of a healthy year of life from polio immunization ranges from $7 to $16 in high-mortality environments, placing it among the most cost-effective health interventions for children.[12]

Even without considering the additional benefits of productivity, strengthened capacity to fight other diseases, and reduced pain and suffering, the polio eradication campaign

FIGURE 5-1 Eradication of wild poliovirus from Latin America and the Caribbean: acute flaccid paralysis, 1969–1995.

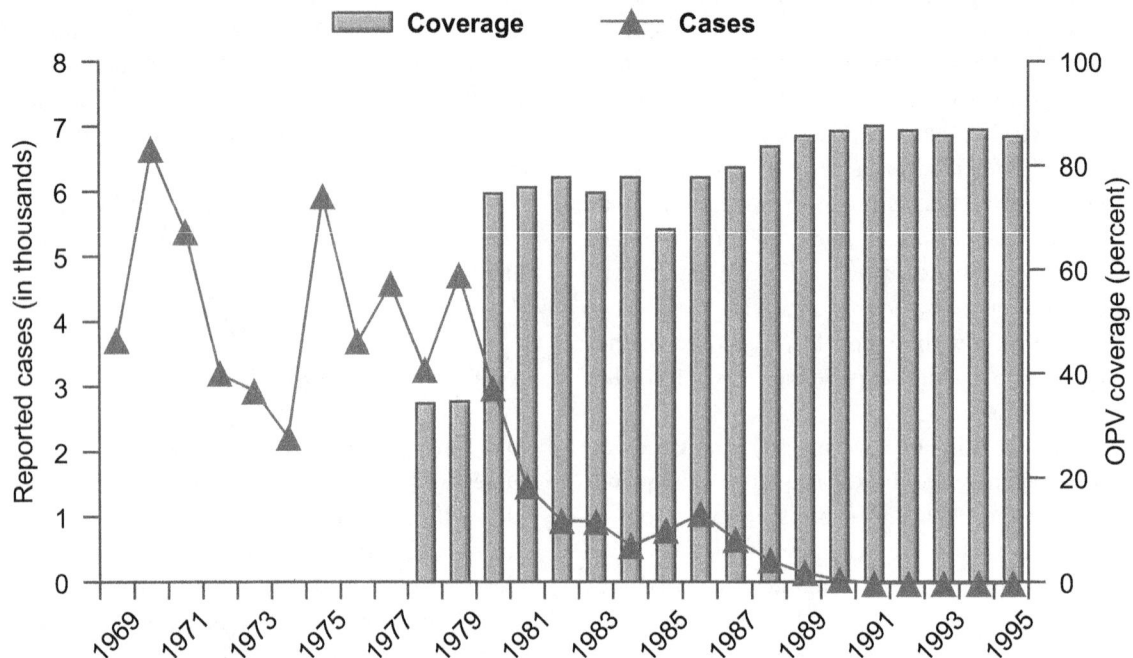

Note: OPV = oral polio vaccine. Bars represent percent of coverage.
Source: de Quadros (1997).

was economically justified based on the savings of medical costs for treatment and rehabilitation alone. The cost of the first five years of the program was reported at $120 million: $74 million from national sources and $46 million from international donors—and $10 million annually from donor sources thereafter.[8] Comparing the savings from treatment costs with the cost of the 5-year program, the net benefit of the eradication campaign (after discounting even at the high rate of 12% per year) in its first five years was $217.2 million. In the 10 years after eradication, the discounted net savings climbed to $264.2 million. Over a 15-year period, donor contributions would pay for themselves. In short, economist Philip Musgrove concluded, "The eradication of polio would actually put money in the coffers of the Ministry of Health, or whoever now pays to treat polio victims."[8]

MAINTAINING AND EXPANDING SUCCESS

The success of the polio eradication campaign was due in large part to exemplary political commitment and inter-agency and regional coordination. Complacency and polio importation from endemic regions, however, pose a risk to the program's achievements. In 2000, these dangers were

realized when incomplete immunization allowed polio to briefly return to Latin America and the Caribbean. A total of 20 cases and two deaths were reported in Haiti and the Dominican Republic after a child developed a rare strain of the disease when the circulating vaccine virus reverted to a more virulent form. Polio was then able to spread quickly because the immunization coverage on the island was inadequate. The outbreak was eventually contained, but not without first illustrating the need for sustained financial support for immunization, sustained political will, and effective surveillance to keep the region polio free.

GOING GLOBAL

Prompted by the success in Latin America and the Caribbean, an effort in 1998 was launched to eradicate polio from the rest of the world. The global campaign, considered the largest public health campaign in history, has been led by the World Health Organization, Rotary International, UNICEF, and the US Centers for Disease Control and Prevention (CDC). More than $3 billion has been rallied from the international community, including private foundations, donor governments, development banks, nongovernmental organizations, and corporate partners. Rotary International has played a particularly instrumental role, raising more than $500 million for the effort and providing volunteers to assist with national immunization days.

The global initiative has employed many of the same effective immunization strategies that proved successful in Latin America and the Caribbean, including national immunization days and "mop-up" campaigns. Since 1988, an estimated two billion children have been immunized against polio, and 5 million children who would have been paralyzed from polio without the vaccine are now walking. Today less than 700 cases have been reported, compared to 350,000 when the initiative began.

The global eradication effort faced a serious setback during 2003 and 2004 when the discontinuation of immunization activities in northern Nigeria due to public fears over vaccine safety led to a regional spread of the virus to 21 previously polio-free countries.[13] Weak routine immunization systems, low vaccine coverage rates, and discontinuation of periodic national immunization days in many of these countries fueled the outbreaks. A series of large-scale supplementary immunization activities was able to dramatically curtail transmission in the countries experiencing importation, except in Somalia.[13] Today, polio transmission has been eliminated from all but four endemic countries: India, Pakistan, Afghanistan, and Nigeria, where just five states contain more than two thirds of all cases.

REFERENCES

1. de Quadros CA. Polio. In: Lederberg J, Alexander M, Bloom BR, et al , eds. *Encyclopedia of Microbiology.* Vol. 3. 2nd. ed. Burlington, VT: Academic Press, Inc.;2000:762–772.

2. Guwande A. The mop-up: eradicating polio from the planet, one child at a time. *New Yorker.* January 2004:34–40.

3. Global Polio Eradication Initiative. Progress report. Available at: http://www.polioeradication.org/content/publications/2003-progress.pdf. Accessed January 12, 2007.

4. Henderson DA, de Quadros CA, Andrus JK, Olivé J-M, Guerra de Macedo C. Polio eradication from the Western Hemisphere. *Annu Rev Public Health.* 1992;13:239–252.

5. Olivé J-M, de Quadros CA. *The Polio Eradication Initiative: An Opportunity for Costing EPI.* Geneva, Switzerland: Expanded Programme on Immunization; 1989.

6. Hinman AR, Foege WH, de Quadros CA, Patriarca PA, Orenstein WA, Brink EW. The case for global eradication of poliomyelitis. *Bull WHO.* 1987;65:835–840.

7. Pan American Health Organization. *Final Report of the Taylor Commission: The Impact of the Expanded Programme on Immunization and the Polio Eradication Initiative on Health Systems in the Americas.* Washington, DC: Pan American Health Organization; 1995.

8. Musgrove P. Is the eradication of polio in the Western Hemisphere economically justified? *Bull Pan Am Sanitary Bureau.* 1988;22(1).

9. de Quadros CA. Global eradication of poliomyelitis. *Int J Infect Dis.* 1997;1(January):125–129.

10. de Quadros CA, Henderson DA. Disease eradication and control in the Americas. *Biologicals.* 1993;21:335–343.

11. de Quadros CA, Andrus JK, Olivé J-M, et al. Eradication of poliomyelitis: progress in the Americas. *Pediatr Infect Dis J.* 1991;10(3):222–229.

12. Brenzel L, Wolfson LJ, Fox-Roshby J, Miller M, Halsey NA. Vaccine-Preventable Diseases. In: Jamison D, Breman JG, Measham AR, Alleyne G, Claeson M, Evans DB, Jha P, Mills A, Mosgrove P, eds. *Diseases Control Priorities in Developing Countries.* 2nd Ed. New York: Oxford University Press; 2006.

13. World Health Organization. *Weekly Epidemiological Record.* 2006;81(7):61–68.

Saving Mothers' Lives in Sri Lanka

ABSTRACT

Geographic area: Sri Lanka

Health condition: In the 1950s, the maternal mortality ratio in Sri Lanka was estimated at between 500 and 600 per 100,000 live births.

Global importance of the health condition today: Pregnancy-related complications annually claim the lives of 585,000 women. Some 99% of these deaths take place in developing countries, where women have a 1 in 8 chance of dying in their lifetime due to pregnancy-related causes, compared with the 1 in 4,800 chance in Western Europe.

Intervention or program: Beginning in the 1950s, the government of Sri Lanka made special efforts to extend health services, including critical elements of maternal health care, through a widespread rural health network. Sri Lanka's success in reducing maternal deaths is attributed to broad access to maternal healthcare, which is built upon a strong health system that provides free services to the entire population, including in rural areas; the professionalization of midwives; the systematic use of health information to identify problems and guide decision making; and targeted quality improvements to vulnerable groups.

Cost and cost-effectiveness: Sri Lanka has spent less on health—and achieved far more—than most countries at similar income levels. In India, for example, the maternal mortality ratio is more than 400 per 100,000 live births, and spending on health constitutes over 5% of GNP. In Sri Lanka, the ratio is less than one quarter of that, and the country spends only 3% of GNP on health.

Impact: Sri Lanka has halved maternal deaths (relative to the number of live births) at least every 12 years since 1935. This has meant a decline in the maternal mortality ratio from between 500 and 600 maternal deaths per 100,000 live births in 1950 to 60 per 100,000 today. In Sri Lanka today, skilled practitioners attend to 97% of the births, compared with 30% in 1940.

The reduction in deaths during pregnancy and delivery has long been held out as a major international public health goal, but many countries have had difficulties making progress toward it. Most observers now agree that there are no quick fixes, and that the solution will come with the strengthening of now-failing health systems in many poor countries, building up the training of professional and paraprofessional health workers, improving access to both basic and higher-level services, and ensuring the availability of basic medical supplies and medications to deal with obstetric problems. The case of Sri Lanka demonstrates how rapidly progress can occur when those fundamental building blocks are in place.

MOTHERS SHOULD NOT DIE IN CHILDBIRTH

Pregnancy and childbirth are natural events and typically require little or no medical intervention for either mother or baby. But in about 15% of all pregnancies, a severe complication affects the woman—for example, maternal diabetes or dangerously high blood pressure sets in, excessive bleeding occurs during childbirth, or the mother suffers from a serious postpartum infection. In about 1% to 2% of the cases, women often require major surgery and may die without effective treatment of these complications.

Over and above the baseline risk of pregnancy, women are in danger of dying during pregnancy and childbirth if their general health is poor. Malnutrition, malaria, immune system deficiency, tuberculosis, and heart disease all contribute to maternal mortality. In addition, use of unsafe abortion services is a major risk factor for maternal death.

Maternal mortality,* the death of a woman while pregnant or within about two months after the end of the pregnancy, echoes through families for many generations. Women who die are in the prime of their lives and are likely to be leaving behind one or more children—a loss that places at risk those children's social development, health, education, and future life chances. The death of a woman in childbirth is highly correlated with the survival of the child she is bearing; the risk of a child dying before age 5 is doubled if the mother dies in childbirth. At least one fifth of the burden of disease for children under 5 is associated with poor maternal health.[1] Because poor women are far more likely to die than better-off women, maternal mortality is one of the factors contributing to the transmission of poverty from one generation to the next.

Interventions to detect pregnancy-related health problems before they become life threatening, and to manage major complications when they do occur, are well known and require relatively little in the way of advanced technology. What is required, however, is a health system that is organized and accessible—physically, financially, and culturally—so that women deliver in hygienic circumstances, those who are at particularly high risk for complications are identified early, and help is available to respond to emergencies when they occur. Although some maternal deaths are unavoidable even under the most favorable circumstances, the vast majority can be prevented through systematic and sustained efforts.

Because of overall high health risks and weak health systems, almost all maternal deaths take place in developing countries. Ninety-nine percent of the 585,000 maternal deaths each year occur in poor nations.

The extremes tell the story: Women in the poorest sub-Saharan countries have a 1 in 8 chance of dying during their lifetime because of pregnancy; Western European women have a risk of 1 in 4,800. And in the developing world, maternal death is very much the tip of the iceberg: For each maternal death, somewhere between 30 and 50 other women experience serious injury or infection because of pregnancy and childbirth. In developing countries, more than 40% of pregnancies lead to complications, illness, or permanent disability in the mother or child.[2]

During the past several decades, as child health indicators have generally improved in the developing world and even as fertility rates have fallen, the WHO estimates that maternal mortality has remained relatively unchanged at a high level. Some countries, however, have been able to make significant and sustained progress toward making pregnancy safer for women, even beyond what would be expected with general improvements in living conditions and female health. The lessons from those settings are now informing the approaches international agencies promote.

SRI LANKA'S PUBLIC HEALTH TRADITIONS

Sri Lanka, an ethnically diverse country of almost 20 million people living on a densely populated island in South Asia, has a storied history of public-sector commitment to human development. Although it is (and always has been) a poor country, with a current average annual per capita income of $740, the development of social services even before independence in 1948 has far exceeded the gains made in countries at similar economic levels. Access to public education was rapidly expanded during the first half of the 1900s, and schooling of girls has long been much more common in Sri Lanka than in neighboring countries in the region. As a result, 89% of Sri Lankan adult women are literate, compared with a South Asian average of 43%.[3]

Health services, too, have benefited from strong public-sector leadership. Going back to the 1930s, the government focused on expanding free health services in rural areas, with attention given to preventive services and especially control of major communicable diseases. Financing for this effort was derived largely from income taxes. Currently, life expectancy in Sri Lanka is 71 years for men and 76 for women,

---

* The official definition of the maternal mortality ratio is the number of maternal deaths for every 100,000 live births. "Maternal" death refers to a death during pregnancy or within 42 days after the end of the pregnancy from a cause related to the pregnancy or its management. Thus, the death of a pregnant woman from an accident or an infectious disease not specifically related to the pregnancy would not count in the numerator.

compared with 57 for men and 58 for women on average in low-income countries.[3]

One unusual asset to which Sri Lanka lays claim is a good civil registration system, which has been in place since 1867. This system, which first started recording maternal deaths around 1900, has provided valuable information for planning and monitoring progress. So, unlike in most poor countries where maternal mortality estimates are based on very imperfect sources and methods, Sri Lanka benefits from relatively good data and a tradition within the public administration of using it.

ELEMENTS OF SUCCESS

Sri Lanka's success in reducing maternal deaths is attributed to widespread access to maternal healthcare, which is built upon a strong health system that provides free services to the entire population, the professionalization and broad use of midwives, the systematic use of health information to identify problems and guide decision making, and targeted quality improvements. These elements have been introduced in steps, with emphasis first on improving overall (and particularly rural) access to both lower- and higher-level facilities, then on reaching particularly vulnerable populations, and later on quality improvements.[†]

Access

The first challenge in this country that is largely rural was access. The creation of a basic health service infrastructure, starting in the 1930s, extended access across rural areas to a range of preventive and curative services, enabling initial improvements in maternal health. At the lowest level, the infrastructure consisted of health units staffed by a medical officer, who was responsible for serving the population within a given area. Within each of these health areas, public health midwives provided care for all pregnant women.

A viable referral system for both pregnancy-related and other health problems was established from the early days. The health units were—and continue to be—supported by cottage hospitals designed to offer very basic services; rural hospitals and maternity homes at a primary level; district hospitals and peripheral units at the secondary level; and tertiary provincial hospitals with specialist services, teaching hospitals, and specialist maternity hospitals.

At both the lower and higher levels, the number of facilities was expanded rapidly, increasing from 112 government hospitals in 1930 (about 182 beds per 100,000 people) to 247 hospitals in 1948 (close to 250 beds per 100,000). The secondary and tertiary institutions also underwent expansion in the 1950s.

No referral system works without accessible transportation—a need that was identified relatively early in Sri Lanka's health system development. Between 1948 and 1950, the national ambulance fleet was increased from 12 to 67 ambulances. All provincial hospitals had between three and five ambulances each, as did major district hospitals and those in more remote areas.[4]

Professionalization of Midwifery

While the basic health infrastructure was being developed, specific attention was paid to the problem of who would deliver what type of services and, in particular, how maternal health services would be delivered. The path chosen was to depend on a large number of clinically qualified midwives. This strategy has proved successful both in Sri Lanka and elsewhere (see Box 6-1).

From early days, public health midwives have underpinned the health unit network. Each midwife serves a population of 3,000 to 5,000 and lives within the local area. Midwives' duties include visiting pregnant women at home, registering them for care, encouraging them to attend antenatal clinics, and working with the doctor who runs those clinics. The midwives are considered to be one of the most important elements in the excellent health performance of the country. Supervision and a referral network back up midwives, who undergo an 18-month training program. They report to supervisors, typically nurse-midwives, who have nursing training in addition to the basic midwife preparation; the supervisors then report to the medical officer. Established procedures for service delivery and supervision, along with frequent in-service training, help midwives stay current and deliver high-quality services.

Importantly, public health midwives are part of both the health system and their local communities and thus provide a valuable link between the women and the health units. Even when a midwife does not attend a birth, the family knows how to find her in the event of a problem. It is widely maintained that the public health midwives are key to sustaining the population's confidence in and satisfaction with the public maternal health care services.

The growth in the number of midwives was rapid, while at the same time fertility was falling. As a result, while in 1935 there were 219 live births per government midwife

---

† Our understanding of the pace and causes for decline in maternal mortality is due to a study by Pathmanathan and colleagues (2003), which sheds light on the main factors of success. Unless otherwise noted, information in this case study is drawn from that source.

on average, by 1960 the ratio had fallen to 143 live births per midwife and by 1995 to 51 live births per midwife (see Table 6-1).

Largely because of the focus on midwifery—combined with access to higher-level services—more than in many other countries, women in Sri Lanka rapidly became accustomed to the notion of attended births and, increasingly, births in hospitals. Up until 1940, skilled attendants assisted only about 30% of the births. By 1950, after the implementation of policies to introduce and expand the cadre of public health midwives, this percentage had doubled. Concurrently, the

BOX 6-1
The Midwife Approach

The relationship between low maternal mortality and extensive use of professional midwives to deliver antenatal, birthing, and postpartum services, which is seen in the developing world today, has been observed historically in the industrialized world. In countries where doctors predominantly assisted births in the period around 1920, such as the United States, New Zealand, and Scotland, the maternal mortality ratio was 600 or more per 100,000 live births. During the same period, in countries where doctors and midwives equally attended births, including France, Ireland, Australia, and England, maternal mortality was lower, averaging around 500 per 100,000 live births. And strikingly, during the same period, in countries where midwives attended most births—Norway, Sweden, the Netherlands, and Denmark—the maternal mortality ratio was very low, between 200 and 300 per 100,000 live births.

Professional midwives have special training to acquire clinical competence, are licensed or registered by public authorities, and are given support, in the form of regular supplies as well as supervision. They also are linked to a functional referral system, so they know precisely where higher-level care can be obtained when women face obstetric emergencies.

Midwives are trusted frontline workers who have the distinct advantage of being close to where births are taking place—within the community—and thus even if they are not called in for each normal birth, they are available when the unexpected occurs.

Moreover, because midwives can be trained and supported at relatively low cost, and have salaries that are far lower than medical doctors, the effective use of this cadre of health workers is one of the keys to saving mothers' lives within a modest budget.

proportion of babies delivered in government health care facilities increased from 6% in 1940 to 33% 10 years later. Currently, skilled practitioners attend to 97% of the births, and the majority are in hospitals.

Information and Organization

Effective management, including the use of information for monitoring and planning, reinforced the two early building blocks of Sri Lanka's success in reducing maternal deaths—access to basic health services and professional midwifery. In the 1950s, the health education division was formed within the Ministry of Health, and medical officers of maternal and child health were designated to coordinate maternal and child health services in each district.

Quality Improvements, Including Targeting of Vulnerable Groups

In part because of the information and close monitoring provided, in the 1960s and 1970s the government identified several ways to improve the system. The Ministry of Health systematically used maternal death inquiries to identify problems in the delivery of care—for example, the reason a problematic delivery was not detected in time to save a life. The Ministry of Health would then circulate information about how to prevent similar problems.

The government's program to reach women on the tea estates—farming operations that contracted South Asian labor in large numbers—provides another example of a targeted effort to ensure good quality services for all. Women on the large, privately owned tea estates were particularly isolated, socially and physically. Once the estates were nationalized in the 1970s, the government assumed responsibility for health services, and medical officers (with transport) and public health nurses established a network of polyclinics to provide integrated maternal and child health services, including family planning services, to the tea estates. Estate management gave the women paid leave to attend the monthly polyclinics.

Bringing these women into the public health system paid off. Between 1986 and 1997, the number of women from the estates delivering in hospitals increased dramatically, from 20% to 63%.

STEADY, IMPRESSIVE DECLINES

While the maternal mortality ratio (the number of deaths during pregnancy or immediately afterward divided by the number of births) has persisted at high levels in many poor countries, Sri Lanka has been able to halve the maternal deaths (relative to the number of live births) every 6 to 12 years since 1935.

TABLE 6-1 Development of Government-Employed Birth Attendants, Sri Lanka, 1930-1995

Year	Live Births per Government Midwife	Population per 1,000 Government Doctors	Government Nurses per Government Doctor	Specialist Obstetricians in Government Hospitals per 100,000 Live Births
1930	405	15.4	n.a.	n.a.
1935	219	n.a.	n.a.	n.a.
1940	n.a.	14.8	n.a.	n.a.
1945	186	n.a.	n.a.	n.a.
1950	163	11.4	1.7	n.a.
1955	157	9.2	2.3	n.a.
1960	143	8.4	2.8	n.a.
1965	n.a.	7.5	2.4	n.a.
1970	n.a.	6.5	2.9	n.a.
1975	n.a.	6.4	2.7	n.a.
1980	125	7.2	3.3	14.0
1985	85	7.4	3.8	15.0
1990	68	7.0	2.7	20.0
1995	51	4.0	2.9	23.0

Note: n.a. = not available
Source: Pathmanathan, Liljestrand, Martins, et al. (2003).

In the 1930s, the maternal mortality ratio in Sri Lanka was estimated to be over 2,000 per 100,000 live births. By the 1950s, the rate had declined to less than 500 per 100,000. Although data limitations prevent a full explanation of the source of these improvements, it is widely believed that successful efforts to combat malaria and the introduction of modern medical practices deserve much of the credit during this phase.

The steep decline in the maternal mortality ratio that was observed from the 1930s to the early 1950s has been attributed largely to the all-out war on malaria.[5] DDT spraying commenced in 1945 and led to a rapid decline in malaria incidence within a few years. In addition to the highly successful malaria control program, control of hookworm infection and general improvements in sanitation might also have contributed to improvements in maternal health before 1950.[6] Moreover, the rapid decline in maternal mortality during the early 1950s could be attributed to the introduction of modern medical treatment, such as antibiotics, through a health service network established in the pre-1950s era and having considerable reach in rural areas.

The maternal mortality ratio was halved again during the following 13 years, up until 1963, when the government made special efforts to extend health services, including critical elements of maternal healthcare, through a widespread rural health network. In the decades that followed, the public sector systematically applied stepwise strategies to improve organizational and clinical management, reducing the maternal mortality ratio by 50% every 6 to 12 years. And among women working on tea estates, the maternal mortality ratio declined from 120 in 1985 to 90 in 1997 as the polyclinic system was developed.

In total, this has meant a decline in the maternal mortality ratio from between 500 and 600 maternal deaths per 100,000 live births in 1950 to 60 per 100,000 today.[7]

DID TARGETED EFFORTS MAKE THE DIFFERENCE?

The declines in maternal mortality are clear, as is information about efforts the government made to build the overall health system and to address the problem of maternal deaths in particular. A reasonable question to ask, then, is whether the system changes caused the health improvements, or just happened at the same time. Tackling this question—using data that span some 60 years—requires piecing together several types of epidemiologic evidence. And doing so yields a convincing answer.

One way to answer the question of whether system changes caused declines in maternal deaths is to compare the overall decline in female deaths with deaths due to maternal causes. Such a comparison is enlightening because overall female mortality can be assumed to be related, in large measure, to improvements in living conditions and in the general health system. In 1950, maternal deaths accounted for 19% of deaths among women aged 15 to 49 years. By 1996, while both maternal and all female deaths declined, maternal causes accounted for only 1.2% of all female deaths in the reproductive age range.

Another way to understand the cause–effect relationship is to look at the changes in maternal deaths due to individual causes known to be associated with specific health care delivery strategies. So, for example, deaths due to hypertensive disease and sepsis—two causes that are associated throughout the world with lack of access to skilled attendance—declined dramatically during the 1940s, when emphasis was being placed on increasing the availability of midwives and skilled attendants at birth. In contrast, hemorrhage did not decline significantly during the early years studied (1930–1950), when the major approaches the government took were the overall development of an accessible health care system, the control of malaria, and decreasing the proportion of home births. But between 1950 and 1970, as the government emphasized blood transfusion services and other strategies to address the problem, maternal deaths due to hemorrhage decreased from 113 to 45 per 100,000.

The main conclusion from this type of analysis is that the actions of the health system, rather than improvements in general living conditions, led to a large share of the improvements in maternal health that occurred over 60 years in Sri Lanka. The finding is reinforced by a parallel analysis of a similar trajectory of maternal mortality decline in Malaysia, which was similarly successful in achieving a sustained, long-term reduction in maternal deaths over several decades (although starting from a lower initial level). In the case of Malaysia,[8] public health researchers have drawn the link between overall and cause-specific changes in maternal mortality and implementation of a similar set of strategies: professionalizing midwifery, expanding access, mobilizing women and communities, and improving management and the ability to reach the poorest.

In Sri Lanka, the story of improvement in maternal health goes far beyond the health system itself. Mothers' health significantly benefited from effective public investment in basic health services, in improving basic living standards, and in high levels of female education. But the Sri Lankan case, like a very different experience in Honduras (see Box 6-2), reveals ways in which specific strategies to address the problem of maternal deaths greatly augmented the health benefits that would have resulted solely from broad improvements in welfare.

RELATIVELY LOW COST

Sri Lanka has achieved much better health status and steeper declines in maternal mortality than countries at comparable income and economic growth levels—and it has done so while spending relatively little on health services, compared with those same countries. In India, for example, the maternal mortality ratio is more than 400 per 100,000 live births, and spending on health constitutes over 5% of GNP. In Sri Lanka, the maternal mortality ratio is less than one quarter of that, and the country spends only 3% of GNP on health.

Major expenditures, aside from the health infrastructure that served a variety of purposes other than maternal care, are on skilled labor. In Sri Lanka, as in other poor countries, labor is relatively cheap, and in fact, salaries for civil servants have been declining in relative terms. The country could afford widespread access to maternal healthcare by using a mix of health personnel: Most of the maternal health workers are well-trained but low-cost midwives who are described as extremely dedicated. They are closely supervised by nurse-midwives, who in turn are supported by a small number of medical doctors.

Most remarkably, Sri Lanka's success was achieved on a decreasing budget. Between 1950 and 1999, the proportion of the national budget spent on maternal health services has steadily fallen, from 0.28% of GDP in the 1950s to 0.16% in the 1990s. Originally, this was due to efficiency gains made in the 1950s and 1960s. More recently, because salaries of government health staff have been falling, overall expenditures have declined. In addition, expenditures on private services have become relatively more important in the health sector as a whole: In 1953, an estimated 38% of total expenditures were private; by 1996, about half of the total spending was from private sources.[9]

MAJOR LESSONS

Sri Lanka's achievements in reducing the toll of pregnancy have been impressive and correspond to a setting where the public sector has for many decades placed priority on the population's health and education. But others can take inspiration from the country's record: In the late 1950s, when the first efforts were made to address the problem of maternal deaths, the GNP of Sri Lanka was equivalent, in constant dollars, to the national income of Bangladesh, Uganda, and Mali today and far lower than that of Pakistan, Egypt, or the Philippines. In relative terms, Sri Lanka has

BOX 6-2 The Honduran Experience

In Honduras, one of the poorest countries in the Western Hemisphere, the maternal mortality ratio declined by 38% between 1990 and 1997, from 182 to 108 maternal deaths per 100,000 live births. This remarkable achievement, which surprised many observers, was the result of a concerted effort by government officials and development agencies to address maternal mortality.

Although expanding access to essential health services had been a government priority since the 1980s, a study of maternal health in the early 1990s that revealed a serious problem of maternal mortality served as a "rude awakening" to the Ministry of Health, according to Dr. Isabella Danel, US Centers for Disease Control and Prevention expert on maternal health, now posted at the World Bank. This study stimulated a new focus on safe motherhood programs and the inclusion of specific maternal health priorities in the national health policy. Importantly, the government used information about differentials among geographic areas to target its efforts.

By the mid-1990s, a three-part strategy was well into implementation. The first part of the strategy was a reorganization of health services, intended to increase access to skilled care for pregnant women. This included the inauguration of community health clinics, with traditional birth attendants supervised by auxiliary nurses; the construction of maternity waiting homes attached to public hospitals; the establishment of birthing centers supervised by nurse-midwives in rural areas; and the expansion of the basic health center and hospital infrastructure.

As a result of these efforts, between 1990 and 1997, Honduras' health infrastructure was expanded by 7 new area hospitals, 13 birthing centers, 36 health centers, 266 rural health centers, and 5 maternity waiting homes.

The second dimension of the strategy was the training of health workers in specific areas: Traditional birth attendants and public health system staff were trained to recognize high-risk pregnancies and deal with both routine births and obstetric emergencies. Traditional birth attendants were encouraged to accompany women with emergencies to the hospital. The final part of the strategy was community participation, in which local communities were provided with the opportunity to describe and identify solutions to their own health problems and, through newly implemented decentralization policies, were given more decision-making authority. Although this was very much a government strategy, resources from a variety of donors were channeled into its support.

Between 1990 and 1997, maternal mortality across Honduras declined, with the biggest reductions in some of the poorest and most remote areas. So while overall skilled birth attendance changed little during the period, the number of maternal deaths declined from 381 in 1990 to 258 in 1997 due to better referral of women with complications before, during, and after delivery.

The experience of Honduras, like that of Sri Lanka, challenges the notion that little can be done to act on the problem of poor maternal health in poor countries. Success depends neither on major technological innovation nor on high levels of spending, but rather on a combination of three factors: government commitment, which is often spurred by quantifying the problem; targeted actions to improve referrals and emergency services in hospitals; and expanded access to well-trained birth attendants within the community, supported by higher levels of care.[10]

spent less on health—and achieved far more—than any of these countries.

The gains that Sri Lanka made were reinforced in many ways by good education, an emphasis on gender equity, and broad health system development—but the specific actions that were taken to solve the problem of maternal deaths had a separate and identifiable positive impact. In Sri Lanka, the basic health system served as an essential platform from which to work but did not itself generate the impressive results. Those were due to a step-by-step strategy to provide broad access to specific clinical services, to encourage utilization of those services, and to systematically improve quality.

REFERENCES

1. World Bank. *Safe Motherhood and the World Bank: Lessons from 10 Years of Experience*. Washington, DC: World Bank; 1999.

2. World Health Organization. *Maternal Mortality in 1995: Estimates Developed by WHO, UNICEF, and UNFPA*. Geneva, Switzerland: World Health Organization; 2001.

3. World Bank. *World Development Indicators*. Washington, DC: World Bank; 2003.

4. Wickramasinghe WG. *Administration Report of the Director of Medical and Sanitary Services for 1951*. Colombo, Sri Lanka: Ceylon Government Press; 1952.

5. Abeyesundere ANA. *Recent Trends in Malaria Morbidity and Mortality in Sri Lanka: Population Problems of Sri Lanka*. Colombo, Sri Lanka: Demographic Training and Research Unit, University of Colombo; 1976.

6. Wickramasuriya GAW. Maternal mortality and morbidity in Ceylon. *J Ceylon Branch British Med Assoc*. 1939;36(2):79–106.

7. United Nations. *Human Development Report*. New York, NY: United Nations; 2003.

8. Pathmanathan I, Liljestrand J, Martins JM, et al. *Investing in Maternal Health: Learnings from Malaysia and Sri Lanka*. Washington, DC: World Bank; 2003.

9. Hsiao W. *A Preliminary Assessment of Sri Lanka's Health Sector and Steps Forward*. Cambridge, Mass: Harvard University and Institute of Policy Studies; 2000.

10. Danel I. *Maternal Mortality Reduction, Honduras, 1990–1997: A Case Study*. Washington, DC: World Bank, Latin America and Caribbean Region; 1999.

Controlling Onchocerciasis (River Blindness) in Sub-Saharan Africa*

* The first draft of this case was prepared by Jane Seymour and Molly Kinder; significant contributions to the current version were made by Bruce Benton.

ABSTRACT

Geographic area: Sub-Saharan Africa

Health condition: In 11 west African countries in 1974, nearly 2 million of the area's 20 million inhabitants were infected with onchocerciasis, and approximately 200,000 were blind.

Global importance of the health condition: Onchocerciasis, or river blindness, afflicts approximately 42 million people worldwide, with well over 99% of its victims in sub-Saharan Africa. An estimated 600,000 people are blind, and an additional 1.5 million Africans are visually impaired due to onchocerciasis.

Intervention or program: The Onchocerciasis Control Program (OCP) was launched in 1974 in 11 west African countries. Weekly aerial spraying with environmentally safe insecticides helped control the disease vector—blackflies that bred in fast-moving waterways—thereby halting transmission of the disease. In 1995, a second program, the African Programme for Onchocerciasis Control (APOC), was established to control the disease in 19 central, east, and southern African countries. Through a broad international partnership and the participation of 115,000 remote, rural communities, APOC and OCP distributed a drug donated by Merck & Co., Inc., Mectizan (ivermectin), to more than 45 million people in sub-Saharan Africa in 2005. The drug prevents and alleviates the symptoms of the disease with one annual dose.

Cost-effectiveness: OCP operated with an annual cost of less than $1 per protected person. Commitments from 27 donors during the 28-year project totaled $600 million. The annual return on investment was calculated to be about 20%, primarily attributable to increased agricultural output; about $3.7 billion will be generated from improved labor and agricultural productivity. The annual cost of APOC operations, taking into account the donation of all needed drugs, is approximately $0.58 per person treated.

Impact: OCP produced an impressive change in health between 1974 and 2002: Transmission of the disease-causing parasite was halted in 11 west African countries, 600,000 cases of blindness were prevented, and 22 million children born in the OCP area are now free from the risk of contracting river blindness. About 25 million hectares of arable land—enough to feed an additional 17 million people per annum—is now safe for resettlement. APOC is expanding this success to central, east, and southern Africa, where 54,000 cases of blindness are expected to be prevented each year.

At the headquarters of the World Bank, the WHO, the Carter Center, the multinational pharmaceutical firm Merck, and the Royal Tropical Institute of the Netherlands, as well as in a prominent square in Ouagadougou, Burkina Faso, visitors see a distinctive statue of a child leading a blind man—a symbolic reminder to passersby of the part each partner played in the control of one of Africa's most devastating diseases. The Onchocerciasis Control Program (OCP) has earned its place as one of the signal achievements of international public health, demonstrating the power of collaboration across countries and agencies, the importance of long-term funding from the donor community, and the benefits of public–private partnership to bring pharmaceutical innovation into large-scale use in developing countries.

THE DISEASE

Onchocerciasis, or "river blindness," is a pernicious disease that afflicts approximately 42 million people worldwide, with well over 99% of its victims residing in sub-Saharan Africa. Primarily a rural disease, onchocerciasis disproportionately burdens the inhabitants of some of the poorest and most remote areas in Africa. Small, isolated areas in Latin America and Yemen also are affected. In the most endemic areas, more than one third of the adult population is blind, and infection often approaches 90% of the population.[1]

The disease is caused by a worm, *Onchocerca volvulus,* which enters its human victim through the bite of an infected blackfly. In the arable riverine areas where the flies breed, residents are bitten as many as 10,000 times a day. Once inside a human, the tiny worm grows to two to three feet in length, each year producing millions of microscopic offspring called microfilaria. These tiny worms are so abundant that a simple snip of the skin can expose hundreds of writhing worms.

The constant movement of the microfilarie through the infected person's skin causes a wide range of debilitating symptoms, including disabling and torturous itching, skin lesions, rashes, muscle pain, weakness, and, in its most severe cases, blindness. The disease is spread when a new blackfly bites an infected person and then bites another person, thus repeating the infection cycle. Today, an estimated 600,000 people are blind due to onchocerciasis, and nearly 1.5 million are severely visually impaired.[2]

Beyond the disabling health burden, onchocerciasis inflicts tremendous social and economic damage on individuals and entire communities. Self-esteem and concentration suffer, and the disease reduces marriage prospects for both women and men. Infected individuals often earn less money as a result of decreased productivity and spend a large portion of their income on extra health costs.[3]

On a community level, the disease has hindered economic growth. The threat of the disease has led people to abandon more than 250,000 square kilometers of some of the best arable land in west Africa. In the words of Dr. Ebrahim Samba, OCP's director from 1980 to 1994, "Onchocerciasis therefore is a disease of human beings and also of the land. It directly retards development and aggravates poverty."

COMBATING THE DISEASE: THE ONCHOCERCIASIS CONTROL PROGRAM

Colonial and ex-colonial entomologists attempted for many years to control the disease in the hardest hit areas, but achieved mixed results. Lasting results proved elusive because the blackflies cover long distances (exceeding 400 kilometers with the wind currents) and cross national boundaries, rendering uncoordinated national control efforts ineffective.

The small-scale control efforts of the 1950s and 1960s provided the seeds for the first regional OCP, which were codified at an international conference in Tunisia in 1968.[4] The disease, concluded conference participants, would be controlled if it could be addressed on a sufficiently large scale. Scientists from WHO and other experts contributed to the preparation of a regional control plan. Several donors expressed mild interest, but none was able to commit alone what was expected to be a 20-year, $120 million program covering at least seven countries.

Serendipity intervened. In 1972, the then-president of the World Bank, Robert McNamara, visited west Africa to observe the impact of a long drought that was under way. While visiting the rural areas of Upper Volta (now Burkina Faso), he witnessed the devastation caused by onchocerciasis; he saw many children leading blind adults, and communities in which nearly all the adults were blind. McNamara decided to spearhead an international effort to control the disease, committing his own institution to a catalytic financing role.[1]

The OCP was launched in 1974 under the leadership of the WHO, the World Bank, the Food and Agriculture Organization (FAO), and the United Nations Development Program (UNDP). Financing and donor support were mobilized through the World Bank from a wide range of donor countries, multilateral institutions, and private foundations.

The program, the first large-scale health program ever supported by the World Bank, set out to eliminate the disease first in 7—and eventually in 11—west African countries.[†] The primary intervention was vector control of the disease-spreading blackflies, with the goal of ultimately halting

---

† Benin, Burkina Faso, Côte d'Ivoire, Ghana, Guinea, Guinea-Bissau, Mali, Niger, Senegal, Sierra Leone, and Togo.

disease transmission. Helicopters facilitated the weekly spraying of larvicides during rainy seasons on the riverine areas most heavily populated by blackflies. The aerial treatment, as well as hand spraying of breeding grounds, persisted even through civil and regional conflicts and coups.

Up-to-date information was a key element in program implementation. Detailed mapping of the 12,000 miles of remote rivers and epidemiological mapping of onchocerciasis prevalence facilitated these efforts. A significant operational research budget was built into the program to respond to emerging challenges and problems and to investigate effective prevention and treatment options.

The duration of the program and its phasing were special features. Because of the time needed for the adult worms in the human population to die off, which at the time was thought to be at least 18 years,[‡] the program was expected to last 20 years. The administrative and financial agreements were broken into 6-year phases, allowing for both firm commitment and flexibility in planning cycles. Most of the original nine donors supported the program for 28 years, and the number of bilateral and multilateral donors increased threefold over that period.

STRIKING SUCCESS IN WEST AFRICA

The OCP's success in controlling onchocerciasis in west Africa has been remarkable. At the start of the program in 1974, nearly 2.5 million of the program area's 30 million inhabitants were infected, and approximately 100,000 were blind. Today, transmission of the disease has been virtually halted, and some 1.5 million people who once were infected with the disease no longer experience any symptoms. An estimated 600,000 cases of blindness have been prevented, and 22 million children born in the area since the program's inception are free from the risk of river blindness.

The economic impact has also been impressive. An estimated 25 million hectares of unusable arable land—enough to feed an additional 17 million people per annum—has become available for agricultural production and resettlement.[5] In Burkina Faso, for example, 15% of the country's land that had been deserted because of the disease has been completely reclaimed, and its new residents now enjoy a thriving agricultural economy.[6]

The program, which formally concluded in December 2002, was extremely cost-effective and had a yearly cost of less than $1 per person protected. Total commitments from 27 donors during the 28-year project amounted to $600 million. The World Bank calculated the annual return on investment (attributable mainly to increased agricultural output)

to be 20%, and it is estimated that $3.7 billion will be generated from improved labor and agricultural productivity.[4]

A MEDICAL BREAKTHROUGH: MECTIZAN IS DISCOVERED

While OCP was proving its success in controlling onchocerciasis in the 11 designated west African countries during the 1970s and 1980s, the disease remained endemic in 19 central, east, and southern African countries not covered by OCP.[§] Controlling the disease was technically and organizationally more complex, because aerial spraying—the only control option available at the time—was considered neither technically feasible nor cost-effective given the area's longer distances and thick forests.[5]

An important scientific breakthrough brought new hope to these 70 million people at risk in the region. In 1978, Dr. William Campbell, a veterinary researcher at Merck & Co., Inc., discovered that the new antiparasitic agent he had developed to treat gastrointestinal worms in cattle and horses was also effective against the family of worms responsible for onchocerciasis. Clinical trials in Africa sponsored by Merck and the WHO demonstrated that just one dose of Mectizan (ivermectin) could relieve the disabling symptoms of river blindness and kill up to 95% of the tiny worms—offspring of the adult worm—for up to a full year.[7] Dr. Kenneth Brown, one of the developers of the drug, explained the significance of this new one-dose medicine: "Most drugs for the treatment of tropical diseases have to be given in multiple doses over days, weeks, even years. The ability to treat and control an important disease, such as river blindness, with a single dose each year is nothing short of spectacular."

GETTING THE DRUGS TO AFRICA: MERCK DONATES MECTIZAN

The battle against river blindness now had a powerful new weapon in its arsenal. The great challenge facing Merck and the public health community, however, was to make sure that those most in need of the drug—and also the least able to pay—could access this critical medicine. Even at a discounted price of $1.50 per treatment, it was clear that the drug would be out of reach to the developing countries where onchocerciasis was endemic. Moreover, resources from the donor community were unable to cover the additional cost for the drug, which would have more than doubled program costs.

---

‡ Later determined to be 14–15 years.

§ Angola, Burundi, Cameroon, Central African Republic, Chad, Democratic Republic of the Congo, Republic of Congo, Equatorial Guinea, Ethiopia, Gabon, Kenya, Liberia, Malawi, Mozambique, Nigeria, Rwanda, Sudan, Tanzania, and Uganda.

Merck was eager to donate Mectizan, but the company's initial attempts to find a partner organization to manage the drug's distribution were unsuccessful. After neither the WHO nor the US Agency for International Development accepted Merck's offer, the company turned to Dr. William Foege, then executive director at the Carter Center. Foege, a veteran of the smallpox eradication effort, agreed to lead the donation program at the Task Force for Child Survival and Development, an affiliate of Emory University, only when Merck pledged that its donation would be long term. In 1987, Ray Vagelos, then CEO of Merck, made the historic announcement that his company would donate Mectizan "to anyone who needed it, for as long as it was needed"—marking the launch of the world's longest ongoing medical donation program, and one of the largest public-private partnerships ever created.[7]

Dr. Foege explained that the program's goal was to "reach as many people with Mectizan as possible, and to make the rules reasonable but not too difficult" (personal communication, June 2004). The Mectizan Expert Committee—a group of experts in tropical medicine, epidemiology, and public health—was established to lay the rules for how the drug would have to be delivered and who would receive it. The committee set up an annual application process through which requests for the drug would be granted based on the applicant's capacity to distribute the product for at least three years. The ministries of health had to endorse the applications, which were submitted mostly by international nongovernmental organizations (NGOs), medical mission groups, foundations, and the ministries of health themselves.[8]

On the ground, the task of reaching millions of residents of remote villages in east, central, and southern African countries with the drug was daunting. Public health systems were either weak or nonexistent in these countries, health workers were in short supply, and combating onchocerciasis was not seen as a public health priority.

Two important factors aided the NGO effort: more than $30 million in grants from the River Blindness Foundation,[9] and the popularity that Mectizan acquired because of its effectiveness in combating many troublesome parasites, including intestinal worms, head lice, and scabies, as well as *O. vovulus*. The drug rapidly alleviates incessant itching and is nearly 100% effective in treating round worms and whipworms, so improvement in quality of life is observable almost immediately after the first dose. So, despite the fact that the drug must be taken annually for nearly 20 years to interrupt transmission of the disease, Mectizan proved popular and uptake across endemic villages was fast.

The Mectizan Donation Program far exceeded its initial goal of 6 million treatments in six years. Since 1988, the program has provided more than 472 million annual treatments.[10] Merck recommitted to indefinite donation of the drug, and in 1998 extended its pledge to also treat lymphatic filariasis (also known as elephantiasis). Transmission of lymphatic filariasis, which WHO has designated as the fourth largest cause of long-term disability in the world, can be successfully interrupted with Mectizan from Merck and albendazole, donated by Smith-Kline Beecham.

Two important economic factors have helped to reinforce Merck's decision to make its contribution, which is estimated to have a value of over US$1.5 billion: US tax benefits that reduce the net cost of the program, and successful marketing of the drug in the veterinary field, which have offset the upfront research and development costs.[11] In 1984, Mectizan was the highest selling animal product and ranked as Merck's second best-selling drug in 1987.[12] The donation program, made more feasible by these economic offsets, represents an important milestone in the global effort to eliminate onchocerciasis and helped pave the way for later donations from multinational pharmaceutical companies.

REACHING THE 19 REMAINING COUNTRIES: APOC IS LAUNCHED

By 1995, however, onchocerciasis still persisted in 19 endemic countries not covered by the OCP. To meet the scale of the problem there, it was clear that more resources were needed to support the efforts of the organizations working on the ground, and that a more cost-effective, affordable, and sustainable approach than the clinic-based Mectizan delivery was necessary.[13]

Building on the work of the NGOs in central and east Africa, a new program was launched in 1995 with the goal of "eliminating onchocerciasis as a disease of public health and socio-economic importance throughout Africa." The African Programme for Onchocerciasis Control (APOC) was designed as a 15-year partnership under the leadership of the World Bank, WHO, UNDP, and FAO, which would build on the success of the OCP and extend its reach to the remaining 19 endemic countries in Africa. The program aimed to treat 86 million people a year by 2010, eventually scaling up to about 90 million treatments annually; to prevent 54,000 cases of blindness per year; to protect the OCP area from reinvasion; and to make an estimated 7.5 million additional years of productive adult labor available for the region's developing countries.[6]

APOC involved the participation of a wide range of organizations and groups, many of which were also involved in the OCP, including the same 4 sponsoring agencies, the governments of 19 developing countries, 21 bilateral and multilateral donors, more than 30 participating NGOs, Merck, and more than 100,000 rural African communities. The primary role of the program was to build the capacity of local communities supported by the NGOs and the ministries of health to deliver Mectizan and to increase the efficiency and sustainability of drug treatment at the local level.

Unlike the OCP, which involved very limited local participation, APOC was not a vertical program but rather was integrated within the national health systems of the participating African countries.[5] Ultimate ownership for controlling the disease would be the responsibility of the affected communities themselves. The fundamental strategy would be based on community empowerment with training, oversight, and supervision provided by the local health services and collaborating NGOs.

This donor-funded program is scheduled to end shortly after 2010. Effectively interrupting transmission of the disease requires annual drug treatment for some 15 to 20 years after outside donor funding ceases. Hence, APOC has placed a strong emphasis on long-term sustainability.

To achieve the program's goal of developing a self-sustainable, fully African-owned and managed program in the post-2010 period, APOC has pioneered a system of Community-Directed Treatment with Mectizan (ComDT). Through this framework, many hundreds of thousands of communities effectively organize and manage the local Mectizan treatment, taking full responsibility for developing and implementing the strategy for comprehensive drug distribution and thus enhancing prospects for long-term sustainability of the program after donor funding ends.[14] The communities select the community-directed distributor, and the distribution efforts are adapted to the local culture and conditions. Community volunteers receive training and supervision from the national public health systems and from the program's NGO partners.

The ComDT system has demonstrated its value not only as a cost-effective intervention but also as a successful framework for delivering treatment with high coverage rates to remote populations. In 2000, the WHO estimated that the ComDT network achieved an average treatment coverage rate of 74%, exceeding the minimum 65% rate necessary to eventually interrupt transmission and thereby eliminate the disease as a major public health problem throughout Africa.[1] A further indicator of the strong prospects for the program's long-term sustainability is the increasing rates of coverage in subsequent rounds of treatment, a trend that illustrates the popularity of the drug and the success of both the education campaigns and the locally run distribution systems.[5]

APOC'S SUCCESS IN CENTRAL, SOUTHERN, AND EAST AFRICA

Approximately 41 million people were treated in the 19 APOC countries with Mectizan by APOC in 2005 alone. The WHO estimates that the program prevents approximately 54,000 cases of blindness each year. As it extends its coverage, the benefits will spread over a wider population and encompass a number of additional positive impacts. These include an 80% reduction in the incidence of optic nerve disease, a 50% reduction in severe itching, and a 45% reduction in visual deterioration for those with atrophied optic nerves.[13] By the time the program begins to phase out at the end of the decade, it is expected that the sight of more than 800 million individuals will have been saved in the 19 APOC countries alone.[15]

Furthermore, the impact of the successful ComDT system extends beyond the treatment and prevention of river blindness. The system offers a valuable entry point for other community-directed health interventions in neglected communities with little or no access to traditional health services.[14] In the Central African Republic, for example, ComDT has provided a stimulus for expanded primary healthcare, where the coordinators of the Mectizan distribution program are often the only health workers to reach every village.[16] Suggestions for health interventions that could utilize the ComDT framework include long-lasting vitamin A capsules to save lives of children under 5 by 25% to 35%, improve maternal health, and prevent deaths; the antibiotic azythromycin, donated by Pfizer to prevent trachoma; albendazole and Mectizan to halt transmission of lymphatic filariasis; and praziquantel to cure schistosomiasis.

THE COST

APOC bears a total price tag of $180 million. Donor funding accounts for 75% of this figure, and African governments and NGOs contribute the remaining 25%.[5] Merck's donation of Mectizan and its coverage of shipping costs of the drug have kept the program's cost below US$0.60 per person treated per year. Because the World Bank and the WHO waive all administrative fees, 100% of donor funds reach country operations with minimal overhead costs.

A preliminary analysis prepared by the World Bank demonstrated that the economic rate of return for the program is 17% for 1996 through 2017.[17] This rate is comparable to World Bank projects in the most productive sectors, such as industry, transportation, and agriculture.

LESSONS LEARNED FROM THE CONTROL OF ONCHOCERCIASIS THROUGHOUT AFRICA

Bruce Benton, manager of the Onchocerciasis Coordination Unit in the World Bank from 1985 to2005, attributes the success of the programs to a number of factors that he believes provide lessons for other disease control programs.

A Comprehensive Regional Approach

Given the natural history of the disease, characterized by the movement of blackfly vectors across national borders, a comprehensive regional approach has been essential. The participating African countries were prepared to contribute to the achievement of a common objective provided all would benefit and the burden would be shared relatively equitably. Frequent multicountry deliberations have exerted peer pressure on the countries and their professional staff to deliver results. The comprehensive approach employed, and the well-defined exit strategies, have helped reassure the donors that the efforts would come to a successful conclusion.

Effective Long-Term Partnership

Regional collaboration among partners was based upon comparative advantage, combined with grassroots community empowerment, and have proved to be highly effective models. The transparent delineation of partners' roles in a memorandum of agreement has maximized effectiveness, minimized turf battles, and helped instill trust among partners. To maintain the partners' commitment and sustain the large coalition over a long period of time, communication has been active and credit has been shared liberally.

Community Participation and Grassroots Empowerment

ComDT, a unique feature of APOC, has been integral to the program's goal of eliminating river blindness as a public health problem throughout Africa. ComDT has given ownership of Mectizan distribution to the communities where the disease is endemic. The communities decide their strategies for ensuring the highest compliance with Mectizan treatment and select distributors in which they have highest confidence. This system has proven extremely cost-effective, given the donated drugs and the practice of compensating community distributors with food or other nonmonetary means. Both ownership and cost-effectiveness have increased the likelihood that the Mectizan treatment network will be sustainable over the long term—a prerequisite for eventual elimination of the disease. Furthermore, the system of community distributors has addressed the paucity of trained health staff in the remote, rural areas where onchocerciasis is most burdensome. Finally ComDT provides a platform for controlling other diseases, particularly those for which free drug treatment or other simple solutions can be "piggy-backed" onto the Mectizan distribution network.

Capacity Building and Africanization

The OCP and APOC programs have made deliberate efforts to strengthen African management and technical capacity. In the mid-1970s nearly 75% of OCP's roughly 30 professional staff were expatriate. Today 99% of program staff for both OCP and APOC is African, and every director has been African since the early 1980s. More than 100,000 community distributors have been trained and retrained since APOC was launched in 1995, and more than 500 former OCP staff members have returned to their home countries in west Africa, bringing advanced degrees, and the scientific, technical, and logistical capacity required to sustain the program's gains. Some of these staff will work on efforts to improve one of the notoriously weakest links in Africa's health system: surveillance of outbreaks, epidemics, and other diseases such as HIV/AIDS, malaria, cerebral spinal meningitis, and possibly avian influenza.

Operational Research

An important contributing factor to the successful control of the highly unpredictable biological agent was the program's emphasis on operational research. Funding for operational research was substantial, always exceeding 10% of the annual budgets. This research proved critical to sustaining OCP in 1985, when the blackfly vector became resistant to the principal insecticide used by the program since 1974. Fortunately, the program had developed seven backup insecticides, which it began to use in rotation until the resistance to the original chemical was overcome after several years, marking the first time that any program completely reversed resistance.

Operational research was also vital in determining whether ComDT would be cost-effective and achieve the program's objectives. The Tropical Disease Research (TDR) Program of WHO conducted extensive social surveys in the affected communities and concluded that ComDT would be cost-effective and reach a high enough portion of the population to eliminate onchocerciasis over time. It also determined that a much higher proportion of women community distributors would have to be recruited and trained if all members of the community were to be reached. Finally, TDR developed a system of rapid mapping of hyperendemic villages that allowed APOC to map the disease throughout Africa in less than 10 years. As a result, APOC operations could be scaled up much more rapidly than otherwise would have been possible.

Dr. Ebrahim Samba, winner of the 1992 Africa Prize for his contribution to the control of onchocerciasis, highlighted the importance of long-term financial commitments as a factor contributing to the programs' success. "Many programs in Africa last three to five years," Samba explained. Such short-term efforts are a "waste of time" because "this is the time one requires to study the situation, install, and start. One needs more time to get going, consolidate, and evaluate." The donor commitments of a minimum of 20 years, most of which lasted 30 years, combined with the commitment from Merck to donate Mectizan indefinitely, are an essential element of the effort's long-term success.[18]

A HEALTH PROGRAM WITH A DEVELOPMENT OUTCOME

In the final year of its operations in 2002, Robert McNamara described the success of the OCP he helped pioneer: "[OCP] has been an enormously effective program: a health program with a development outcome; it has empowered rural communities to banish this burden and thrive." Samba stated, "It proves it can be done—effective aid programs deliver lasting results. African member-states contributed in cash and kind, and donors have been steadfast in their support. This was achieved through hard work, transparency, and accountability."

BOX 7-1 Success in the Western Hemisphere: The Onchocerciasis Elimination Program for the Americas (OEPA)

Onchocerciasis is a threat to the health of more than 500,000 people living in Central and South America. Six countries (Brazil, Colombia, Ecuador, Guatemala, Mexico, and Venezuela) are home to some 2,000 communities in 13 foci or areas particularly affected by the disease. To address this situation, the Pan American Health Organization (PAHO) passed Resolution XIV in 1991 calling for the elimination of onchocerciasis in the Americas (WHO 1999). To achieve that goal, the Onchocerciasis Elimination Program of the Americas (OEPA) was formed in 1993. Now in its 14th year, OEPA is well on its way to accomplishing its objective through regular treatment of at-risk populations with Mectizan (ivermectin).

The Santa Rosa focus in Guatemala is an example of OEPA's success. Based on scientific information indicating that transmission of onchocerciasis has been interrupted and that there are no cases of eye disease attributable to onchocerciasis, the Minister of Health of Guatemala made the historic decision in November 2006 to end Mectizan treatment in the Santa Rosa focus. This is the first of the 13 endemic foci in the Americas where such a decision has been made. In 5 of the remaining 13 foci, transmission of onchocerciasis is also suspected to be supressed.[1] The continuing success of OEPA is due in large part to the strong partnership and cooperation between national Ministries of Health, The Carter Center, PAHO, Lions Clubs International Foundation, Merck & Co., Inc. and the Bill and Melinda Gates Foundation.

1. The Carter Center, *Eye of the Eagle*, Vol 7 number 2, pp 3 6, July 2006.

REFERENCES

1. Benton B, Bump J, Sékétéli A, Liese B. Partnership and promise: evolution of the African river blindness campaigns. *Ann Trop Med Parasitol.* 2002;96(suppl 1):S5–S14.

2. Uche Amazigo, Director, African Programme for Onchocerciasis Control, personal correspondence, July 14, 2006.

3. Kim A, Tandon A, Hailu A, et al. *Health and Labor Productivity: The Economic Impact of Onchocercal Skin Disease (OSD).* Washington, DC: World Bank; 1997. Policy Research Working Paper 1836.

4. Hopkins DR, Richards F. Visionary campaign: eliminating river blindness. In: Bernstein E, ed. *Medical and Health Annual.* Chicago: Encyclopaedia Britannica. 1997 8–23.

5. African Programme for Onchocerciasis Control. Defeating onchocerciasis in Africa. Available at: http://www1.worldbank.org/operations/licus/defeatingoncho.pdf. Accessed December 13, 2006.

6. OPEC Fund. Onchocerciasis Control Program nears completion. Available at: http://www.opecfund.org/publications/ar01/boxes/box5.htm. Accessed December 13, 2006.

7. Merck & Co Inc. The story of Mectizan. Available at: http://www.merck.com/about/cr/mectizan/. Accessed December 13, 2006.

8. Dull HB, Meredith SEO. The Mectizan donation programme—a 10-year report. *Ann Trop Med Parasitol.* 1998;92(suppl 1):S69–S71.

9. Drameh PS, Richards FO Jr, Cross C, Etya'ale DE, Kassalow JS. Ten years of NGDO action against river blindness. *Trends Parasitol.* 2002;18(9):378–380.

10. Thylefors B. 2005 onchocerciasis achievements. *2005 Annual Highlights of the Mectizan Donation Program.* Decatur, Ga: Mectizan Donation Program Secretariat; 2006.

11. Coyne PE, Berk DW. *The Mectizan (Ivermectin) Donation Program for River Blindness as a Paradigm for Pharmaceutical Industry Donation Programs.* Washington, DC: World Bank; 2001.

12. Eckholm E. River blindness: conquering an ancient scourge. *New York Times Magazine,* January 8, 1989:20-29 .

13. Sékétéli A, Adeoye G, Eyamba A, et al. The achievements and challenges of the African Programme for Onchocerciasis Control (APOC). *Ann Trop Med Parasitol.* 2002;96(suppl 1):S15–S28.

14. Amazigo UV, Brieger WR, Katabarwa M, et al. The challenges of community-directed treatment with ivermectin (CDTI) within the African Programme for Onchocerciasis Control (APOC). *Ann Trop Med Parasitol.* 2002;96(suppl 1):S41–S58.

15. Uche Amazigo, Director, African Programme for Onchocerciasis Control, personal correspondence, July 14, 2006.

16. Hopkins DA. Mectizan delivery systems and cost recovery in the Central African Republic. *Ann Trop Med Parasitol.* 1998;92(suppl 1): S97–S108.

17. Benton B. Economic impact of onchocerciasis control through the African Programme for Onchocerciasis Control: an overview. *Ann Trop Med Parasitol.* 1998;92(suppl 1):S33–S39.

18. Akande L. Victory over river blindness. *Africa Recovery.* 2003;17(1):6.

Preventing Diarrheal Deaths in Egypt*

* Case drafted by Molly Kinder

ABSTRACT

Geographic area: Egypt

Health condition: In 1977, diarrheal disease among children, which results in life-threatening dehydration, was identified as the cause of at least half of all infant deaths in Egypt.

Global importance of health condition today: Diarrheal disease is estimated to cause 2 million deaths in the developing world each year; the vast majority of those are among children younger than 2 years. Currently, 1 out of every 200 children who contract diarrhea will die of its consequences, including particularly dehydration. Almost all of these deaths could be prevented with the timely use of a simple and low-cost treatment for dehydration.

Intervention or program: The National Control of Diarrheal Disease Project of Egypt was established to promote the use of locally manufactured oral rehydration salts, which reverse the course of dehydration. The program sought to distribute the salts, along with information about the appropriate treatment of children with diarrhea, through public and private channels; the program reached mothers through mass media, including television. Training of all types of health workers also was integral to the program, as many physicians and nurses had to reorient their understanding of the optimal treatment of diarrhea.

Cost and cost-effectiveness: The average cost per child treated with oral rehydration therapy was estimated at $6. The cost per death averted was between $100 and $200. The program cost a total of $43 million, approximately 60% of which was financed under a grant from the US Agency for International Development, with the United Nations Children's Fund and the World Health Organization collaborating on technical aspects of the program.

Impact: The program succeeded in increasing the production of oral rehydration salts, increasing mothers' correct use of these salts, and changing feeding behavior. During the peak of the program in the mid-1980s, the program had achieved a fourfold increase in the distribution of oral rehydration salts, compared with the 1979 baseline. Virtually all mothers in the country were aware of oral rehydration salts, and most women could correctly mix the solution. Between 1982 and 1987, infant mortality declined by 36%, and child mortality fell by 43%. Mortality attributed to diarrhea during this same period fell 82% among infants and 62% among children. Because of the reduction in diarrheal deaths between 1982 and 1989, 300,000 fewer children died.

Diarrheal disease is one of the leading killers of children, causing nearly 20% of all child deaths. This represents one of the world's great failures, because the life-threatening complications can be so easily prevented. Worldwide, dehydration from diarrhea kills between 1.4 million and 2.5 million babies each year, and the vast majority of these deaths occur in developing countries.[1] Children born in developing countries suffer from an average of three episodes a year, and nearly 20 out of every 1,000 die of the disease before they reach the age of 2. In total, diarrhea causes a billion episodes of illness annually and in high-incidence regions is responsible for more than 30% of all hospital admissions of children. Virtually all the deaths from dehydration associated with diarrhea could be prevented with the timely use of a simple treatment that parents can provide at home.

Egypt is among the countries that have succeeded in disseminating knowledge about life-saving treatment of dehydration to both health workers and parents through modern communication methods. The result: dramatic declines in mortality associated with diarrhea—enough to contribute to an overall large improvement in infant and child survival.

HOW DIARRHEA STEALS LIVES

Diarrhea is an intestinal disorder characterized by abnormally frequent and watery stools. Acute watery diarrhea lasts just a few hours or days and can quickly become deadly. Bacteria (such as *E. coli* and salmonella), protozoa, and viruses can all cause diarrhea; of these, rotavirus is the leading cause in developing countries.

Unclean water, eating with dirty hands, and spoiled food are primary sources of transmission. Children are most vulnerable, particularly those from poor families living in unclean surroundings. Thus, the most effective modes of prevention include the improvement of the water supply and sanitation, the promotion of personal and domestic hygiene, and immunization against measles. Vaccines against rotavirus do exist but are not yet in widespread use.

Dehydration is diarrhea's most acute effect. During an episode of diarrhea, the body expels electrolytes (sodium, chloride, potassium, and bicarbonate) and water—all of which are necessary for life. Life-threatening dehydration ensues when the loss of the essential fluids is not replaced quickly and the body begins to "dry up." Symptoms of dehydration include thirst, restlessness, sunken eyes, rapid breathing, heart failure, bloated stomach, convulsions, and fainting. When fluid loss reaches 10%, dehydration turns fatal. In cases that are not immediately deadly, dehydration can leave a child more susceptible to infections.

Avoiding death from dehydration requires the swift restoration of lost fluids and electrolytes. Until the development of oral rehydration therapy (ORT) in the 1960s, the only effective treatment available was through intravenous infusions in a hospital or clinic that "rehydrated" patients. Intravenous therapy is far from a treatment of choice in the developing world because of its high cost, the hardship patients experience in traveling to clinics from remote areas, and the shortages of both trained personnel and supplies. Many people instead turn to popular drugs, including antibiotics, which can stop diarrhea but still expose the child to the risk of dehydration. The majority of these drugs demonstrate no proven health benefit and in some cases cause dangerous side effects.

ORAL REHYDRATION THERAPY: "THE MOST IMPORTANT MEDICAL DISCOVERY OF THE 20TH CENTURY"

A massive cholera outbreak in refugee camps on the border of India and Bangladesh in the 1970s exposed the limitations of intravenous treatment and paved the way for a radically different approach to treating dehydration. In 1971, the war for independence in what is now Bangladesh prompted 10 million refugees to flee to the border of West Bengal, India. The unsanitary conditions in the overcrowded refugee camps fueled a deadly cholera outbreak characterized by fatality rates approaching 30%.[2] Health officials from the Indian and West Bengal governments and relief agencies faced a daunting task: Conditions were squalid and chaotic, intravenous fluid was in scarce supply, treatment facilities and transportation were inadequate, and trained personnel were limited.[2] Mass treatment with intravenous therapy alone would not halt the impending crisis.

Dr. Dilip Mahalanabis, a cholera expert at the Johns Hopkins Centre for Medical Research and Training in Calcutta and head of a health center at one of the refugee camps, proposed an alternative to the intravenous treatment. He suggested the camp use a new method of oral replacement of fluid, known as oral rehydration therapy, that had been developed in the 1960s in Bangladesh and Calcutta.

The science was as ingenious as it was simple: A solution of water, salt, and sugar was found to be as effective in halting dehydration as intravenous therapy (see Box 8-1). Mahalanabis's team recognized the many advantages of oral therapy over the intravenous rehydration: It is immensely cheaper, at just a few cents per dose; safer and easier to administer; and more practical for mass treatment. ORT, however, had still not been tested in an uncontrolled setting, and skeptical health specialists cautioned that only

BOX 8-1 Oral Rehydration Therapy

Oral rehydration therapy (ORT) is the oral application of fluids to treat diarrhea. Since 1993 ORT has been defined by the WHO as "increased fluids plus continued feeding." The science is based on research that shows that glucose helps the body quickly replace the electrolytes and fluid expelled by diarrhea. Two strategies have been recommended for increasing fluids.

The first element is use of oral rehydration salts or "recommended home fluids." Oral rehydration salts are prepared by dissolving in water a ready-made packet with the following formula:

- 2.6 grams sodium chloride (common salt)
- 2.9 grams trisodium citrate dehydrate
- 1.5 grams potassium chloride
- 13.5 grams glucose

The formula was updated in 2004 by WHO and UNICEF based on new studies demonstrating improved effectiveness of reduced osmolarity (ORS) solution, especially for children with acute, noncholera diarrhea.[3]

A homemade treatment draws on a tradition dating back thousands of years in which spiritual leaders and health practitioners used various fluid combinations to treat diarrhea. Recommended home fluids are homemade solutions of water, glucose (or a carbohydrate substitute), and sodium. Variations include salt-and-sugar solutions, salted rice water, cereal-based solutions, and traditional soups.

Increased feeding is the second element of ORT. Withholding food is a dangerous practice that can increase a child's chance of becoming malnourished and can accelerate a life-threatening cycle of malnutrition and severe diarrhea.

---

health professionals and doctors should administer the new therapy.[4]

Mahalanabis's team moved quickly to introduce the treatment to the 350,000 residents of the camp. Packets of table salt, baking soda, and glucose were prepared in Calcutta at the diminutive cost of one penny per liter of fluid.[2] The solution was widely distributed, with instructions about how to dissolve it in water. Despite the shortage of trained health personnel, large numbers of patients were treated, with mothers, friends, and patients themselves administering the solution.

The results were extraordinary: At the height of the outbreak, cholera fatalities in the camp using ORT dropped to less than 4%, compared with 20% to 30% in camps treated with intravenous therapy.[4]

The success of ORT in the refugee camps demonstrated that diarrhea could be treated effectively and inexpensively even in the world's most impoverished and isolated regions. Thus, ORT, heralded by *Lancet* as "potentially the most important medical discovery of the 20th century," gave the world a powerful tool to reduce the estimated 5 million annual deaths from diarrhea recorded in the 1970s. In 1972, one year after Mahalanabis's results from the refugee camps, the WHO made ORT the world's standard treatment for diarrhea, setting in motion a revolution that would drastically cut diarrheal deaths in the following decades.

EGYPT: A PIONEER IN ORT

Egypt was one of the pioneers of national-level administration of ORT, and its experience represents a tremendous public health success story. In the 1970s, as the efficacy of ORT was being proved, diarrhea posed a serious public health problem in the North African country. In 1977, diarrhea caused at least half of the large number of infant deaths in Egypt (the infant mortality rate at the time was 100 per 1,000 live births).[5] That year, the Egyptian Ministry of Health introduced packets of Oralyte, oral rehydration salts (ORS) packaged for the United Nations Children's Fund (UNICEF), in its public clinics; soon after, a parastatal company began manufacturing ORS packets called Rehydran for sale at pharmacies.

Despite the availability of ORS, progress by the early 1980s was disappointing. Few mothers were aware of the new treatment and even fewer used it. In 1982, only 10% to 20% of diarrhea cases used ORS,[6] and most of the ORS lay untouched in warehouses and clinics.[5] Instead, the most widespread treatments were ineffective antidiarrheal medicines, and physicians commonly recommended that mothers withhold fluids and food and suspend breast-feeding—dangerous advice that was at odds with the effective use of ORT.[5]

Health officials recognized that the success of Egypt's ORT promotion efforts depended almost entirely on the active involvement of mothers and physicians. To test how these important groups could be persuaded to use and promote ORT, community trials were held in 29 rural villages in 1980 through the Strengthening of Rural Health Delivery Project. Nurses taught mothers at their homes how to use ORT, and public physicians were educated about the therapy. ORT use rose dramatically, and as a result, overall child mortality was 38% lower than in control villages, and diarrhea-associated mortality during the peak season was 45% lower.[7]

Based on the success of the community trials, Egypt undertook a massive promotion of ORT use among the country's 41 million residents. The National Control of Diarrheal Diseases Project (NCDDP) was established in 1981 with financial support from the US Agency for International Development (USAID) and a technical team from John Snow Incorporated. The program involved the entire Ministry of Health as well as other branches of government, the private sector, professional societies, and international organizations including WHO, and UNICEF. In 1984, the program became fully operational and set out to achieve the following goals:

- Reduce diarrhea mortality in children under 5 by at least 25%.
- Increase awareness of ORT to at least 90% of mothers.
- Increase understanding of ORT use to at least 75% of mothers.
- Decrease hospital mortality from diarrhea to at least 5%.
- Increase the number of severe diarrhea cases treated with ORT in the health system to at least 50%.

THE NCDDP IN ACTION

To achieve its ambitious objectives, the national program had to change the behavior of mothers and physicians and ensure an adequate supply of ORS. Mothers needed to understand the value and proper use of ORT, and physicians needed to be convinced of its efficacy over competing treatments (intravenous therapy, drugs, and fasting). The program began with a pilot study or "rehearsal" to test the various approaches and gather baseline data; it was then scaled up based on this information. Rather than providing the ORT services directly, the national program worked through the existing health infrastructure to strengthen the capacity of the health service delivery units to produce, promote, and explain ORT. The four main components of the program included product design and branding, production and distribution, training, and promotion and marketing.

Product Design and Branding

Based on market research, the program chose to supply ORS packets in a 200-milliliter size, rather than the standard one-liter pack distributed by UNICEF in most countries. Surveys found that mothers generally lacked an appropriate liter container at home, and many felt that a full liter was too much to give to a child to drink. So 200-milliliter plastic measuring cups were designed with the project logo for distribution through pharmacies and public health centers. Mothers were also encouraged to use a small soda bottle as a replacement for the measuring container.

Because ORS helps halt dehydration but does not stop diarrhea as popular antidiarrheals do, appropriate branding and product positioning were essential to promote the product competitively. The brand name selected for ORS was "Mahloul Moalgett et Gafaff," meaning "solution for treating dehydration," and was referred to simply as "the solution." The brand name used the word "gafaff," Arabic for drought, which was intended to help mothers make the link between the symptoms of dehydration and the oral therapy. The project logo—a seated mother feeding her small child—became the most recognized product label in Egypt.

Production and Distribution

An uninterrupted supply of ORS was vital to the program's success, and this rested on local production. An extensive tracking system was established to help the project forecast demand and meet its goal of a 3-month supply of ORS. A parastatal company, Chemical Industries Development, played a large role in the production of ORS. The company sold the packets at cost to the project, and the solution was then distributed through public-sector stores. NCDDP and UNICEF subsidized both public and private production. With an average of 6 million liter-equivalents of ORS produced each year, local production met demand, and Egypt even began exporting surplus production to the Middle East and Africa.

Distribution was accomplished through both public and private channels. The public sector received the ORS packets through a network of 5 main distribution centers and 37 subbranches. In rural areas, where the death rates from diarrhea were twice that in urban centers, long distances between homes and health centers inhibited distribution. To reach the more remote rural areas, 3,000 "depot holders" were recruited to hold ORS packets at their homes and distribute them to villagers for either a small price (about two cents) or for free. Depot-holders included community leaders, traditional birth attendants, or health workers who were trained in the use of ORS.

Private-sector distribution posed a significant challenge. There, ORS had to compete with the more profitable antidiarrheal drugs. To create financial incentives for pharmacies to promote ORS, the NCDDP provided pharmacies with free measuring cups that the pharmacy could sell with ORS packets, thus raising profit margins to a more competitive 30%.

Training

The program set out to train health workers to accurately diagnose diarrhea and dehydration and to teach mothers how to use ORT. The program distributed audiovisual and print materials, held seminars, and conducted 6-day training courses covering practical and theoretical aspects of diarrhea and ORT, emphasizing that ORT should be the primary tool to manage cases of diarrhea; that the use of antidiarrheal drugs should be limited; and that breast-feeding and good hygiene can help prevent diarrhea.

By 1990, 47 rehydration training centers had been established at university and central hospitals, teaching hospitals, urban clinics, and various other health centers. Between 1984 and 1990, nearly 14,000 practicing nurses and 10,000 physicians underwent the training course.[6] The program also persuaded medical and nursing schools to include rehydration and ORT in their curricula to train future generations of health professionals.

Promotion and Marketing

The most pivotal component of the program was the social marketing and mass media campaign. The primary audience for the outreach was mothers of children under 3 years; health professionals, pharmacists, and media reporters also were targeted.[8] In 1984, the first national media campaign was launched, emphasizing several basic messages about the dangers of diarrhea, its causes, and the means to reduce its impact.

The program's launch coincided with an important new phenomenon in Egypt: television. The share of households with a television had skyrocketed to 90% by 1984, from just 38% in 1980. Television became the primary media outlet of the campaign and provided a powerful vehicle to spread the program's core messages and to reach even rural, illiterate households that would have been inaccessible through print media. The television spots were designed to have a wide appeal and were particularly targeted at poorer audiences. The language was simple, employing expressions commonly used by mothers, with a theme of maternal love.

In Egypt, the recruitment of a well-liked, motherly soap opera star as spokesperson bolstered the campaign's popularity. More than 63 television spots were aired between 1984 and 1990, and billboards, magazine ads, and posters in pharmacies and health centers also were used to spread the core messages. (Far different approaches are required to reach mothers in countries where the penetration of mass media is lower; see Box 8-2.)

The media campaign was extraordinarily successful. Following the first national campaign in 1984, more than 90% of the mothers knew of ORS, and ORS use rose quickly to 60%.

IMPACT: SUCCESS AND LIMITATIONS

By 1991, when the 10-year program ended, virtually all of the goals had been reached. During the peak of the program in 1985 and 1986, the distribution of ORS was four times the level at the start of the program. By 1986, nearly 99% of mothers were aware of ORS, use of the solution was widespread, and most women could correctly mix the solution. The program also succeeded in increasing attendance rates at public health clinics—the number of children with diarrhea who attended a clinic rose from 630,000 in 1983 to 1.4 million in 1985.[5]

Through its success in disseminating both the ORS and the knowledge about how to use it, the program contributed to a reduction in infant and childhood mortality. According to civil registration data, infant mortality dropped by 36% and child mortality by 43% between 1982 and 1987. Diarrhea mortality during this same period fell 82% among infants and 62% among children.[5] Data from national household surveys and local area investigations suggest that the figures are actually an underestimate and that the reduction was even more impressive. By some estimates, the program helped reduce child diarrheal deaths by 300,000 between 1982 and 1989.[6]

Despite this success, some elements of the program were disappointing. The private sector has been slower at converting to ORT than have the public facilities; because private physicians see nearly three quarters of all cases, this gap will need to be addressed. And the market for antidiarrheals remains large—a continued trend that poses a threat to ORT use and to children's lives.

A COST-EFFECTIVE INTERVENTION

The program achieved success with an extremely cost-effective intervention. The average cost per child treated in Egypt with ORT was estimated at less than $6, which includes operational costs,[9] and the program calculated that the cost per death averted was roughly between $100 and $200. Overall, the program cost was $43 million, paid for by $26 million in grants from USAID and $17 million in cash and in kind from the government of Egypt. UNICEF donated $827,000 worth of raw materials for ORS production, and WHO contributed training programs and materials worth about $452,000.[6]

BOX 8-2 Reaching Bangladeshi Children with ORT

As in Egypt, diarrhea and dehydration have posed a formidable health problem in Bangladesh. The setting in Bangladesh, however, was markedly different from that in Egypt when both countries introduced oral rehydration therapy in the early 1980s. Meeting the needs of Bangladesh's population of more than 100 million, nearly 10 times the size of Egypt, would have required a massive production effort of tens of millions of packets of oral rehydration salts each year. Considering that more than 90% of Bangladesh's population lived in rural areas with poor transportation, distribution of salts also posed a serious challenge. And unlike Egypt, where the vast majority of households had a television, very few in Bangladesh even had access to a radio. Hence, a nationwide media campaign mirroring Egypt's successful television campaign was impractical.

Beginning in 1980, the Bangladesh Rural Advancement Committee, a large nongovernmental organization, began a program to promote ORT in rural Bangladesh. The program, the largest nationwide ORT program ever undertaken, trained tens of thousands of oral rehydration workers, or female health workers aged between 20 and 50, who went door to door training mothers about dehydration and ORT. The health workers visited each household in the program area and taught at least one woman in the household the "10 points to remember," including what diarrhea and dehydration are and look like, how to rehydrate through ORT, how to make the solution at home and when to use it, when to call the doctor, and when to continue feeding. The oral rehydration workers demonstrated how to make a homemade oral solution called *lobon-gur* through the "pinch and scoop method" by mixing a 3-finger pinch of salt, a fistful of sugar, and a liter of water. (Today, packaged oral rehydration salts are widely available in most of the country, including the rural areas.)

The program employed an innovative performance-based salary system that provided incentives for oral rehydration workers to accurately and thoroughly teach mothers the 10 points. Approximately one month following the workers' visits, a monitor would randomly select and visit 10% of the households. The monitor would ask the mother questions about the 10 points and test her ability to make the mixture properly. The health worker would be paid based on how much the mothers within the program area had learned.

Because men in Bangladesh are the key decision makers, the program also tried to reach men. Male workers at bazaars, mosques, and schools helped influence the attitudes of men toward ORT. Village healers were also recruited to spread the message about ORT, and a small radio and television education campaign was launched.[10]

Between 1980 and 1990, 13 million mothers were taught to make oral rehydration mixtures in their homes. An evaluation of more than 7,000 households found that between 25% and 52% of cases of "severe diarrhea" used the *lobon-gur* mixture.[11] Today, the usage rate of ORT in Bangladesh is 80%, one of the highest in the world. ORT is now part of the Bangladeshi culture: Studies show mothers are transmitting ORT knowledge to the next generation.[10]

ELEMENTS OF SUCCESS

Two elements of success are worth highlighting: first, the use of scientific investigation, including the research that supported various parts of the program, and the evaluation efforts; and second, the program's flexibility.

Market and anthropological research about consumer preferences and cultural practices played a central role in shaping the communications efforts and the product design and branding. Epidemiological and clinical research, conducted in nearly all Egyptian universities through NCDDP-supported projects, had the dual purpose of increasing knowledge and information about risk factors and proper ORS composition, and keeping the medical community engaged and interested in ORT.

An evaluation component was incorporated into the program's design from the outset. Ongoing evaluation efforts tracked the progress of the interventions, their effects (such as ORS use and attitudes), and the impact on mortality. Evaluation tools included mortality studies, knowledge and practice surveys of mothers, cost-effectiveness studies, national household surveys, and monthly and quarterly reports of diarrheal control activities. The project also benefited from independent, external evaluations, with data used continuously as input into decision making.

The diarrhea control program deliberately applied a flexible approach based on trial and error and data analysis. Interventions were frequently tested first in pilots or rehearsals, with the expectation that mistakes would be made and valuable lessons learned. The work plan was reexamined monthly, and the program elements were frequently adapted. For example, ORS packaging was altered after consumer preferences were expressed, and the media campaign changed the star of the TV ads from a male comedian to a TV actress after audiences disliked the earlier spokesperson's comedic approach.

Thirty years after its resounding success in the Bangladeshi refugee camps, ORT continues to be the most cost-effective means of treating dehydration. An increase in the use of ORT across the globe has helped slash diarrhea mortality rates in children worldwide by at least half. It is estimated that ORT saves the lives of 1 million children each year.[10]

BOX 8-3 Prevention and Treatment of Diarrheal Diseases: Old and New Approaches

In addition to ORT, the portfolio of diarrheal interventions is broad and rapidly expanding, giving countries multiple, complementary options for feasible, cost-effective strategies to reduce diarrheal deaths:
- New innovations in health technologies are paving the way for a vaccine against rotavirus.
- A new use of an old micronutrient provides a cost-effective addition to child health interventions.
- Global advocacy efforts promote the expanded application of a tried and true intervention.
- New efforts to encourage healthy behaviors demonstrate real life-saving potential.

Rotavirus Vaccine
Recent progress to develop a rotavirus vaccine has important potential to drastically decrease diarrheal incidence and deaths. Rotavirus is the most common cause of severe diarrhea in young children and is responsible for nearly 500,000 deaths and many more hospitalizations each year, mostly in developing countries.[12] Vaccination is the only way to prevent severe episodes of rotavirus infection, and the quest for a safe and effective vaccine has proved challenging. However, two new vaccines recently developed by major pharmaceutical companies are making headlines. In clinical trials in Latin America, GlaxoSmithKline's Rotarix decreased hospitalization for diarrhea among children under one year of age by 42%; it was approved in Europe in March 2006. In the United States and Finland, Merck's Rotateq, approved by the US Food and Drug Administration in February 2006, was demonstrated to reduce hospitalizations by 63% among infants.[13] Despite these exciting developments, additional trials of these vaccines must be conducted before recommending their use in other settings.

Zinc Supplementation
Zinc supplementation is another powerful new way to combat diarrheal disease in infants in developing countries. One meta-analysis of zinc supplementation trials demonstrated that zinc can reduce the prevalence of diarrhea and other common childhood infections.[14] When paired with ORS, zinc supplementation also has been shown to reduce the duration and severity of acute and persistent diarrhea.[15] An encouraging study in Tanzania has suggested that combining zinc supplementation with ORT can improve the cost-effectiveness of case management of diarrhea by more than one third.[16]

Exclusive Breast-Feeding
Exclusive breast-feeding, an ancient strategy with wide-ranging nutrition, health, and child development benefits, can effectively prevent and manage diarrhea in infants. According to WHO, six months is the optimal duration of exclusive breast-feeding, when no other food or drink is given to infants. Studies in India[17] and Bangladesh[18] demonstrate that exclusive breast-feeding in the first months of life can substantially decrease the prevalence of diarrhea in infants. This can be explained, in part, by the ability of breast milk to convey vital infection-fighting antibodies from the mother to the infant, and by the reduction in exposure to contaminated foods. Though effective at addressing diarrheal disease, breast-feeding can pose problems in regions with high rates of HIV transmission.

Hand Washing with Soap
Hand washing with soap and clean water and the proper disposal of fecal matter is being increasingly promoted in a number of developing countries to combat diarrheal deaths through the reduced spread of bacteria. A recent systematic review of the available evidence found that the risk of diarrheal diseases can be reduced by 42% through the promotion of hand washing with soap.[19] The Global Public Private Partnership to Promote Hand Washing, initiated in 2001 with funding from the Bank-Netherlands Water Partnership, the World Bank, USAID, and others, promotes the practice of hand washing with soap in developing countries. As part of the initiative, smaller public-private partnerships are currently under way in Ghana, Nepal, Peru, and Senegal. Through mass media and direct consumer contact with target audiences such as new mothers and schoolchildren, these national programs rely primarily upon health education to increase hand washing with soap.

REFERENCES

1. Kosek M, Bern C, Guerrant RL. The global burden of diarrheal disease, as estimated from studies published between 1992 and 2000. *Bull WHO.* 2003;81(3):197–204.

2. Mahalanabis D, Choudhuri AB, Bagchi N, Bhattacharya AK, Simpson TW. Oral fluid therapy of cholera among Bangladesh refugees. *Johns Hopkins Med J.* 1973;132:197–205.

3. World Health Organization, United Nations Children's Fund. *WHO/UNICEF Joint Statement: Clinical Management of Acute Diarrhea.* Geneva, Switzerland: World Health Organization; 2004.

4. Fontaine O, Newton C. A revolution in the management of diarrhea. *Bull WHO.* 2001;79(5):471–472.

5. el-Rafie M, Hassouna WA, Hirschhorn N, et al. Effect of diarrheal disease control on infant and childhood mortality in Egypt: report from the National Control of Diarrheal Diseases Project. *Lancet.* 1990;335(8685):334–338.

6. John Snow, Inc. *Taming a Child Killer: The Egyptian National Control of Diarrheal Diseases Project.* Washington, DC: John Snow Inc; 1995.

7. Gomaa A, Mwafi M, Nagaty A, et al. Impact of the National Control of Diarrheal Diseases Project on infant and child mortality in Dakahlia, Egypt. *Lancet.* 1988(2):145–148.

8. Hirschhorn N. Saving children's lives: a communication campaign in Egypt. *Dev Commun Rep.*1985;51:13–14.

9. Martines J, Phillips M, Feacham RG. Diarrheal diseases. In: Jamison D, Mosely H, Measham A, Bobadilla JL, eds. *Disease Control Priorities in Developing Countries.* Oxford, England: Oxford University Press for the World Bank; 1993.

10. Chowdhury AM, Karim F, Sarkar SK, Cash R, Bhuiya A. The status of ORT in Bangladesh: how widely is it used? *Health Policy and Planning.* 1997;12(1):58–66.

11. Chowdhury AM, Vaughan JP, Abed FH. Use and safety of homemade oral rehydration solutions: an epidemiological evaluation from Bangladesh. *Int J Epidemiol.* 1988;17(3):655–665.

12. Parashar UD, Hummelman EG, Bresee JS, Miller MA, Glass RI. Global illness and deaths caused by rotavirus disease in children. *Emerg Infect Dis.* 2003;9(5):565–572.

13. Glass RI, Parashar UD. The promise of new rotavirus vaccines. *N Engl J Med.* 2006;354(1):75–77.

14. Zinc Investigators' Collaborative Group. Prevention of diarrhea and pneumonia by zinc supplementation in children in developing countries: pooled analysis of randomized controlled trials. *J Pediatr.* 1999;135:689–697.

15. Zinc Investigators' Collaborative Group. Therapeutic effects of oral zinc in acute and persistent diarrhea in children in developing countries: pooled analysis of randomized controlled trials. *Am J Clin Nutr.* 2000;72:1516–1522.

16. Robberstad B, Strand T, Black RE, Sommerfelt H. Adding zinc to treatment for acute childhood diarrhoea could cut costs and save lives. *Bull WHO.* 2004;82:523–531.

17. Bhandari N, Bahl R, Mazumdar S, Marines J, Black RE, Bhan MK. Effect of community-based promotion of exclusive breast-feeding on diarrhoeal illness and growth: a cluster randomized controlled trial. *Lancet.* 2003;361:1418–1423.

18. Arifeen S, Black RE, Antelman G, Baqui A, Caulfield L, Becker S. Exclusive breast-feeding reduces acute respiratory infection and diarrhea deaths among infants in Dhaka slums. *Pediatrics.* 2001;108(4):67–74 .

19. Curtis V, Cairncross S. Effect of washing hands with soap on diarrhoea risk in the community: a systematic review. *Lancet Infect Dis.* 2003;3:275–281.

Improving the Health of the Poor in Mexico

ABSTRACT

Geographic area: Mexico

Health condition: Among the rural poor in Mexico, the incidence of preventable childhood and adult illnesses, poor reproductive outcomes (including low birth weight), and infant mortality are high—the result of unhygienic living conditions, poor nutrition, and social deprivation.

Intervention or program: The Programa de Educación, Salud y Alimentación (Progresa)—now known as Oportunidades—was designed to provide incentives in the form of cash transfers to poor families; to improve use of preventive and other basic health services, nutrition counseling, and supplementary foods; and to increase school enrollment and attendance. The program was designed to affect household-level decisions by providing incentives for behaviors that would result in improved social outcomes. The program was based on a compact of "co-responsibility" between the government and the recipients: The government would provide significant levels of financial support directly to poor households, but only if the beneficiaries did their part by taking their children to clinics for immunizations and other services and sending them to school.

Cost and cost-effectiveness: Expenditures on Progresa totaled about $770 million per year by 1999 and $1 billion in 2000, translating into fully 0.2% of the country's GDP and about 20% of the federal budget. Of that, administrative costs are estimated to absorb about 9% of total program costs.

Impact: A well-designed evaluation revealed that Progresa significantly improved both child and adult health, which accompanied increased use of health services. Children under 5 years of age in Progresa, who were required to seek well-child care and received nutritional support, had a 12% lower incidence of illness than children not included in the program. Adult beneficiaries of Progresa between 18 and 50 years had 19% fewer days of difficulty with daily activities due to illness than their non-Progresa counterparts. For beneficiaries over 50 years, those in Progresa had 19% fewer days of difficulty with daily activities, 17% fewer days incapacitated, and 22% fewer days in bed, compared with similar individuals who did not receive program benefits.

That people with few financial resources tend to be poorly educated, unhealthy, and malnourished has been often observed and frequently bemoaned but rarely tackled head-on. In the case of an antipoverty program in Mexico, however, policymakers chose a comprehensive—and ultimately successful—approach to address the basic causes of social problems (including health) facing many of the country's most underprivileged citizens. The program, which initially was aimed at rural populations, showed such strong positive results in improving health and education outcomes in a rigorous evaluation that the government decided to expand it to cover poor families in urban areas. The story of this program—originally called Progresa, now known as Oportunidades—is one of innovation in social policy, reinforced by research.

STARTING CONDITIONS

In Mexico, an estimated 40% to 50% of the country's 103 million citizens live below the poverty line, and about 15% to 20% are classified as indigent. Although progress was made in the 1960s and 1970s to reduce the incidence of poverty, those gains were quickly eroded during the economic crisis that began in 1982, and since then the government has searched for ways to effectively reduce the extent of poverty and to ameliorate its effects on people's lives.

Although large numbers of poor people can be found in each of Mexico's 32 states, poverty follows a rough gradient toward higher levels with distance away from the Mexico-US border, and from the three massive urban poles of Mexico City, Guadalajara, and Monterrey. In most of the states that are on or close to the US border, fewer than 35% of the families are poor; in 13 states of the country's southwestern region, more than half the families fall below the poverty line.

Throughout the country, poverty is very much a rural phenomenon, with something on the order of three quarters of all rural families falling below the poverty line. Most of Mexico's poorest citizens live in small villages with no paved roads, running water, or modern sanitation, where the only work is hard agricultural labor. Of the poor population, a large share is indigenous in origin and speaks little or no Spanish—disenfranchised, in important ways, from the mainstream of public services and civic participation. For many poor Mexicans, seasonal migration to the United States themselves or by family members, who send money home, represents the only chance at economic survival.

Education and health indicators in rural areas are as poor as the people themselves: Although more than 90% of rural children attend primary school at some time, about half drop out after the sixth grade. Among those who continue, some 42% drop out after the ninth grade. High infant mortality and incidence of preventable childhood illnesses (many linked to poor sanitation), reproductive health problems, malnutrition, violence, and all manner of health problems characterize the lives of Mexico's rural communities.

The use of modern health services in rural Mexico is low, averaging less than one visit per year per person. Poor people, although sicker than their better-off counterparts, use fewer health services: 0.65 visits per year for the poor, compared with 0.8 visits for the nonpoor. Protein-energy malnutrition is widespread, with stunting (low height for age) affecting an estimated 44% of 12- to 36-month-old children in 1998.[1]

CHANGE IN SOCIAL POLICY WITH EACH PRESIDENT

Sweeping changes in Mexican social policies designed to address the problems of poverty have roughly coincided with political moments. In the 1970s, for example, the Lopez Portillo administration invested heavily in the provision of social services and the bureaucracies behind them. About 2,000 rural health clinics were built under the government agency called IMSS-Complamar, and thousands of government-run stores were established to provide basic products to low-income families at subsidized prices.

In 1993, during the Carlos Salinas de Gortari administration, social spending increased dramatically, almost doubling in the case of the health sector. A large share of the social-sector spending was channeled through Pronasol, an umbrella organization that was intended to represent a transition away from general subsidies toward more targeted, cost-effective programs that fostered community involvement.

The sheer scale of the programs was impressive. The federal government provided funds and raw materials for social projects designed by 250,000 grassroots committees, and over the span of six years Pronasol created about 80,000 new classrooms and workshops and renovated 120,000 schools; awarded scholarships for 1.2 million indigent children; established 300 hospitals, 4,000 health centers, and 1,000 rural medical units; and improved water, sanitation, and housing in thousands of localities. Despite this vast investment, however, the government was persistently criticized for merely ameliorating the worst symptoms of poverty, rather than addressing root causes, while at the same time creating bloated bureaucracies.

In the mid-1990s, President Ernesto Zedillo was encouraged by his advisers to think differently about how to help people raise themselves from poverty. Principal among those advisers was the Director General of Social Security, Santiago Levy, an economist who for many years had a vision of how to use the power of public policy to affect the daily choices in poor households that, in combination, help keep those households in poverty. In 1997, under the intellectual leadership of Levy, a new program was initiated—a program that sought to act simultaneously on the causes and consequences of poverty, attempting to break the transmission of economic and social vulnerability from one generation to the next.

On August 6, 1997, President Zedillo traveled to the state of Hidalgo to announce the start of Progresa, saying, "Today we begin a program to break the vicious cycle of ignorance, lack of hygiene, and malnutrition, which has trapped many millions of Mexicans in poverty. For the first time, the Government of the Republic sets in motion a program that will deal with the causes of poverty in an integral manner. With Progresa, we will bring together actions in education, health care, and nutrition for the poorest families in Mexico, centering attention on the family nucleus and the boys and girls, and placing a great responsibility on the mothers."[2]

THE PROGRESA APPROACH

Progresa had the goal of increasing the basic capabilities of extremely poor people in rural Mexico. Progresa, a serendipitous acronym for Programa de Educación, Salud y Alimentación (Education, Health, and Food Program), represented a departure from traditional social programs for the poor in several ways. First, it was principally designed to affect the "demand side"—that is, instead of focusing primarily on the supply of services to the poor, such as health centers, water systems, schools, and so forth, the program provided monetary incentives directly to families to help overcome the financial barriers to health services use and schooling and to induce parents to make decisions that would bring their children more education and better health (see Box 9-1). Second, the program was designed around a compact of "co-responsibility" between the government and the recipients. The government would provide significant levels of financial support directly to households, but only if the beneficiaries did their part by sending children to school and taking them to clinics for immunizations and other services. Third, Progresa was based on the notion that improvements in education, health, and nutrition would be mutually reinforcing; a program affecting all three dimensions of human welfare would equal more than the sum of the parts. In this way, it sought to break from the "silos" of social-sector ministries.[3,4]

The program had three linked components: education, health, and nutrition. In the health component, cash transfers were given if (and only if) every member of the family accepted preventive health services, delivered through the Ministry of Health and IMSS-Solidaridad, a branch of the Mexican Social Security Institute. The relatively comprehensive health service package was aimed at the most common health problems and the most important opportunities for prevention, including basic sanitation at the family level; family planning; prenatal, childbirth, and postpartum care; supervision of nutrition and children's growth; vaccinations; prevention and treatment of outbreaks of diarrhea; antiparasite treatment; prevention and treatment of respiratory infections; prevention and control of tuberculosis; prevention and control of high blood pressure and diabetes mellitus; accident prevention and first aid for injuries; and community training for health care "self-help."[4]

BOX 9-1 Use of Health Services by the Poor

Empirical data generally shows that the poor in poor countries use health services less than their rich counterparts—even when services are available at no direct cost through the public sector and when the underlying health needs among the poor are greater. So, for example, immunization rates, use of oral rehydration therapy, and use of other basic maternal and child health care services are all lower for poor populations than for more privileged ones. The reasons for this have been traced to a complex interaction between supply and demand factors. In general, the services closest to low-income areas are in poor repair, with inadequate supplies of medicines and with health workers who have high rates of absenteeism from their posts. On the household side, many of the basic characteristics that typify poor families—low levels of education, social marginalization, lack of money to pay for transportation, and other costs related to seeking services—prevent the effective use of health services.[5] So, while governments in developing countries typically have depended on the provision of free services to address the needs of the poor, sometimes augmenting fixed-site facilities with extensive outreach to help overcome some of the physical and economic barriers, these efforts have rarely closed the equity gap in the use of health services.

In parallel with the conditional cash transfers, the program sought to improve the quality of services available through public providers. In practice, this meant a steadier flow of medicines to public clinics, more training of doctors and nurses, and, importantly, higher wages for health care providers in Progresa areas.

In the nutrition component, the cash transfer was given if (and only if) children aged 5 years and under and breastfeeding mothers attended nutrition monitoring clinics where growth was measured, and if pregnant women visited clinics for prenatal care, nutritional supplements, and health education. A fixed monetary transfer of $11 per month was provided for improved food consumption. Nutritional supplements also were provided to a level of 20% of daily calorie intake and 100% of the micronutrient requirements of children and pregnant and lactating women.[4]

In the education component, program designers attempted to promote school attendance and performance of children in school by providing monetary education grants for each child under 18 who was enrolled in school between the third grade of primary school and the third level of secondary school—the period when risk of school dropout was the greatest. Because children often dropped out so they could work to supplement the meager family income, the size of the monetary grants was calibrated to partially compensate for the lost wages while they were in school, gradually increasing as the children moved from grade to grade. Thus, monthly grants ranged from $7 for a child in the third grade of primary school to around $24 for a boy in the third grade of secondary school. Examination of school enrollment patterns revealed that girls were more likely to drop out of secondary school than boys, so a slightly higher incentive was provided for girls who remained in school—$28 compared with $24 per month for boys.[4]

The monthly income transfers, received in the form of a wire transfer that could be cashed immediately, significantly increased the monthly income of poor families. The transfers constituted about 22% of household income, on average, thus effectively increasing a family's purchasing power and feeding financial resources into the local economy.[4]

FOCUS ON INCENTIVES

Program designers carefully constructed incentives that would achieve program goals, using state-of-the-art social science research as the foundation for the design. So, for example, the monetary benefits were given directly to adult female beneficiaries because a wealth of social science analysis has shown that mothers in developing countries are more likely than fathers to spend additional household resources on children's health and welfare, rather than on consumption goods like alcohol and cigarettes. In addition, designers capped monthly benefits at $70 per family, recognizing that an unlimited per-child benefit might create an unintended incentive among the poor to have more children. Unlike many cash transfer programs, in Progresa beneficiaries were not penalized if family members got jobs or earned more than they did at the start of the program, which might have discouraged people from looking for employment. Once needs-based eligibility was established at the outset, the family could remain in the program for three years. During that 3-year period, additional income did not make families ineligible. Eligibility was reassessed at the end of the 3-year period.[4]

Although some critics accused the government of patronizing poor people in Progresa because it attempted to encourage choices deemed by social policymakers to be correct, program designers rejected this concern. In the words of Santiago Levy, "Compared with giving a kilo of tortillas or a liter of milk as we used to do in the past, Progresa delivers purchasing power. But even poor parents must invest in their children's futures—that's why the strings are attached."[6]

TIERED TARGETING

As with any cash transfer program, the challenge of targeting was significant. Good targeting means that selection criteria are established so that they permit the inclusion of all those who need the program, yet keep to a minimum "leakage" of benefits to individuals and households who are not the intended program participants. And all this has to be done while keeping the administrative and information costs of the program within a reasonable level.

Progresa employed a 3-stage targeting strategy. In the first stage, geographic targeting was used to select poor localities, or communities, within poor regions of the country. To do this, program designers used data from the 1990 census and the 1995 population count to create a "marginality index," a composite of information about the communities' average levels of adult illiteracy, living conditions (proportions of households with access to water, drainage systems, and electricity; types of building materials; and the average number of occupants per room), and the proportion of the population working in agriculture. Communities were selected for inclusion in Progresa if they ranked as "high" or "very high" in terms of marginality but also had a primary school, a secondary school, and a clinic and were not so small and isolated that it would be virtually impossible for potential participants to reach health services and schools.[7,8]

In the second stage, eligible households were selected using census data on per capita income. All those classified as "poor" were deemed eligible for the program and invited to participate.[7,8]

The third stage tapped into community knowledge and was designed to increase the transparency and fairness of the program. Within each Progresa community, the list of selected families was made public at a meeting, and comment was taken about whether the program had accurately identified the poor families in the area. Families who had not been selected could ask to be reevaluated if they believed they had been excluded unfairly. In practice, this third stage rarely changed the list of households that were eligible but may have contributed to the sense that the program was truly aimed at the poor and was not a program of political patronage.[7,8]

Using this multilevel strategy, Progresa was able to effectively target its considerable resources at the poor and marginalized, although by design it did leave out the relatively small number of people living in very remote areas without access to even the most rudimentary public services.

Progresa beneficiaries were indeed very poor: On average, a beneficiary family had a per capita income of $18 per month, or a mere one quarter of the average Mexican per capita income. Among Progresa beneficiaries who were employed, most were agricultural day laborers earning the minimum wage of $3 per day. Less than 5% of beneficiaries' homes had running water; more than three quarters of beneficiary families had dwellings with a mud floor. Many were of indigenous origin and did not speak Spanish.[9]

Although quantitative measures have shown the targeting strategy to be effective, qualitative studies have identified substantial dissatisfaction. Focus group discussions have revealed that in many rural communities, virtually every person tends to think that she or he is "poor," and making fine distinctions between the "poor" and "nonpoor" based on income and other objective characteristics is unwelcome and seen as unfair. There are some indications that the Progresa approach of household-level targeting may in fact exacerbate social divisions.[10]

EVALUATION, BUILT IN FROM THE START

One of the signature features of the Progresa design was its elaborate monitoring and evaluation. In fact, the two basic ingredients of the program were cash and information. The program itself depended for its day-to-day functioning on up-to-date and accurate information about beneficiary behavior and for its long-term sustainability on credible information about its impact.

Because mothers received a month's benefits only during the previous month if children used the education and health services according to established norms, reliable information about school attendance and health service utilization was essential. And, while school attendance and clinic visits were monitored for individual beneficiary families, overall program implementation was monitored through indicators that were collected and assessed on a bimonthly basis: incorporation of new families, number of children receiving education grants, families who fulfilled their education and health commitments, and other indicators of operation. These indicators were scrutinized at all levels in the program management, with adjustments made when problems appeared.[4]

Among the several unusual aspects of Progresa, the impact evaluation strategy stands out (see Box 9-2). From the start, Levy and others involved in the program design saw

BOX 9-2 The Progresa Evaluation

Researchers at the International Food Policy Research Institute conducted the Progresa evaluation under a contract with the Mexican government. The evaluation employed a quasi-experimental design, in which a sample of 505 of the 50,000 Progresa communities, including more than 24,000 households, formed the evaluation sample and were randomly assigned in 1998 to 320 "treatment" and 185 "control" groups. The program was scaled up so that households in "treatment" communities received benefits immediately; benefits to households in the "control" communities were delayed until close to two years later, although no information was provided to local authorities at the outset about the intention to eventually include those communities.

A preintervention survey was conducted among about 19,000 households, covering more than 95,000 individuals; four follow-up surveys at 6-month intervals of the same households were also conducted during the 2-year experimental period. In addition to the household surveys, service utilization and health data from clinics and test scores, attendance measures, and other data from schools were used for the evaluations, as were observational studies, focus groups with stakeholders, and community questionnaires.[11,12]

This evaluation strategy elegantly took advantage of the fact that no program can reach all beneficiaries simultaneously; randomizing the staged entry into the program and measuring the difference between those "in" and those "not yet in" provided an incomparable base of information for evaluators. Because the "treatment" and "control" communities were randomized, investigators were able to say with confidence that differences observed between the households in the two types of communities were due to the effects of the program and not to unobserved differences between those two groups. At the same time, the fact that the "control" households were deemed eligible for the program at a later stage in implementation helped designers manage a potentially very difficult political situation that occurs when some households or individuals are included in a program while others with similar characteristics are excluded. Together, the randomization approach and the intensive data collection eventually permitted evaluators to end up with analyses that met extraordinarily high quality standards.

the value of an external, independent evaluation employing rigorous methodology; such an evaluation was seen as a way to establish the program's credibility within Mexican (and international) policy circles and to help ensure its continuation—in the event that it was shown to be successful—during future political transitions.

RAPID SCALE UP, HIGH COVERAGE

In 1997, early in its implementation, Progresa had enrolled about 400,000 households. By the end of 1999, Progresa covered 2.6 million families, or one tenth of all families in Mexico. Operating in 50,000 localities in 32 states, the program had a national reach, although it was confined to rural populations. The program was reaching some 40% of the rural Mexican population.[1]

The Mexican government's strong commitment set the stage for rapid scale up. More than that, however, the program could be rapidly expanded because it did not depend on drawing up blueprints, issuing bidding documents, writing contracts, pouring cement, enrolling trainees, developing curricula, and procuring drugs and equipment—in short, all of the time-consuming tasks required when the public sector builds and operates new schools and health centers. Once program managers worked out the basic mechanics of identifying beneficiaries, transferring funds, and maintaining a flow of information, expansion was relatively uncomplicated.

The scale of the program was large, and so was the budget. Expenditures on Progresa totaled about $700 million per year by 1999 and $1 billion in 2000, translating into fully 0.2% of the country's GDP. Of that, administrative costs are estimated to absorb about 9% of total program costs.[3,7,8]

To date, no cost-effectiveness assessments have been conducted on the health interventions—and, in fact, the analytic challenges in doing such studies would be great. Unlike single-intervention programs, Progresa was intended to affect multiple sectors and even generations. These features do not easily lend themselves to comparison with investments that have more limited and time-bound outcomes.

IMPACT ON ADULT AND CHILD HEALTH, EDUCATION, AND NUTRITION

The well-designed evaluation revealed that Progresa resulted in a significant improvement in both child and adult health, which accompanied an increase in the use of health services.

In 1996, before Progresa's implementation began, the utilization of health services was identical in the localities identified as "treatment" and "control," as were measures of health status. During 1998, the first complete year of implementation, health service utilization increased more rapidly in the Progresa "treatment" areas than in the areas where no transfers were provided. Nutrition-monitoring visits, immunization, and prenatal care increased significantly, as did overall average use of health services. Importantly, prenatal care started earlier in pregnancy, on average, in the Progresa areas compared with the others. This trend continued as program implementation expanded.[11]

Child health improved in the Progresa areas. Children under 5 years of age in Progresa, who were required to seek well-child care and who received nutritional support, had a 12% lower incidence of illness than children not included in the program.[11]

Adult beneficiaries of Progresa between 18 and 50 years had 19% fewer days of difficulty with daily activities due to illness than their non-Progresa counterparts. For beneficiaries over 50 years, those in Progresa had 19% fewer days of difficulty with daily activities, 17% fewer days incapacitated, and 22% fewer days in bed, compared with similar individuals who did not receive program benefits.[11]

In addition to a striking impact on health, nutritional status also was better for Progresa children than for those outside the program. Progresa resulted in a reduced probability of stunting among children 12 to 36 months of age; researchers estimated that the impact of the program was equivalent to an increase of 16% in the average growth rate per year among those children.[13] Beneficiaries reported both higher calorie consumption and consumption of a more diverse diet, including more fruits, vegetables, and meat. Iron-deficiency anemia decreased by 18%.[14]

In education, Progresa's impact was even more dramatic. The program caused 11% to 14% increases in secondary school enrollment for girls and 5% to 8% for boys. Transitions to secondary school increased by nearly 20%, and child labor declined.[15]

Although it is possible to imagine interventions that would be as successful in any one of the sectors (education, health, and nutrition), it is not easy to envisage an alternative that could act so effectively in all areas at the same time. Emmanuel Skoufias, who served as coordinator of the International Food Policy Research Institute evaluation, commented, "The results of the evaluation show that after only three years, poor Mexican children living in the rural areas where [the program] operates have increased their school enrollment, have more balanced diets, are receiving more medical attention, and are learning that the future can be very different from the past."[3]

FROM PROGRESA TO OPORTUNIDADES, AND OTHER COUNTRIES

As a result of the favorable evaluation findings, the program survived the transition from the Zedillo administration to the Fox administration. In fact, the Mexican government decided to extend the program to urban areas, assisted by a $1 billion loan from the Inter-American Development Bank.[16] (The program's name also was changed in 2002, from Progresa to Oportunidades, to reflect an expanded mission.) Education grants were extended to the high-school level, and a new component was added. The "Youth with Opportunities" component is a savings plan for high school students, in which savings grow each year from ninth grade through graduation.

The Progresa evaluation also brought the program to the attention of policymakers in other Latin American countries and in major development agencies. Although Progresa was not the first of the so-called conditional cash transfer pro-grams, it is arguably the most well evaluated and thus has inspired similar efforts in Argentina, Honduras, Nicaragua, Colombia, Bangladesh, and other countries.

It now appears that Oportunidades will be a part of Mexican social policy for many years to come and has the potential to make a difference on a massive scale. The program covers more than 4 million families and represents close to 50% of Mexico's annual antipoverty budget.

Just as the program evaluation was hailed for being able to compare those "with" and those "without," it is also important to think about Mexico "with" and "without" the program. Without question, Mexico "with" Progresa has a better future than "without." While no social program can erase centuries of deprivation and structural lack of access to credit and markets—all serious problems that continue to face Mexico's most marginalized populations—Progresa did far better than the traditional supply-side efforts in obtaining genuine results and giving hope.

REFERENCES

1. Skoufias E. *Is PROGRESA Working? Summary of the Results of an Evaluation by IFPRI.* Washington, DC: International Food Policy Research Institute; 2000.

2. Zedillo E. Transcript of speech presenting PROGRESA program. Available at: http://zedilloworld.presidencia.gob.mx/welcome/PAGES/library/sp_06aug97.html. Accessed December 13, 2006.

3. Parker S. *Case Study Summary: Mexico's Oportunidades Program.* Washington, DC: World Bank; 2004.

4. Gomez de Leon J, Parker S, Hernandez D. PROGRESA: a new strategy to alleviate poverty in Mexico. Document prepared for: World Bank Conference on Evaluation and Poverty Reduction; Washington, DC; June 14–15, 1999.

5. Wagstaff A. Poverty and Health Sector Inequalities. *Bull WHO.* 2002;80(2):97–105.

6. Egan J. Mexico's welfare revolution. *BBC News* (Friday, October 15, 1999).

7. Wodon Q, de la Briere B, Siaens C, Yitzhaki S. Mexico's PROGRESA: innovative targeting, gender focus, and impact on social welfare. *En Breve.* 2003;17:1–4.

8. Gundersen C, Yanez M, Kuhn B. Food assistance programs and poverty in Mexico. *Agri Outlook.* 2000;(December):13–15.

9. Behrman J, Davis B, Levy D, Skoufias E. *A Preliminary Evaluation of the Selection of Beneficiary Households in the Education, Health, and Nutrition Program (PROGRESA) of Mexico.* Washington, DC: International Food Policy Research Institute; 1998.

10. Adato M, Coady D, Ruel M. *Final Report: An Operations Evaluation of PROGRESA from the Perspective of Beneficiaries, Promotoras, School Directors, and Health Staff.* Washington, DC: International Food Policy Research Institute; 2000.

11. Gertler P. *Final Report: The Impact of PROGRESA on Health.* Washington, DC: International Food Policy Research Institute; 2000.

12. Behrman JR, Todd PE. *Randomness in the Experimental Samples of PROGRESA.* Washington, DC: International Food Policy Research Institute; 1999.

13. Behrman JR, Hoddinott J. *An Evaluation of the Impact of Progresa on Pre-School Child Height.* Washington, DC: International Food Policy Research Institute; 2000.

14. Hoddinott J, Skoufias E. *The Impact of PROGRESA on Food Consumption.* Washington, DC: International Food Policy Research Institute; 2003. IFPRI FCND Discussion Paper 150.

15. Schultz TP. *Final Report: The Impact of PROGRESA on School Enrollments.* Washington, DC: International Food Policy Research Institute; 2000.

16. Inter-American Development Bank. IDB approves its largest-ever loan for Mexico: US$1 billion for expansion of the PROGRESA poverty-reduction program. [Press release]. January 16, 2002. Available at: http://www.iadb.org/exr/PRENSA/2002/cp1002e.htm. Accessed December 13, 2006.

Controlling Trachoma in Morocco*

* The first draft of this case was prepared by Gail Vines; significant contributions to the current version were made by Molly Kinder.

ABSTRACT

Geographic area: Morocco

Health condition: In 1992, a national survey found that just over 5% of Morocco's population had the blinding disease trachoma. Nearly all the cases were concentrated in five poor, rural provinces in the southeast of the country where 25,000 people showed a serious decline in vision due to trachoma, 625,000 needed treatment for inflammatory trachoma, and 40,000 urgently needed surgery.

Global importance of the health condition today: Trachoma is the second leading cause of blindness in the world, and the number one cause of preventable blindness. More than 84 million people in 55 countries have trachoma. Economic development and improved hygiene have eliminated the disease from North America and Europe. But it plagues millions in hot, dry regions where access to clean water, sanitation, and health care is limited.

Intervention or program: In 1991, Morocco formed the National Blindness Control Program to eliminate trachoma by 2005. Between 1997 and 1999, the program implemented a new strategy called SAFE (surgery, antibiotics, face washing, and environmental change), giving Morocco the distinction as the first national-level test of the 4-part strategy. Mobile teams have performed simple, inexpensive surgeries in small towns across the provinces, 4.3 million treatments of the antibiotic azithromycin have been distributed, health education efforts promoting face washing and hygiene have been conducted, latrines have been constructed, and safe drinking water supplied.

Cost and cost-effectiveness: The Moroccan government has provided the bulk of the financing for the program, with external support from the United Nations Children's Fund and a public-private partnership called the International Trachoma Initiative. Through this partnership, the pharmaceutical company Pfizer has donated over $72 million worth of its antibiotic Zithromax®.

Impact: Overall, the prevalence of active disease in children under 10 has been reduced by 99% since 1997.

Trachoma is the second leading cause of blindness (after cataracts) and the number one cause of preventable blindness in the world. More than 84 million people in 55 countries have trachoma, and some 6 million have been blinded by it.[1] Although the disease is now confined to developing countries where it threatens an estimated 1 in 10 people, just a century ago it was common throughout the world, including the United States (see Box 10-1). With economic development and improved hygiene, however, the disease has been eliminated from North America and Europe.

But those same changes have not benefited the world's poorest. Today trachoma plagues millions of marginalized people living in hot, dry regions of Africa, Latin America, the Middle East, and Asia, where access to clean water, sanitation, and health care is limited. The heaviest burden of blindness from trachoma affects the populations of sub-Saharan Africa. Modern antibiotics, combined with prevention and other treatment methods that can be deployed in low-income countries, hold much promise in the fight against trachoma. Morocco, the first country to start a large-scale campaign against trachoma with a newly developed strategy, is at the threshold of eliminating blinding trachoma.

DISEASE OF POVERTY

Trachoma is highly contagious, marked by chronic conjunctivitis, or "pink eye." Children are its first victims. Active infection is caused when the bacterium *Chlamydia trachomatis* is spread (mainly among young children) through direct contact with eye and nose secretions from affected individuals, contact with contaminated towels and clothing, and through fluid-seeking flies. Disease transmission is rapid and intense in conditions of overcrowding, poor hygiene, and poverty. In endemic areas, prevalence rates in children aged 2 to 5 years can reach 90%.[2]

Active trachoma alone is not immediately threatening to sight. Repeated trachoma infections over many years, however, cause problems that can eventually lead to blindness. The upper lid frequently becomes chronically inflamed, resulting in scarring and a condition called "trichiasis," or in-turning of the eyelash. If this condition is not treated, the eyelash painfully rubs the eye, resulting in corneal scarring, opacity, and blindness. Blindness from trachoma, whose seeds are first sown in early childhood, usually strikes when a person is between 40 and 50 years old.

Trachoma is linked closely with poverty—both as a symptom of underdevelopment and as a cause. The disease disproportionately affects women, who are infected through their close contact with children; women contract trachoma at a rate two to three times more frequently than men.

The economic impact of trachoma on endemic areas is profound, as blindness develops during the most economically productive years. An estimated $2.9 billion worth of potential productivity is lost annually due to the disease.[3]

NEW STRATEGY: SAFE

In the mid-1980s, the Edna McConnell Clark Foundation brought renewed attention to trachoma by funding extensive research on the disease's epidemiology and the viable options for its control. The scientific findings contributed to the development of a new, comprehensive strategy to treat and prevent trachoma. This strategy was called "SAFE," which stands for surgery, antibiotics, facial cleanliness, and environmental change—the four main interventions. The community-based SAFE strategy seeks to confront the underlying causes of the disease as well as the imminent threats of blindness, and differs from earlier approaches by emphasizing the need to effect not just medical but also behavioral and environmental changes.

Surgery

Surgery is needed to halt corneal damage in the later stages of trichiasis and prevent the onset of blindness. Researchers in Oman designed a simple, quick, and inexpensive surgical procedure, which can be applied to treat large numbers of patients at the community level. Health professionals are trained to make a slit in the outer part of the eyelid and restitch it in a way that pulls the edge and lashes away from the eye's surface. The simple procedure has a success rate of approximately 80%, and in low-income countries like Ghana can cost as little as $6 per person.[2]

Antibiotics

Antibiotics are used to treat active trachoma infections and can reduce the community pool of infections and prevent scarring.[4] Until the discovery of the one-dose azithromycin, the available antibiotic was a 1% topical tetracycline eye ointment applied daily in a 6- to 4-week regimen. Because of the time-intensive treatment and its side effects of stinging sensations and blurred vision, however, compliance with the earlier treatment was often poor.

BOX 10-1 Trachoma in the United States

At the end of the 1900s, the threat of trachoma was very real in the United States. The disease was rampant in crowded slums in both the United States and Europe during the Industrial Revolution, and New York newspapers commonly ran public health notices warning about the disease's communicable nature. Trachoma became a criterion for excluding immigrants from the United States, causing more than 36,000 immigrants to be denied entry between 1897 and 1924.

The US Public Health Service launched an ambitious campaign to control the disease in the "trachoma belt" in the southeastern states. A public education campaign was initiated, and hospitals to treat trachoma were established. In the 1960s, after several decades, trachoma was finally eliminated from the United States.[2]

Facial Cleanliness

Studies have shown that clean faces, especially among children, can break the cycle of reinfection and prevent the spread of trachoma-causing bacteria. Washing helps remove the discharge from infected eyes, which attracts disease-spreading flies seeking fluid and salt. Children's faces can be kept clean even with small amounts of water—one liter can clean as many as 30 faces.

Environmental Change

Improving living conditions and community hygiene has reduced the spread of trachoma. Construction of latrines is an important way to reduce the prevalence of the flies associated with trachoma.[4] Health education and the provision of adequate water have also proved effective in reducing the spread of infection.

MEDICAL BREAKTHROUGH AND INTERNATIONAL MOVEMENT

A major advance for the SAFE strategy occurred in the mid-1990s with the discovery of a much more potent antibiotic, which strengthened the strategy's "A" component. Studies showed that a single dose of the antibiotic azithromycin was as effective as (or even more effective than) the 6-week regimen of the widely used tetracycline antibiotic. Pfizer, the global pharmaceutical giant that manufactures the prescription version of the drug (Zithromax®), and the Clark Foundation began pilot tests of the drug in the early 1990s in Africa. Their results established that the drug is a powerful 1-dose cure and a substantial improvement over the tetracycline ointment treatment because it assures a higher adherence rate.

With the discovery of azithromycin and the development of a comprehensive strategy to prevent and treat the disease, the global health community now had powerful weapons in the fight against trachoma. The mounting evidence demonstrating the feasibility of eliminating trachoma was first outlined in a 1996 WHO global scientific meeting.

Momentum was boosted further in 1998 when Pfizer and the Clark Foundation announced the formation of a public-private partnership called the International Trachoma Initiative (ITI) aimed at eliminating blinding trachoma worldwide. The initiative was first financed with $3.2 million grants from each of the two main partners and set out to help governments of endemic countries start national trachoma programs based on the SAFE strategy.

Pfizer's pledge to contribute $60 million worth of Zithromax® was key to ITI's strategy and represented a shift in the company's philanthropy. Zithromax® has a broad consumer market and is the most prescribed branded oral antibiotic in the United States, accounting for more than $1 billion annually of the company's revenues.[5] The company donated large quantities of the drug, despite the risk that the donated drugs could be sold on the black market.

With funding, leadership, momentum, and a strategy in place, the international movement embarked in 1999 on the first national-level test of the SAFE strategy, choosing Morocco as the site.

MOROCCO LEADS THE FIGHT AGAINST TRACHOMA

Morocco, a North African country of just under 32 million people, has a long history of trachoma control efforts. The country's fight against the disease began nearly a century ago, when the disease ravaged all parts of the country. Dr. Youssef Chami Khazrazi, head of Morocco's National Blindness Control Program (NBCP), wrote, "There is not a single Moroccan among two to three generations who does not remember the years where the fight of [trachoma] represented one of the major and permanent activities of the Ministry of Health."[6]

Initially, the disease was regarded as primarily a medical problem, and in the 1970s and 1980s it was tackled by treating schoolchildren in the most-affected provinces with tetracycline eye ointment twice a year. Medical treatment was not yet integrated with improvements in sanitation and standard of living among the rural poor. Therefore, while economic development led to the virtual disappearance of trachoma from most urban areas in the previous few decades, the disease pervaded many of the country's poorer, rural areas.

A national survey in 1992 found that approximately 5.4% of the population showed signs of trachoma, with virtually all of these cases concentrated in five rural provinces in the southeast of the country: Errachidia, Figuig, Ouarzazate, Tata, and Zagora. These five arid provinces constitute a quarter of the total area of the country and have a widely dispersed population of approximately 1.5 million people. Poverty, scarce water, agricultural subsistence, and weak infrastructure and sanitation characterize the region. There, the problems of trachoma were great: 25,000 people showed a serious decline in vision due to trachoma; some 625,000 needed treatment for inflammatory trachoma; and surgery was urgently needed for 40,000 people with trichiasis.

Morocco's political leaders were committed to eliminating trachoma by 2005, and in 1991 formed the National Blindness Control Program (NBCP). Between 1997 and 1999, the SAFE strategy was integrated into the program. "We now recognized," says Dr. Khazrazi, "that trachoma at the level of these regions is not strictly a medical problem; it is essentially the reflection of a socioeconomic problem." The "real enemies," he explains, "are the disfavored rural communities, illiteracy, family overcrowding, lack of water, the accumulation of animal wastes, and the proliferation of domestic flies. In sum, the enemy to combat is not *Chlamydia* but poverty."[6]

To address the disease's wide-ranging causes, the NBCP formed a comprehensive partnership including five government divisions (Ministry of Health, Ministry of National Education, Ministry of Employment, Ministry of Equipment, and National Office for Potable Water), international organizations (ITI, UNICEF, WHO, and Helen Keller International), bilateral and multilateral agencies, and local nongovernmental organizations. With scientific evidence, political resolve, and financial support in place, the NBCP was launched.

PUTTING SAFE IN MOTION

Each of the four elements of the SAFE strategy was mobilized.

Surgery

Government officials in the Ministry of Health moved quickly to decentralize surgery so that eyelid correction was readily available in small towns and villages. Before surgical teams arrived in the countryside, village leaders and outreach workers were briefed so that they could publicize the procedure and explain its benefits. In partnership with the Hassan II Foundation of Ophthalmology, the ministry deployed mobile surgical units staffed by doctors and specialist nurses trained to carry out the vision-saving procedures. Forty-three physicians and 119 nurses have worked in 34 centers throughout the five provinces. Between 1992 and 2005, more than 40,000 people underwent eyelid surgery. At the same time, education campaigns were launched to motivate infected individuals to come forward for treatment.

Antibiotics

Azithromycin was first field tested in Morocco during the mid-1990s, when 10,000 patients were successfully treated. Widespread treatment with the donated drug began in the five southeastern provinces in 1999, and approximately 4.3 million doses have been distributed to date (ITI statistics through December 2005). A successful strategy was soon developed, built on the recognition that trachoma is a community disease and reinfection is very likely to occur if only isolated cases are treated. Different approaches were developed depending on the prevalence. When more than

one fifth of the children under 10 showed signs of active trachoma, everyone in the community was treated. Where infection rates were lower—between 10% and 20%—treatment focused on affected children and their families; at less than 10%, infections were treated individually. Treatment campaigns were launched annually, between the months of September and December.

Facial Cleanliness

Health education has proven effective in increasing awareness and changing attitudes, thus increasing clean faces and preventing disease transmission. Campaigns promoting individual and community hygiene have centered on information, education, and communication to explain the causes of the disease and the means of prevention. Outreach workers, health professionals, and teachers have used slide shows, videos, films, community theater, meetings, photos, notices, pamphlets, and even megaphones to communicate the messages. Newspaper articles and radio and television broadcasts have also been effective. To educate children, the primary carriers of the disease, the Ministry of Education designed a model lesson on trachoma that was incorporated into the curriculum of primary schools in the five provinces.

The education campaigns depend in large part on the active engagement of the local community. Mosques, lodgings for young women, local associations, and schools have proved to be ideal venues for communicating the campaign's message.

Environmental Change

The National Office for Potable Water has overseen the construction of latrines in 32 villages. Supporting these efforts are 350 local village associations that have drilled wells, built latrines, and found safe ways of storing animal dung, so that this valuable natural fertilizer does not spread flies through the village. The national office is also leading the provision of drinking water: 74 villages in Errachidia and Zagora have been supplied with water, and access to potable water is reported to have increased from 13% of all rural communities in 1992 to 60% in 2000 to at least 80% in each trachoma endemic region as of 2005.

Interventions to reduce poverty and improve literacy among women are now acknowledged to be central to the fight against trachoma. In Zagora, for example, the work of the Ministry of Employment and Helen Keller International has helped 8,500 women learn to read. Helen Keller International has also implemented economic programs aimed at increasing the incomes of women.

BLINDING TRACHOMA NEARLY ELIMINATED

The implementation of the SAFE program has had a dramatic impact in Morocco and represents the most rapid elimination of blindness due to trachoma in a single country in history. Prevalence has fallen 99% since 1997, from 28% to just less than 2.5% in 2005.[7] Acute infections have been significantly reduced in children and in some places, such as Figuig and Ouarzazate, eliminated. In Zagora province, which remains the hardest hit, annual epidemiological surveys beginning in 1997 revealed a drop in prevalence from 69% to 3.3% in 2004. In Tata, Ouarzazate, and Figuig provinces, no cases of active infection have been reported since 2003. Overall, the intervention has achieved a 99% reduction in the prevalence of active disease in children under 10 since 1997 (see Figure 10-1).

Morocco has reached its "ultimate intervention goals" and has reduced the burden of disease to the trachoma elimination target levels set by the WHO: less than 5% prevalence of active disease in children 1 to 9 years of age and less than 0.1% trichiasis in adults over the age of 15. The next phase is surveillance of the disease to ensure that levels remain below these targets. Once this is sustained, Morocco will apply for WHO certification of elimination of blinding trachoma.

COST

The elements of the SAFE strategy that are most expensive are improving environmental infrastructure and providing the drugs. Although quantitative information about total spending on the initiative is unavailable, to date the Moroccan government has provided the bulk of the funds to improve village sanitation—supplemented with grants worth over $2 million from ITI between 2001 and 2004.

The dramatic reduction in trachoma achieved in Morocco over the past few years would probably have been impossible without Pfizer's donation of the antibiotic, valued at around US$72 million. The company has also provided grants for public education to support other components of the SAFE strategy.

The US Fund for UNICEF has supported the implementation of the face cleanliness and environmental change components of the SAFE strategy with a grant of $225,000. Total costs for surgical treatment have been estimated at $15 to $25 per person, with funding from the Moroccan government as

FIGURE 10-1 Prevalence of active disease in five provinces in Morocco, 1997–2005.

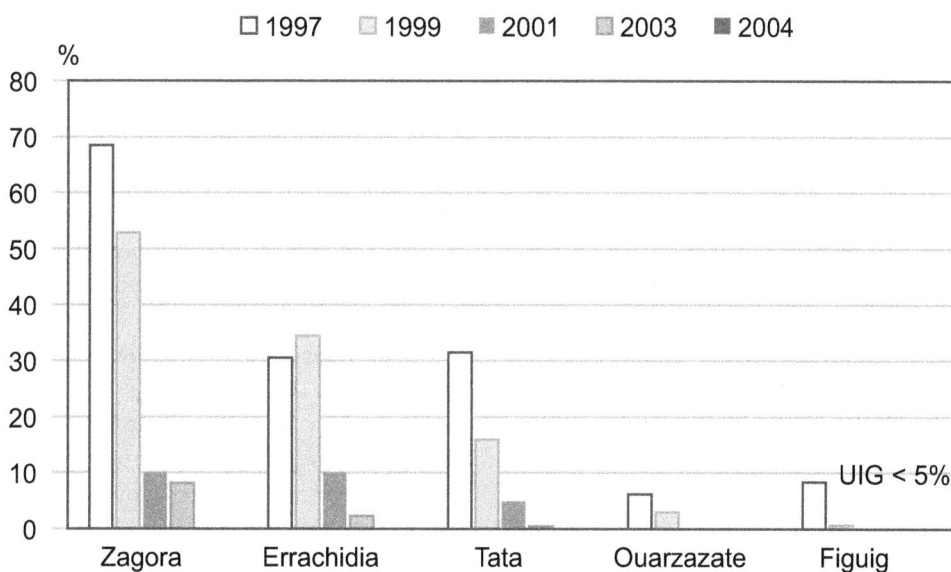

Note: In Morocco, the prevalence of active disease in children under 10 has been reduced by 99%.
Source: Ministry of Health, Morocco (2006).

well as ITI, worth between US$440,000 and US$730,000. A further grant from ITI— $180,000 from 2000 to 2004—supported the Moroccan Ministry of Health's evaluation of the impacts of interventions.

THE FINAL STAGES: MAINTENANCE AND SURVEILLANCE

Morocco's SAFE program has succeeded in slashing the prevalence rate of active trachoma among children and clearing the backlog of surgeries. The effort to eliminate blinding trachoma from Morocco has thus entered its final, and crucial, stage: maintenance and surveillance before being certified by WHO as having eliminated blinding trachoma. This entails the early identification of active trachoma cases and prompt treatment of those infected in order to prevent spread of the disease. Identification of infected patients can occur during health visits, such as at maternal and child health clinics; through sentinel site activities; and through the reporting of suspected cases to local partners in trachoma control, such as local NGOs, teachers, health personnel, and the Red Crescent Society. Immediately following the diagnosis of an active trachoma case, a visit is made to the household where all members are examined for infections and, if needed, treated with antibiotics.

It can often take years of repeated infections to cause scarring of the upper lid and trichiasis, or inversion of the upper lid that precedes blindness, so surgery cases will continue to emerge even after active trachoma is interrupted in Morocco. Community leaders and organizations such as the Red Crescent Society will continue to play an important role in locating and reporting trichiasis cases to district surgical teams.

Because of the expected emergence of a limited number of new cases of active trachoma and trichiasis, the need for an effective epidemiological surveillance system for trachoma is great. All new cases are reported to the district health departments by village sentinel sites and health facilities. Periodic reviews are conducted, with the results shared with provincial and central authorities. Unless unforeseen epidemics occur, this surveillance phase is expected to continue until 2009.

ELEMENTS OF SUCCESS

Dr. Jacob Kumaresan, the president of ITI, has identified three factors as the keys to Morocco's success in the elimination of blindness due to trachoma, which can be an inspiration for other trachoma endemic countries.[8] First, government buy-in exists at all levels of the national blindness control program. Second, the program developed strong public-private partnerships, including a network of NGOs and local associations; and third, the government has taken an aggressive approach to provision of safe drinking water and improved sanitation for at-risk populations.

Dr. Khazrazi also reported that the solid support of the government of Morocco was invaluable. "One of the major assets is commitment and political will. Political will is, first of all, the commitment of the Ministry of Health." This support is evidenced by frequent periodic visits of ministry officials to endemic areas to affirm the government's commitment to the disease's elimination.

CATALYST FOR GLOBAL EFFORTS

The success of the trachoma program in Morocco has provided a catalyst for efforts to eliminate the disease worldwide. Robert L. Mallett, senior vice president of corporate affairs of Pfizer's international philanthropy department, explained that Morocco's program "made history by completing their mass antibiotic and surgical campaigns, signaling the beginning of the end for a disease that has plagued the country for centuries."

In 2000, after data demonstrated that prevalence rates in Morocco had been reduced by more than half in just one year, the ITI accelerated its international efforts. Pfizer committed to donating 10 million additional doses of Zithromax® and $6 million in operational funding, the Clark Foundation contributed another $6 million, the UK Department for International Development provided approximately $1.8 million, and the Bill & Melinda Gates Foundation awarded $20 million over five years—the foundation's largest donation to date to international blindness. With the additional funding in place, the SAFE strategy was initiated in Tanzania, Mali, Sudan, Ghana, Vietnam, Ethiopia, Nepal, Niger, Mauritania, Senegal, and Kenya. In these countries, representing one quarter of the global burden of trachoma, 221,000 surgeries have been performed and around 36.7 million doses of Zithromax® were distributed (ITI statistics, through December 2005).

In November 2003, recognizing the effectiveness of the SAFE strategy and the need to scale up programs, Pfizer announced that it would donate up to 135 million doses of Zithromax® over the next five years.[9] Pfizer's contribution represents one of the largest donations of a patented drug in history. According to Pfizer's Chairman and CEO Hank McKinnell, "By 2020 we hope to have all of (the endemic countries)." Thus, ITI and its many partners have helped ensure that Morocco's success with SAFE, like the disease that it has nearly eliminated, is contagious.

REFERENCES

1. Mariotti S. New steps toward eliminating blinding trachoma. *N Engl J Med.* 2004;351;19:2004–2007.

2. Mecaskey J, Knirsch C, Kumaresan J, Cook J. The possibility of eliminating blinding trachoma. *Lancet Infect Dis.* 2003;3(11):728–734.

3. Frick K, Hanson C, Jacobson G. Global burden of trachoma and economics of the disease. *Am J Trop Med Hygiene.* 2003;69(suppl 5):1–10.

4. West S. Blinding trachoma: prevention with the SAFE strategy. *Am J Trop Med Hygiene.* 2003;69(suppl 5):S18–S23.

5. Barrett D, Austin J, McCarthy S. *Cross-Sector Collaboration: Lessons from the International Trachoma Initiative.* Paper presented at: Workshop on Public-Private Partnerships in Public Health; Endicott House, Dedham, MA; April 7–8, 2000.

6. Khazraji YC. Revival in the fight of trachoma: ten years of fight in the Kingdom of Morocco, 1991–2001. 2002 report of the French League Against Trachoma and International Organization Against Trachoma. Available at: http://www.cgdev.org/doc/millions/Trachoma_in_Morrocco .pdf. Accessed December 13, 2006.

7. Ministry of Health, Morocco. Presentation at the Global Elimination of Blinding Trachoma 2020 meeting, Geneva, Switzerland; April 10, 2006.

8. Donnelly J. Pfizer to donate US$500 million in drugs. *Boston Globe.* November 12, 2003.

9. Kumaresan J, Mecaskey J. The global elimination of blinding trachoma: progress and promise. *Am J Trop Med Hygiene.* 2003;69(suppl 5): S24–S28.

Reducing Guinea Worm in Asia and Sub-Saharan Africa*

* Case drafted by Molly Kinder.

ABSTRACT

Geographic area: 20 countries in Asia and sub-Saharan Africa

Health condition: Before the start of the campaign in 1986, an estimated 3.5 million people in 18 endemic countries in Africa and Asia were infected with guinea worm, and 120 million were at risk.

Global importance of the health condition today: In 2005, fewer than 11,000 cases of guinea worm were reported in the nine remaining endemic countries. Just three countries have reported more than 1,000 cases—and the vast majority of the cases are in Sudan, where civil war has impeded progress.

Intervention or program: With the technical and financial support of a global coalition of organizations led by the Carter Center, the United Nations Children's Fund, the US Centers for Disease Control and Prevention, and the World Health Organization, 20 countries implemented national guinea worm eradication programs, run through their ministries of health. The primary interventions of the campaign include the provision of safe water (through deep well digging, applying larvicide, and purifying water through cloth filters); health education; and case containment, management, and surveillance.

Cost and cost-effectiveness: The total cost of the program between 1986 and 1998 was $87.4 million. The estimated cost per case was $5 to $8. The World Bank determined that the campaign has been highly cost-effective and cost-beneficial. The economic rate of return based on agricultural productivity alone has been estimated at 29%. The estimated cumulative cost of the campaign as of 2004 was approximately $125 million.

Impact: The eradication efforts have led to a 99.7% drop in guinea worm prevalence. In 2005, fewer than 11,000 cases were reported, compared with an estimated 3.5 million infected people in 1986. By 1998, the campaign prevented between 9 million and 13 million cases of guinea worm. As of 2005, the campaign has prevented more than 63 million cases of guinea worm disease, reduced the number of endemic villages by 91%, and stopped the transmission of the disease in 11 of the 20 endemic countries.

Dracunculiasis, or guinea worm disease, is an ancient scourge that once afflicted much of the world, including parts of the Americas. Documented in Egyptian medical texts as early as the 15th century BC, it is thought to be the "fiery serpent" referenced in the Old Testament. One of the most preventable of all parasitic diseases, guinea worm disease has vanished from developed countries since the introduction of safe drinking water. Today it is truly a disease of the poor, debilitating many of the most remote and disadvantaged communities in Africa, where access to potable water is limited and health care and education are lacking. In 1986, an estimated 3.2 million people in 20 endemic countries in Africa and Asia were infected with the disease,[†] and an estimated 120 million remained at risk.[1] Estimates of cases of disease prevalence in India and Pakistan during 1986 raised the annual global burden to 3.5 million cases.

The fight against guinea worm disease represents one of the most successful international collaborations and is particularly interesting because the intervention is, at its heart, behavior change. Success depended on the campaign's ability to reach poor, isolated communities and convey essential messages about how to handle water and prevent the disease. This was possible because of the steady commitment of donors and technical supporters, as well as national governments.

HOW THE WORM TURNS

Guinea worm disease is contracted when a person drinks stagnant water from a well or pond that is contaminated with tiny freshwater copepods carrying guinea worm larvae. Once inside the human, the stomach acid kills the copepods allowing the larvae to migrate into the small intestine, where they penetrate the intestinal wall into the abdominal cavity. After 60 to 90 days, male and female larvae mate and, unbeknown to their host, grow to an average of two to three feet in length. A year later, the fully grown female worm rises to the skin in search of a water source to lay her larvae. A painful blister forms, usually in the person's lower limbs, although the worms can emerge from any part of the body. To ease the burning pain, infected individuals frequently submerge the blister in cool water, causing the blister's rupture and the release of hundreds of thousands of larvae into the water. A vicious cycle of reinfection occurs when sufferers inadvertently contaminate sources of drinking water and set the stage for themselves and other residents to contract the infection.

The worm, about the width of spaghetti, gradually emerges from the blister in a painful process that can last 8 to 12 weeks. Numerous worms can emerge simultaneously or may emerge sequentially over a period of many weeks. Lesions caused by guinea worms invariably develop secondary bacterial infections, which exacerbate the pain and duration of disability. The most common treatment used by infected individuals during this agonizing period is a rudimentary technique that dates back to ancient times. Worms are coaxed out of the blister by being slowly wound

around a narrow stick, a few centimeters each day—a process that is represented in the Caduceus—the symbol of medicine. The patient must take extreme caution to avoid breaking the worm, or they risk painful inflammation caused when a broken worm retreats into the body. No medication is available to treat guinea worm disease, and there is no vaccine to prevent it.

DISEASE OF THE EMPTY GRANARY

Guinea worm disease takes its toll not through death, as the disease is rarely fatal, but rather through devastating disability, pain, and infection. Two studies in Nigeria, for example, reported that 58% to 76% of patients were bedridden for at least one month following the worm's emergence. The pain is also long lasting, evidenced by the fact that in one study 28% of infected individuals in Ghana experienced pain 12 to 18 months later.[2] The disease's other symptoms, including nausea, vomiting, diarrhea, and dizziness, further exacerbate this burden. Secondary bacterial infections occur in about half of all cases and can lead to arthritis, "locked" joints, tetanus, and permanent crippling.[3]

Although the disease afflicts all age groups, it particularly harms children. The likelihood of a child under the age of 6 years in Sudan being malnourished is more than three times higher when the adults in the household are infected with the disease. School absenteeism rises when the debilitating symptoms render children incapable of walking the often long distance to school and when children forgo school to take on the agricultural and household work of sick adults. As a result, schools in endemic areas frequently shut their doors for a month each year.[2]

Guinea worm disease is not only a symptom of poverty but also a perpetrator. The economic burden inflicted on poor rural communities is severe and is compounded by the seasonal nature of the disease and its high prevalence in affected communities. Cyclical weather patterns and harvesting and planting seasons lead to peak periods when water in contaminated ponds and wells is widely consumed. A year later, an entire community can be debilitated and unable to work—a period that often cruelly coincides with the busiest agricultural seasons. This phenomenon explains the disease's nickname among the Dogon people in Mali—"the disease of the empty granary."

The economic damage is extreme. The annual economic loss in three southern rice-growing states in Nigeria was calculated at $20 million. Further research in Mali found that overall production in that country of sorghum and peanuts, two critical subsistence crops grown in northeast Mali, was reduced by 5%.[2]

---

† The 20 endemic countries included Benin, Burkina Faso, Cameroon, Chad, Côte d'Ivoire, Central African Republic, Ethiopia, Ghana, India, Kenya, Mali, Mauritania, Niger, Nigeria, Pakistan, Senegal, Sudan, Togo, Uganda, and Yemen.

PLANTING THE SEEDS OF ERADICATION

In 1980, the US Centers for Disease Control and Prevention (CDC) first planted the seeds of the global guinea worm eradication campaign. At the time, many in the global health community considered the disease to be an unlikely candidate for eradication. Unlike the eradication campaign that successfully wiped out smallpox, a guinea worm campaign would not have in its arsenal a vaccine to prevent the disease; the campaign also lacked a medical cure to treat a person once he or she had been infected. Instead, eradicating guinea worm would require the disruption of the worm's transmission for one year through the principal interventions: provision of safe sources of drinking water; treatment of unsafe sources of drinking water with larvicide; and health education and social mobilization to keep those infected from contaminating sources of drinking water and to ensure filtration of household drinking water; and surveillance and monthly case reporting.

Skeptics pointed out the numerous challenges facing the implementation of the interventions in Asia and Africa. First, the construction and maintenance of safe water sources is a time- and resource-intensive process requiring considerable external financing. Furthermore, many of the remote, endemic villages were outside the national public health infrastructure and in some instances were not even known to the government. The task, then, of coordinating an effort to change the behavior of millions of poor, illiterate, and geographically isolated villagers throughout Asia and Africa appeared exceptionally daunting.

In 1981, an important event prompted the CDC to spearhead eradication efforts. The launch that year of an international initiative to provide universal access to safe drinking water presented an unprecedented opportunity for the fight against guinea worm. Dr. Donald Hopkins and his colleagues at the CDC recognized the implications of the International Drinking Water Supply and Sanitation Decade for the prospects for guinea worm eradication and persuaded the initiative to include the eradication of the disease as a subgoal of the decade. The decision ensured that priority would be placed on the construction and maintenance of safe water sources in endemic communities and provided an important foundation for further eradication efforts. With the prospects for eradication now considerably stronger, the CDC launched a more than 10-year advocacy campaign to catalyze a global eradication effort.[2]

Momentum was extremely slow to build. Initially, lack of data on disease prevalence, inadequate funding, and weak political commitment impeded progress. Skepticism mounted in the public health community and among African leaders when, after recognizing the slow pace of the water decade in providing safe water to endemic communities, the campaign began emphasizing the important role of public health campaigns and behavior change in the eradication efforts. By the end of the water decade in 1991, just 4 of the 20 endemic countries (Ghana, India, Nigeria, and Pakistan) had initiated full-scale national guinea worm eradication programs, which were to have formed the backbone of the global campaign.

TURNING THE TIDE

Key events in the 1980s helped overcome these obstacles and turn the tide in the fight against guinea worm. In 1986, the World Health Assembly (WHA), the highest governing body of the WHO, passed a resolution that set the elimination of guinea worm as a goal of the organization and bestowed greater international legitimacy to the campaign. That same year, a meeting of public health leaders from 14 African countries helped make important strides toward filling the gaps in data, awareness, and political commitment on the continent.

A major turning point in the campaign occurred later in 1986 when US President Jimmy Carter began his nearly 20-year involvement in the campaign and became a powerful advocate for eradication, with the Carter Center taking the role of lead nongovernmental organization providing financial and technical assistance to national eradication programs. That year, President Carter persuaded Pakistan's head of state, General Zia ul Haq, to follow India as the second country to launch a national eradication effort. He then focused on Africa and in 1988 attended a regional conference in Ghana of African guinea worm program coordinators. His high-profile presence and personal persuasion helped propel the campaign forward in Africa and prompted the involvement of Ghana's president, Jerry Rawlings. Rawlings subsequently toured highly endemic villages in northern Ghana and launched the first African eradication program.

Political commitment in Africa was firmly consolidated thanks to the advocacy efforts of two popular former African leaders whom President Carter recruited to the campaign. In 1992, General Amadou Toumani Touré, the former head of state of Mali, began an extensive campaign to raise awareness and to persuade the nine other endemic Francophone countries in Africa to also launch eradication programs. Nigeria's former head of state, General Yakubu Gowon, was recruited in 1999 and has played an important role in galvanizing political support for efforts in Nigeria, a country that then had the highest number of guinea worm cases outside of Sudan. General Gowon has visited villages in all the major endemic regions in Nigeria and mobilized the commitment of political and public health leaders.

As national commitment was being harnessed, the essential technical and financial resources of the donor community were also successfully marshaled. By 1995, national eradication programs had been established in all 20 endemic countries and a global effort to eradicate the disease was fully under way. Under the stewardship of Hopkins and in close collaboration with the United Nations Children's Fund (UNICEF), the CDC, and the WHO, the Carter Center has led the eradication effort and has worked directly with and through the ministries of health in each endemic country to provide support to the national eradication efforts. The global partnership has drawn on the participation of an impressive range of groups: donor countries, international agencies, foundations, NGOs, African governments, the private sector, village volunteers, and even the infected individuals themselves.

THE ERADICATION CAMPAIGN

The goal of the national campaigns, operated by the ministries of health, has been to wipe out the disease by stopping the worm's transmission from every locality where it occurs, effectively bringing the case incidence to zero. Because there are no nonhuman carriers of the disease, guinea worm would thereafter be eradicated. The primary interventions of the campaign include village-based surveillance and monthly case reporting; health education to prevent infected persons from contaminating sources of drinking water and to use free cloth filters to filter all drinking water; applying larvicide to contaminated sources of drinking water; and advocacy for the provision of safe water.

SAFE WATER

To improve the safety of water in endemic regions, the national programs facilitated the construction and maintenance of accessible water sources (mainly wells) and the selective application of ABATE larvicide, which can effectively kill the copepods, or "water fleas," in ponds and other stagnant sources of drinking water. Construction of safe water sources is the most expensive and long-term option of all the available interventions and has received sizable financial support from UNICEF and the government of Japan. Because the cost of this intervention can exceed $40 per person (plus additional maintenance costs), and the cost of constructing a borehole well can exceed $10,000, it is not considered cost-effective in many villages with small and/or nomadic populations and instead has been most effective in areas with higher population density. Voluntary participation has allowed hundreds of endemic communities to improve their water supply; in southeast Nigeria alone, villagers hand dug more than 400 wells.[4]

One of the most cost-effective ways of improving the safety of drinking water (to prevent guinea worm disease) is by passing it through a cloth filter. At the start of the eradication campaign, efforts relied on filters made of local fabrics. However, the cloth fabric clogged frequently, and these filters often were used instead as decorations.[2]

A new nylon cloth that was less prone to clogging was developed in the early 1990s. Through the Carter Center, Precision Fabrics and DuPont donated several million square yards of nylon for filters, valued at more than $14 million.[2] More user-friendly filters made from cotton-polyester cloth with nylon mesh filters in the center have been in use since 1999. Health education campaigns have promoted the use of filters and explained the health benefits of the simple intervention, helping bolster their popularity and use.

HEALTH EDUCATION

Essential to the campaign has been the voluntary participation of the residents of endemic communities in preventing, treating, and containing the disease. As President Carter explained in 1999, "It is the affected villagers who must act in order to free themselves of this disease." Despite the initial skepticism, one of the most remarkable accomplishments has been the success of the locally targeted public education campaigns, which Hopkins considered to be the "fastest and most effective intervention."[5]

The public education interventions have convinced individuals and communities that they can prevent the disease and its spread. Individuals are encouraged to clean drinking water by passing it through a nylon filter, to avoid recontamination of ponds, and to report infestations. An extensive social marketing campaign has been employed with the goal, in the words of Hopkins, that "No individual would be able to approach a drinking water source without thinking of guinea worm disease." The simple, targeted messages are communicated through radio, t-shirts, posters, banners, stamps, sides of vehicles, and videos.

A popular communications tool has been "worm weeks"—weeks of intensive health education and community mobilization in the most highly endemic communities during which local and international volunteers (including those from the US Peace Corps) perform plays, arrange ceremonies with prominent officials, and demonstrate how to use cloth filters and prevent the disease.[6] Research in Ghana demonstrated the success of the worm weeks: The communities that had participated in worm weeks showed an 80% decrease in cases versus a 45% reduction in neighboring villages without the intervention.[6]

SURVEILLANCE AND CASE MANAGEMENT

The 1-year incubation period leaves little room for mistakes, so the campaign has required careful case identification, management, and containment of transmission. Because many of the remote endemic villages lack primary health care workers, these efforts have relied heavily on the help of "village volunteers" in more than 23,000 communities at its peak in 1993.[7] Trained and supervised by representatives from the ministry of health, the village volunteers form the bulk of the eradication staff and perform a range of key functions including daily detection of cases, case management, containment of transmission, distribution and replacement of nylon cloth or pipe filters, and social mobilization and public awareness campaigns. These village volunteers are the keys to success of the monthly reporting system that provides national coordinators with data necessary for tracking the disease and monitoring the campaign's progress. The village-based reporting system, virtually nonexistent in countries such as Ghana and Nigeria at the start of the campaign, is now considered a model for the surveillance of other diseases such as tetanus, lymphatic filariasis, and leprosy.[5]

A 99% DROP IN GUINEA WORM PREVALENCE

The result of the campaign's efforts has been a 99% drop in the prevalence of guinea worm. In 2005, only 10,674 cases of the disease were reported, compared with an estimated 3.5 million infected people in 1986. All three countries in Asia are now free of guinea worm: Pakistan (1993), India (1996), and Yemen (1997). As of 2005, 11 of the original 20 endemic countries halted transmission of the disease; 4 reported fewer than 100 cases each, and just 2 had more than 1,000 each. The vast majority (89%) of the cases reported in 2005 were from Sudan (5,569 cases) and from Ghana (3,981 cases) (see Box 11-1). In the absence of the eradication campaign begun in 1986, a total of 3.5 million cases of the disease would have presumably occurred annually. Therefore, the eradication campaign can be said to have prevented at least 63 million cases of guinea worm disease since 1987.

COST AND ECONOMIC RETURNS

The estimated cost of the global campaign between 1987 and 1998 is $87.5 million.[3] The effort received major financial support and donor support from the governments of Canada,

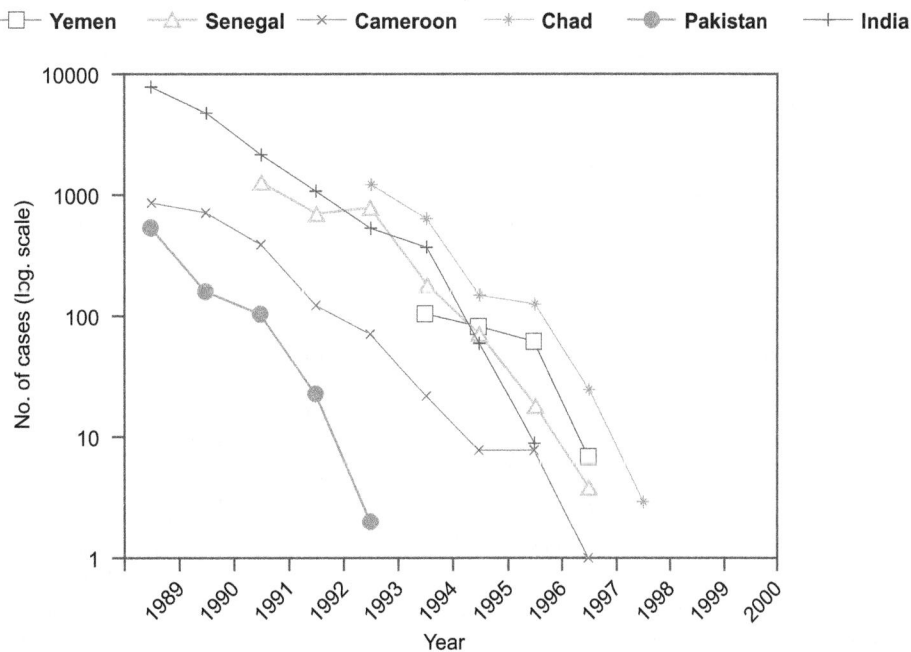

FIGURE 11-1 Countries that have interrupted transmission of guinea worm disease.

Source: Cairncross S, Muller R, Zagaria (2002).

Denmark, Finland, Japan, the Netherlands, Norway, Qatar, Saudi Arabia, Spain, Sweden, United Arab Emirates, the United Kingdom, and the United States.[8] The private sector also contributed to the campaign: BASF (formerly American Home Products) donated more than $2 million worth of insecticide to the campaign, and E.I. DuPont Corporation donated more than $14 million worth of cloth for filters. The announcements of a grant from the Bill & Melinda Gates Foundation in 2000 worth $28.5 million and, more recently, a $25 million matching grant, has helped ensure that the campaign remains funded through 2010.

A World Bank study determined that the financial investment made by the campaign has yielded considerable financial returns. According to the study, the economic rate of return based on agricultural productivity alone has been estimated at 29%—an impressive figure many consider to be an underestimate, especially if the goal of eradication is achieved and the benefits accrue in the future at no additional cost. The cost per case prevented was estimated at $5 to $8.[3]

KEYS TO SUCCESS

Hopkins identified the following strategies that contributed to the campaign's impressive success:

- **Coordination**—Interagency meetings, held three to four times a year, and annual meetings of coordinators of national eradication programs facilitated exemplary coordination of major partners and donors.
- **Power of data**—The data provided by the village volunteers through the monthly reporting system helped with what Hopkins calls the "Disneyland effect"—that people will stand in long lines if they see that the line is moving and that no one is "cutting" ahead of others. Data published in the CDC's monthly publication, *Guinea Worm Wrap-Up*, demonstrating the progress and success of the national programs, has helped keep countries motivated and focused on the efforts—and has pressured countries lagging behind. The campaign has actively promoted competition between rivals such as Ghana and Nigeria, and India and Pakistan.
- **High-level advocacy and political leadership**—High-level advocacy and political leadership from current and former heads of state helped prevent the "problem" of success—resources and support tend to dwindle as time passes and progress is made. The political support of President Carter, General

BOX 11-1 Sudan: The Final Bastion

The biggest obstacle facing the guinea worm eradication campaign is not the tenacious parasite but rather the civil strife in Sudan—a country that is home to more than three of every four remaining cases of guinea worm disease. The challenge of eliminating the disease in what may soon be its final bastion has been exacerbated by the more than 20-year civil war that has divided Sudan, particularly in the south, where disease prevalence is highest. Ernesto Ruiz-Tiben, technical director of the Carter Center's Guinea Worm Eradication Program, explains that "The war and the absence of infrastructure in southern Sudan make it very difficult to organize a program in endemic villages."

Despite the constraints, some progress has been made. In 1995, President Carter negotiated a 4-month "guinea worm cease fire," which allowed health workers to distribute more than 200,000 cloth filters to nearly 2,000 villages. (The cease-fire also provided a precious window for providing other life-saving health interventions: 100,000 people at risk of river blindness were treated; 41,000 children were vaccinated for measles; 35,000 received a polio vaccine; 35,000 doses of vitamin A were distributed; and 9,000 children were treated with oral rehydration therapy.[4]) Since the cease-fire, government authorities, the United Nations, the Carter Center, and more than 20 NGOs have focused on combating the disease in the south. An estimated 600,000 cloth filters have been distributed each year, and in 2001, nearly 8 million pipe filters—a strawlike tube with a nylon filter cloth that can be worn around the neck and used when farming or traveling—were distributed. These efforts have been assisted by political commitment from the highest levels of Sudan's government and from the advocacy of President Carter, who visited parts of the rebel-controlled region in 2002.[6,9] Success in Sudan is not believed possible without an end to the conflict. Until then, the persistence of guinea worm there jeopardizes the residents, the populations of the neighboring countries, and the success that the national eradication programs have worked so hard to achieve.

Toumani Touré, General Gowon, and others brought sustained attention and awareness to the remaining challenge—the cases that are the most difficult to reach—and kept programs on track. For example, General Gowon visited all the major endemic foci in Nigeria, extracted promises of action, and revisited the areas later to check on their progress. Largely thanks to his efforts, the number of cases in Nigeria fell by half.

The success of the guinea worm eradication campaign is remarkable and places the disease in line to be eradicated. As Cairncross and colleagues summarize, the guinea worm eradication campaign demonstrates that "It is possible, at affordable expense, to control and even eliminate a disease at a national level, even in the remotest and most neglected areas of some of the poorest countries in the world and in spite of the fact that the key interventions involve substantial changes in behavior."[2]

REFERENCES

1. Watts SJ. Dracunculiasis in Africa in 1986: its geographic extent, incidence, and at-risk population. *Am J Trop Med and Hyg.* 1987;37:119–125.

2. Cairncross S, Muller R, Zagaria N. Dracunculiasis (guinea worm disease) and the eradication initiative. *Clin Microbiol Rev.* 2002;15(2):223–246.

3. Kim A, Tandon A, Ruiz-Tiben E.*Cost-Benefit Analysis of the Global Dracunculiasis Eradication Campaign.* Policy Research Working Paper 1835. Washington, DC: World Bank, Africa Human Development Department; 1997.

4. Hopkins DR. Perspectives from the dracunculiasis eradication programme. *MMWR.* 1999;48(SU01):43–49.

5. Hopkins DR. The guinea worm eradication effort: lessons for the future. *Emerg Infect Dis.* 1998;4(3).

6. Hopkins DR, Ruiz-Tiben E, Diallo N, Withers PC Jr, Maguire JH. Dracunculiasis eradication: and now, Sudan. *Am J Trop Med Hyg.* 2002;67(4):415–422.

7. Ruiz-Tiben E, Hopkins DR. Dracunculiasis (guinea worm disease) eradication. *Adv Parasitol.* 2006;61:275–309.

8. Carter J. The power of partnership: the eradication of guinea worm disease. *Cooperation South.* 1999;2:140–147.

9. Hopkins DR, Withers PC Jr. Sudan's war and eradication of dracunculiasis. *Lancet Suppl.* 2002;260(December):21–22.

Controlling Chagas Disease in the Southern Cone of South America*

* The first draft of this case was prepared by Gail Vines.

ABSTRACT

Geographic area: Seven countries in South America's southern cone: Argentina, Bolivia, Brazil, Chile, Paraguay, Uruguay, and Peru

Health condition: In the early 1990s, Chagas disease was ranked as the most serious parasitic disease in Latin America. The disease was endemic in all seven countries of the southern cone, and wavering political commitment and reinfestation of the insect vectors across borders hampered efforts to control the disease.

Global importance of the health condition today: Today an estimated 11 million people in 15 Latin American countries are infected with Chagas disease. The disease also plagues northern South America, Central America, and Mexico, as well as the remaining pockets in the southern cone.

Intervention or program: The Southern Cone Initiative to Control/Eliminate Chagas was launched in 1991 under the leadership of the Pan American Health Organization. Spray teams operated by ministries of health have treated more than 2.5 million homes across the region with long-lasting pyrethroid insecticides. Houses in poor rural areas have been improved to eliminate the insect's hiding places, and blood is screened for Chagas disease.

Cost and cost-effectiveness: Financial resources for the regional program, provided by each of the seven countries, have totaled more than $400 million since 1991. The intervention is considered among the most cost-effective interventions in public health, at just $37 per disability adjusted life year saved in Brazil.

Impact: Incidence in the seven countries covered by the initiative fell by an average of 94% by 2000. Overall, the number of new cases on the continent fell from 700,000 in 1983 to fewer than 200,000 in 2000. Furthermore, the number of deaths each year from the disease was halved from 45,000 to 22,000. By 2001, disease transmission was halted in Uruguay, Chile, and large parts of Brazil and Paraguay.

If ever there were a good example of a problem calling for a regional solution and steady sustained leadership, Chagas disease is it. Chagas disease, or American trypanosomiasis, is a debilitating and deadly infection that afflicts rural communities throughout Latin America. The poorest people living in rural areas, particularly those with inadequate housing, are the most vulnerable. In the early 1990s, Chagas disease was ranked as the most serious parasitic disease in Latin America, with a socioeconomic impact greater than that of all the other parasitic infections combined.[1] An estimated 16 million to 18 million people in Latin America were infected with the disease a decade ago, with 50,000 deaths each year.[2] An additional 120 million people—one quarter of the population of Latin America—were thought to be at risk of infection. Today, thanks to large regional efforts to control the disease, just over 11 million are infected, and incidence across the continent has fallen 70%.[3] However, unsteady commitment at the highest levels has jeopardized the achievements at various times, demonstrating how the very result of success—fewer people infected—can undermine long-term sustainability.

"KISSING BUG" DISEASE

The disease is named after Carlos Chagas, the Brazilian doctor who first described it in 1909 and subsequently discovered its cause: a protozoan parasite, *Trypanosoma cruzi*. The parasites are harbored within the feces of "kissing bugs," several species of blood-feeding insects in the subfamily *Triatominae*. In many rural areas, these insects live within the walls of houses and emerge at night to suck human blood. The parasites enter the bloodstream when the insect bites are rubbed or scratched or when food is contaminated. The second most common route of infection is infected blood, a risk that is heightened when rural hardship forces people to migrate to cities. The disease also can be spread from an infected mother to her fetus.

Two phases mark the course of Chagas disease. First comes the acute phase, during which symptoms are relatively mild. A small sore that frequently develops around the bite is the first sign of infection. Within a few days, the parasite invades the lymph nodes, and fever, malaise, and swelling may develop. This first phase can be fatal, especially in young children. In most cases, however, infected individuals enter the second, chronic stage and show no symptoms for several years. During this period, the parasites spread throughout the major organs of the body, damaging the heart, intestines, and esophagus. Complications associated with the disease include congestive heart failure, abdominal pain and constipation, and swallowing difficulties that can lead to malnutrition.[4] In nearly one third of all cases, the damage to the heart and digestive system proves fatal.

The lost years of productive lives of Chagas disease victims, combined with the expense of treating patients, make it an extremely costly disease. The estimated economic loss due to premature deaths between 1979 and 1981 in Brazil alone topped $237 million, and $750 million would have been needed each year to treat the cardiac and digestive problems from Chagas disease in Brazil.[3]

Chagas is endemic in 15 countries in Latin America. These countries fall into two broad ecological zones. The first is the southern cone—Argentina, Brazil, Bolivia, Chile, Paraguay, Peru, and Uruguay—where the species of blood-sucking insects that spread the parasites lives entirely inside houses. The second zone embraces northern South America, Central America, and Mexico, where the insect vectors are harder to eradicate because reinfestations can occur from hardier species that can survive outside homes.

Unfortunately, no vaccine currently exists to prevent the disease, and treatment strategies remain poorly developed. Acute infections in newborns and young children and infections in the chronic phase can, during the first few years, respond to the drugs nifurtimox and benznidazole in at least half the cases. However, because these drugs are of little use in later chronic infections, have serious side effects, and are prohibitively expensive, their use is limited. Long-term symptomatic treatment of chronic disease requires specialized clinics, which are beyond the means of most patients. As a result, control efforts require the prevention of new infection—by eliminating the vector and screening the blood supply.

EARLY ATTEMPTS TO TACKLE THE DISEASE

Beginning with the pioneering insights of Carlos Chagas and his colleagues in Brazil, many generations of workers have searched for effective ways of destroying the insect vectors that live within homes. Early attempts entailed dousing the walls of houses with kerosene or scalding water and even scorching walls with military flamethrowers. More effective, but equally impractical on a large scale, were schemes to enclose houses in canvas tents and fill them with cyanide gas.[1] During the 1940s, the introduction of synthetic insecticides offered a more plausible solution. Although DDT was quickly found to be ineffective against the insects, two other organochlorine insecticides, dieldrin and lindane, did kill the insects. Spraying campaigns began in several countries in the 1950s and 1960s.

A major breakthrough occurred in the early 1980s when synthetic pyrethroid insecticides were developed. These new chemicals proved even more effective than the earlier insecticides—at lower doses and even in single applications. The new treatments were more cost-effective and significantly easier to use than earlier methods. They were more attractive to both sprayers and residents because they left neither unpleasant smells nor stains on the walls of infected homes.

Armed with this improved technology, Brazil's Ministry of Health initiated a national eradication campaign in 1983, which showed promising results. The campaign set out to eradicate the main vector, the kissing bugs, through nationwide spraying programs. Community vigilance schemes staffed by volunteers ensured that all infected houses were sprayed. Residents who spotted insects were encouraged to alert the local volunteer post known as Posto de Informacao sobre Triatomineos, or PIT. By 1986, almost three quarters of the infested localities had been mapped, sprayed, and placed under the scrutiny of local PIT volunteers.[1]

Brazil's early success with the program demonstrated the technical feasibility of vector control efforts. However, the program also exposed two challenges facing the fight against Chagas disease: border-crossing insects and wavering political commitment. Despite the diligent mapping and control efforts within its borders, Brazil's campaign faced disease transmission from neighboring countries. The insect vector can easily cross borders and is thought to have originated in Bolivia and spread across a large swath of the continent, hidden in people's belongings as they moved from one place to another. As such, Brazil's experience demonstrated that unilateral control efforts would be unable to defeat the disease. Furthermore, attention in 1986 was suddenly shifted away from Chagas disease to a new threat in Brazil: the return to coastal cities of the insect vector of yellow fever and dengue. Urban populations were suddenly at risk, generating widespread alarm in the media and political circles. As the focus shifted to urban concerns, the rural Chagas disease campaign was sidelined, and political commitment waned. As a result, the program's earlier achievements eroded.[1] The malaria control program in Brazil experienced similar challenges around the same time (see Box 12-1). For both Chagas and malaria, new strategies were needed.

A UNITED FRONT: THE SOUTHERN CONE INITIATIVE IS LAUNCHED

In 1991, a new control program, known as the Southern Cone Initiative to Control/Eliminate Chagas (INCOSUR) addressed these challenges and marshaled the commitment of the countries of the southern cone region where Chagas was an endemic threat. The initiative was a joint agreement among the governments of Argentina, Bolivia, Brazil, Chile, Paraguay, Uruguay, and later Peru, which set out to control Chagas disease through the elimination of the main insect vector. Led by the Pan American Health Organization (PAHO), the initiative was designed to bolster national resolve and prevent cross-border reinfestations.

Within the INCOSUR, each country finances and manages its own national program. However, regional cooperation has proved essential to the program's success and has been coordinated by PAHO. Each year, representatives from the collaborating nations share operational aims, methods, and achievements at a PAHO-sponsored annual meeting of the Intergovernmental Commission of the Southern Cone. A series of intercountry technical cooperation agreements has fostered the sharing of information among scientists throughout the region and among their respective government organizations.

Additional scientific support has been provided by a network of research groups in 22 countries and has had "a decisive influence on our understanding of the biology and evolution of domestic vectors of disease," says Chris Schofield, a leading Chagas disease researcher at the London School of Hygiene and Tropical Medicine.[5] WHO's Special Programme for Research and Training in Tropical Diseases has provided additional support.

SUCCESSFUL STRATEGIES IN PRACTICE

Elimination of the insect vector in infested homes was a vital first step, and the technical and operational procedures for achieving this goal are now demonstrably successful and cost-effective. The professional treatment of houses with long-lasting pyrethroid insecticides has eliminated or greatly reduced the insect vector population throughout the southern cone. Spray teams operated through the ministries of health treat each house in municipalities where the vector's presence has been confirmed. Between 1992 and 2001, more than 2.5 million homes were sprayed. Canisters that release insecticidal fumes when lit also have been made available to households. In many areas, house improvement schemes for the rural poor are also under way to eliminate hiding places for vector insects. Cracks and crevices in poor-quality houses have been fixed, adobe walls have been replaced with plaster, and metal roofs constructed.

The spread of the disease through the unwitting transfusion of contaminated blood is also being tackled throughout the southern cone. A decade ago, most countries in Latin America had laws or decrees mandating the screening of blood donors for infectious diseases, but enforcement was usually lax.[6] However, the HIV/AIDS epidemic heightened awareness of the need for universal screening, and technical expertise in each country has been strengthened through workshops and expert visits sponsored by the INCOSUR.[1] Blood donors have increasingly been tested to prevent the transfusion of parasite-infected blood. Today the screening of blood donors for the parasite is virtually universal in 10 South American countries.[7]

MAJOR IMPACT

To date, the INCOSUR has achieved tremendous success, and elimination of the disease as a public health problem is now close at hand in several countries. Incidence in the seven countries covered by the INCOSUR fell by an average of 94%, contributing to a continent-wide reduction of 70% by 2000. Overall, the number of new cases on the continent fell from

BOX 12-1 Combating Malaria in Brazil

As more effective means of combating the Chagas vector were being deployed in Brazil in the late 1980s, the country was also facing a mounting death toll from malaria, another disease borne by an insect vector.

In Brazil, as elsewhere, the fight against malaria has been characterized both by periods of optimism and moments of defeat. By the late 1970s, most of Brazil was malaria free, thanks largely to the application of insecticides through in-house spraying. But the traditional control approach, which had succeeded elsewhere in the country, was failing in the Amazon basin, home to the largest tropical rain forest in the world. Thick vegetation, scattered and sometimes temporary human settlements—including migrating miners who slept in improvised tents that could not retain insecticide—impeded vector control and case-finding measures. In the Amazon, malaria prevalence and fatality rates were high and, at the time, growing fast. Between 1977 and 1988, the deaths from malaria per 100,000 population had more than quadrupled, and by the end of the period incidence had reached almost half a million cases.[8]

Recognizing the special problems of malaria in the region, the government of Brazil obtained financing and technical support from the World Bank for the Amazon Basin Malaria Control Project. The project, which was designed to last four years and eventually took seven, started operations in late 1989. It was intended to help the government deal with the malaria problem in the Amazon basin, prevent spread into uninfected areas, and increase the capacity of public health authorities involved in malaria control.

The program's technical strategy evolved as new challenges arose. Observing the results of early *Plasmodium falciparum* vaccine trials in Colombia and Ecuador, Renato Gusmao and other advisors from PAHO noticed that when health care personnel were dedicated to early detection and immediate treatment of every *P. falciparum* case—as was ethically required during the trials—the *P. falciparum* transmission was interrupted. Although this complicated the vaccine trials, it provided new insights for those fighting malaria. Together with Agostinho Marquez and Carlos Catão of the Brazilian Ministry of Health, and consultant Hernando Cardenas, PAHO developed the strategy to shift the emphasis of the *P. falciparum* control. It moved away from a single-minded focus on vector control and toward the expansion of basic health services for early detection and prompt treatment: "Emphasis shifted from the mosquito to the people" (R. Gusmao, personal communication, July 2006). With good health service coverage, as basic health facilities increased from about 400 to about 35,000 in a few years, the program was able to interrupt *P. falciparum* transmission.

At the same time, Brazilian public health officials detected an increase in the resistance of *P. falciparum* to the traditional, quinine-based antimalarials. Thus, the program introduced new antimalarials (mefloquine plus artemisinin) and new diagnostic procedures. Because one form of the disease, *P. vivax,* was still sensitive to older, cheaper antimalarials, and program managers were keen to reserve the newer products for those suffering from *P. falciparum,* the deadlier form of the disease, emphasis was placed on the introduction of dipsticks, a new diagnostic procedure.

Although the oscillatory pattern of malaria incidence complicates the task of estimating the program's net effects, clear gains were made against the problem of malaria in the Amazon basin over the course of the World Bank–financed program. By 1996, the program had shown a decrease in malaria morbidity, from 557,787 cases in 1989 to 455,194 in 1996. Of all cases, the share attributable to *P. falciparum* declined from 47% to 29%. One analysis estimated that about 1.8 million cases of malaria and 230,000 deaths were averted by the program, with equal credit for health gains due to preventive and curative activities.[8,9]

Brazil's ability to combat malaria and to adapt the program strategy through an expansion of case finding and treatment with new antimalarials yield inspiration for those working on the vast challenge of fighting malaria in sub-Saharan Africa, where the disease claims nearly a million lives each year.

700,000 in 1983 to fewer than 200,000 in 2000.[3] Furthermore, the number of deaths each year from the disease was halved, from 45,000 to 22,000.

The number of endemic countries has also fallen, from 18 to 15. Uruguay was declared virtually free of vectoral transmission in 1997, and Chile followed in 1999. Children no longer suffer from acute infections in the two countries, demonstrating that disease transmission has been interrupted. Six Brazilian states where the disease had been endemic were declared free of transmission in March 2000, and another state was certified a year later. By 2001, disease transmission had been virtually halted in Uruguay, Chile, and large parts of Brazil and Paraguay, and house infestation rates decreased in Bolivia.[1]

The full social impact of Chagas disease control in Latin America has yet to be fully calculated, but it has been profound, particularly for the poorest rural communities, which have long suffered from a disproportionate burden of morbidity and mortality from the disease. In regions where vectors have been eliminated, surveys have indicated an improved sense of well-being, domestic pride, and security. Researchers suggest that a greater sense of citizenship and social inclusion may also ultimately promote the stability of rural communities.

HIGH COST BUT HIGHER BENEFITS

Since the INCOSUR began in 1991, the countries involved have invested more than $400 million in the fight against Chagas disease. Brazil's experience demonstrates that each dollar spent has resulted in tremendous health gains and considerable savings. Between 1975 and 1995, Brazil invested $516 million, of which 78% was for vector control and 4% for housing improvement. This investment is estimated to have prevented 2,339,000 new infections and 337,000 deaths.[3] In total, Brazil's effort prevented the loss of nearly 11.5 million disability adjusted life years (DALYs). At $39 per DALY, Chagas disease control efforts in Brazil are among the most cost-effective interventions in public health.[3]

The regional program's financial return on investment has been impressive: In Argentina, taking into consideration the reduced morbidity and the savings in medical costs, the return exceeded 64%. In Brazil, the benefits of the program, from savings of medical costs and disability insurance, amounted to $7.5 billion.[3] Thus, for each dollar spent on prevention in Brazil, $17 was saved from reduced medical and disability costs.[10]

KEYS TO SUCCESS

International scientific and political cooperation has contributed to the notable progress against Chagas disease. Political commitment has been vital to sustained success and has ensured continued vigilance. The INCOSUR has succeeded, says Chris Schofield, for three reasons: "It was big and designed to reach a definitive end point", "it had a simple, well-proven technical approach"; and a strong scientific community, in close contact with the government authorities, helped ensure political continuity. These lessons are now being applied in Africa in the development of the Pan African Tsetse and Trypanosomiasis Eradication Campaign.[1]

Alfredo Solari, Uruguay's former minister of health, expanded on the key elements of the program's success:

- **Peer pressure** by neighboring countries was a very positive factor. "I participated as minister of health

of Uruguay in some of the annual meetings of the initiative," explained Solari. "I listened very carefully at the presentations of Argentina and Brazil, since our final success in Uruguay was dependent on their effectiveness. There was a clear sense of joint responsibility and commitment by countries with common borders. Furthermore, I know directly of at least one instance—Argentina and Bolivia in the mid-1990s—where the process was kept alive in one country by the direct involvement of a neighboring country to avoid reinfestation."

- The existence of an **international cooperative** commitment by all the countries concerned, backed up by international organizations (PAHO and WHO) able to promote trust and provide technical expertise and administrative support, was integral to the initiative's effectiveness.

- **An international technical secretariat** was also key to the initiative's success. The secretariat at PAHO was in charge of verifying surveillance, sharing information about progress of neighboring countries, processing requests to the WHO for certification of interruption and eradication, and preparing the annual meetings.

- Finally, a **favorable economic and institutional environment** in the southern cone contributed to success. The Mercado Comun del Sur (Mercosur), or Southern Cone Common Market, had just been created in 1990, and although the INCOSUR was not officially part of it, the Mercosur process favored policy coordination in other health areas among southern cone countries. "The economies of all countries in the region were growing quite strongly," explained Solari, "thus, enabling the fiscal resources needed to sustain these expensive national public health programs."

LOOKING AHEAD

The success of the INCOSUR to date has helped revitalize control campaigns in Paraguay and Bolivia, which are beginning to show tangible signs of progress.[11] At present, Central America and the Amazon region remain as the next major challenges. "Here, Chagas disease surveillance and control are in their infancy," says Joao Carlos Pinto Dias of the René Rachou Research Center at the Oswaldo Cruz Foundation in Brazil. The Andean countries of Colombia, Ecuador, Peru, and Venezuela, which currently are home to 5 million infected individuals, began a regional effort in 1997 to halt transmission. Similarly, the governments of the Central American countries Belize, Costa Rica, El Salvador,

Guatemala, Honduras, Mexico, Nicaragua, and Panama also pledged in 1997 to work toward elimination of the vector.[3]

Although the INCOSUR has achieved impressive success, sustaining the achievements will take vigilance. With success comes the inevitable tendency to relax surveillance and withdraw resources, with a subsequent loss of awareness and expertise. To ensure long-term success in the southern cone, existing programs need continued political support over the next decade so that achievements can be consolidated rather than reversed. Projections during the initial planning of the INCOSUR showed that premature curtailment of active surveillance could cause a radical decline in the total benefits, reaching zero after just 11 years. As with many diseases, the battle against Chagas disease is a long one, requiring persistent support after the first gains have been made.

REFERENCES

1. Dias JCP, Silveira AC, Schofield CJ. The impact of Chagas disease control in Latin America—a review. *Memorias do Instituto Oswaldo Cruz.* 2002;97:603–612.

2. World Health Organization. *Control of Chagas Disease. Report of a WHO Expert Committee.* WHO Technical Report Series: 811. Geneva, Switzerland: World Health Organization; 1991.

3. Moncayo A. Chagas disease: current epidemiological trends after the interruption of vectorial and transfusional transmission in the southern cone countries. *Memorias do Instituto Oswaldo Cruz.* 2003;98(5):577–591.

4. US Centers for Disease Control and Prevention. Fact sheet: Chagas disease. Division of Parasitic Diseases. Available at: http://www.cdc.gov/ncidod/dpd/parasites/_chagasdisease/factsht_chagas_disease.htm. Accessed January 12, 2007.

5. Schofield CJ, Dias JCP. The southern cone programme against Chagas disease. *Adv Parasitol.* 1998;42:1–25.

6. Schmunis GA. Prevention of transfusional *Trypanosoma cruzi* infection in Latin America. *Memorias do Instituto Oswaldo Cruz.* 1999;94(suppl 1):S93–S101.

7. Schmunis GA, Zicker F, Cruz J, Cuchi P. Safety of blood supply for infectious diseases in Latin American countries, 1994–1997. *Am J Trop Med Hyg.* 2001;65:924–930.

8. Akhavan D, Musgrove P, Abrantes A, Gusmao R. Cost-effective malaria control in Brazil: cost-effectiveness of a malaria control program in the Amazon basin of Brazil, 1988–1996. *Soc Sci Med.* 1996;49:1385–1399.

9. Barat L. Four malaria success stories: how malaria burden was successfully reduced in Brazil, Eritrea, India, and Vietnam. *Am J Trop Med Hyg.* 2006;74(1):12–16.

10. Moncayo A. Progress towards interruption of transmission of Chagas disease. *Memorias do Instituto Oswaldo Cruz.* 1999;94:401–404.

11. Feliciangeli MD, Campbell-Lenrum D, Martinez C, Gonzalez D, Coleman P, Davies C. Chagas disease control in Venezuela: lessons for the Andean region and beyond. *Trends Parasitol.* 2003;19:44–49.

Reducing Fertility in Bangladesh

ABSTRACT

Geographic area: Bangladesh

Health condition: In the mid-1970s, a Bangladeshi woman had more than six children on average. In combination with poor nutrition and lack of access to quality health services, this high fertility rate jeopardized the health of both the woman and her children. Beyond the health impact, high fertility and rapid population growth represented a major constraint to the country's economic development and social progress.

Global importance of the health condition today: More than 150 million women in the developing world who would like to limit or space their pregnancies do not currently use a contraceptive method. So, for example, about 16% of married women in India have this "unmet need." In sub-Saharan Africa, where services are in relatively short supply, the unmet need is the greatest.

Intervention or program: The Bangladesh family planning program has depended on a large cadre of female outreach workers going door to door to provide information, motivate clients, and provide commodities; the program has used mass media to stimulate a change in attitudes about family size. The program both contributed to and benefited from improvements in women's status in Bangladesh during the past 30 years.

Cost and cost-effectiveness: The program is estimated to cost about $100 million to $150 million per year, with about one half to two thirds of the funding coming from external donors. Cost-effectiveness has been estimated at about $13 to $18 per birth averted, a standard measure for family planning programs.

Impact: As a result of the program, virtually all women in Bangladesh are aware of modern family planning methods. The current use of contraceptives among married women increased from 8% in the mid-1970s to about 60% in 2004, and fertility decreased from an average of more than six children per woman in 1975 to slightly more than three. Although social and economic improvements have played a major role in increasing demand for contraception, the provision of services and information has been shown to have had an independent effect on attitudes and behavior.

Whether or not couples can limit the number of children they have has profound consequences. For the couples, having the family size they want can mean the difference between economic security and a precarious existence. For a woman and her current and future offspring, the level and pattern of childbearing are central determinants of health status because with each pregnancy and delivery come health risks, particularly in the poorest countries. For societies at large, demographic patterns, particularly fertility rates, are among the most important factors affecting long-term prospects for economic growth and social development.

Modern contraceptive methods make it relatively easy and safe for couples to limit the total number of children they bear and to time their pregnancies. Both permanent methods, including male and female sterilization, and temporary methods, such as hormonal methods (oral contraceptive pills, injectable hormones, and others) and barrier methods (condoms and diaphragms), have advantages and drawbacks for individual couples. But all are reasonably effective at reducing the chances of unintended pregnancy, and they confer few health risks, particularly compared with the baseline hazards associated with pregnancy and childbirth.

Combined with changes in attitudes about the ideal family size, the availability of effective contraceptive methods through both public and private family planning services has changed the world. In the past 30 to 40 years, the average number of children borne by each woman (also known as the total fertility rate, or TFR) has declined steadily in the developing world, although with major differences in the rate of decrease across world regions. Between 1970 and 2000, the TFR in Latin America and the Caribbean decreased by half, from about 5 to 2.5 children per woman. In East Asia, the TFR declined from 5 to 2; and in South Asia, from 5.6 to 3.3.[1]

Much of the decline in childbearing can be directly attributed to the use of contraception. About 30 years ago, less than one fifth of married women worldwide used contraception; now about 60% use either modern or traditional contraceptive methods. Contraceptive use varies widely by demographic group as well as by region—in many countries of sub-Saharan Africa, only about 10% to 20% of women use contraception, while in China upward of 80% do.[2] In general, contraceptive use is highest among well-educated women, those living in urban areas, and those in higher-income households. So, for example, only 16% of married women in Kenya with no education use contraception, compared to about 46% of married women with the highest level of education.[2]

UNMET NEED

Despite the existence of a range of good family planning methods, not all women who are sexually active and who wish to limit childbearing or delay their next pregnancy use contraception. Surveys of women in developing countries indicate that a large share of women who want to limit childbearing—somewhere between 10 and 40%, depending on the country—do not use contraception.[3] Researchers estimate that more than 123 million women in their reproductive years who would like to limit or space their pregnancies do not currently use a contraceptive method—a situation termed the "unmet need for contraception."[4] So, for example, about 16% of married women in India have this unmet need. In sub-Saharan Africa, where services are in relatively short supply, the unmet need is greatest. In Rwanda, some 36% of married women who wish to limit or space their pregnancies are not using contraception; in Malawi, it is 30%.[5]

For many of these women, the absence of an effective family planning program is the problem. An analysis of data from 13 countries found that many women with this unmet need lacked knowledge about contraceptive methods, had health concerns, or could not afford or did not have easy access to services.[3]

As a consequence of the unmet need for contraception, couples are having more children than they ideally would like, and the women and their babies are exposed to major health risks. In developing countries—and particularly the types of settings where the unmet need is the greatest—the risk of death and disability from pregnancy is high (see also Case 6). Importantly, the 20 million unsafe abortions that occur in the developing world annually result in 80,000 preventable deaths. It is estimated, in fact, that each year family planning could prevent fully one quarter of the more than 500,000 maternal deaths in developing countries. In addition, more than 7 million newborns die each year because of inadequate or inappropriate care in pregnancy and around the time of delivery.[6]

UNLIKELY SETTING FOR SUCCESS?

Of all the possible settings for success in family planning, Bangladesh would not be the first place to come to mind. It is the ninth most populous country in the world, with a per capita income of about $250 per year in the mid-1990s and close to 80% of the population living in poverty. Population density in Bangladesh is among the highest in the world, at more than 2,000 persons per square mile.[7–9] The economy is primarily agricultural and faces increasing population pressure, with ever-increasing use of marginal lands; the per hectare agricultural yield is among the lowest in the world.[10]

Given low levels of education—more than half of all Bangladeshi women are illiterate—and cultural traditions among both Hindu and Muslim populations, which favor large families, high fertility would be expected. It is not surprising, then, that in the mid-1970s the average Bangladeshi woman was bearing about seven children during her lifetime, and the annual rate of population growth reached almost 2.5%.

A PROGRAM MOTIVATED BY DEMOGRAPHIC GOALS, TEMPERED BY EXPERIENCE

The history of successful family planning in Bangladesh started with resounding failure. In the early 1960s, when Bangladesh was an eastern province of Pakistan—the result of the 1947 partition of India—the Pakistani government instituted a heavy-handed family planning program that went against local needs and preferences. The coercive approaches used eventually led to a popular backlash, contributing to the 1968 collapse of the government. It was not until 1975, after a deadly famine and growing concerns about the demographic pressure on the country's natural resources and economic prospects, that the now-independent Bangladesh embarked on a renewed family planning program. As it did so, leaders recalled the cautionary tale of how attempts to affect the most profound decisions in families and communities led to political conflict.

The main challenges facing the program at the start, in 1975, were low levels of knowledge about family planning, a prevailing belief that large families were best (typical of agrarian societies), low levels of women's status, and lack of access to family planning services among the predominantly rural population—particularly among women who had limited mobility. Each of these constraints was addressed through the program and through complementary public sector actions.

While the program evolved substantially over time with the application of operations research (see Box 13-1 on the Matlab population laboratory), in general it was characterized by four elements:

- The deployment of young, married women as outreach workers
- The provision of as wide a range of methods as possible to meet a range of reproductive needs
- The establishment of family planning clinics in rural areas to provide clinical contraceptive services
- The provision of information, education, and communication activities

Young, married women were deployed as outreach workers and were trained to conduct home visits with women, offering contraceptive services and information. The number of these outreach workers, referred to as family welfare assistants (FWAs), eventually reached about 25,000 in the public sector; another 12,000 field workers were from nongovernmental organizations (NGOs). An additional 4,500 male outreach workers also were recruited.

Each FWA was expected to cover an area corresponding to three to five villages, visiting each household once every two months. This way, each FWA could serve about 850 rural women.[11] The reach of the program was staggering: Virtually all Bangladeshi women were contacted at least once by an FWA, and more than one third were reached at home every six months. The FWAs were well-recognized village visitors and constituted the main link between the government program and rural women.

BOX 13-1
The Matlab Contribution

Throughout the evolution of the Bangladesh family planning program, planners and program implementers, as well as donors, have benefited from the existence of the Matlab Health Research Center, which has operated for more than 35 years as a site for large-scale operations research on health programs. The Matlab center has maintained decades worth of demographic surveillance data on all births and deaths for a rural population of more than 220,000 people in about 142 villages in Bangladesh. Within the Matlab villages, researchers have tested various approaches to delivery of reproductive, child, and other health services, using rigorous methods for field tests—and then been able to closely monitor the results through high-quality information systems. The knowledge generated through the Matlab evaluations has been instrumental in shaping both Bangladesh's health programs and maternal and child health programs throughout the developing world. In fact, much of what is known about the impact of family planning programs on behavior and health is derived from research at Matlab.

Since the 1970s, Matlab has been the testing ground for a variety of new approaches to delivery of family planning services, many of which the national program later adopted. So, for example, Matlab researchers were able to compare the impact on contraceptive use of different combinations of outreach services and fixed sites for delivery of care, of vertical family planning services versus integrated maternal and child health care, and of limited contraceptive choices versus the provision of a broad range of methods available.

This type of outreach was seen as particularly important in the Bangladesh setting, where cultural practices (the tradition of *purdah*) restrict women's mobility. Even where *purdah* was not strictly enforced, geographic isolation and difficult transport limited women's ability to go to fixed sites for services (see Box 13-2).

The second element of the program was the provision of as wide a range of methods as possible to meet a range of reproductive needs. With this "cafeteria approach," the program offered a range of temporary methods as well as sterilization services for individuals with two living children, where the youngest child was at least 2 years old.[12] To support the work of the outreach workers, family planning commodities were provided through a well-managed distribution system.

The third element of the program was the family planning clinics established in rural areas to provide clinical contraceptive services, to which outreach workers could refer clients who wished to use long-term or permanent methods such as sterilization. Eventually, about 4,000 government facilities and 200 nongovernment clinics were established. (Nongovernmental organizations cover something on the order of one fifth of family planning clients.)

In the early days of the program, most of the clinics were dedicated only to the provision of family planning services. More recently, efforts have been made to develop an integrated approach, where health workers provide both family planning and basic maternal and child health services, such as immunization services.

The fourth element was the information, education, and communication activities that were intended to change norms about family size and provide information about contraceptive options. In particular, state-of-the-art use of mass media proved to be effective (see Box 13-3).

COSTS, FINANCING, COST-EFFECTIVENESS—AND THE SEARCH FOR A MORE SUSTAINABLE MODEL

With the goal of reducing the rate of population growth foremost in their minds, Bangladeshi policymakers at the highest levels were willing to spend considerable sums on the family planning program—and donors were, too.

In 1995, the program cost some $120 million to operate, and to meet increasing demands caused by population growth alone it was estimated that an additional $10 million would be needed each year, reaching $220 million by 2005.[15]

With most program financing coming from external donors, including the US Agency for International Development, the United Nations Development Program (UNDP), the World Bank, and other agencies—and the government now financing only about half of program costs—donors are encouraging the government to find ways to increase the program's efficiency. Dependence on a large cadre of fieldworkers has long been recognized to be an expensive way to go. Thus, the government has considered alternative and potentially less costly approaches to provide family planning services. Through research, analysts determined that the most cost-effective strategy was the provision of an integrated package of health and family planning services from clinics, complemented with targeted outreach to hard-to-reach clients. The fixed site approach cost $13 per birth averted (a standard measure of cost-effectiveness of family planning programs), compared with $18 for the doorstep strategy.[15] This information has contributed to reconsideration of the optimal (and most financially sustainable) strategy.

MAJOR PROGRAM IMPACT, FACILITATED BY SOCIAL CHANGE

Bangladesh's family planning program demonstrated success in reaching its objectives of informing couples about

BOX 13-2 Debate About the Outreach Approach

One topic of ongoing debate in the Bangladesh family planning program is about the approach of using female outreach workers for door-to-door visits—an element of the program some view as essential and others as costlier, less useful, and leading to poorer social outcomes than other approaches.

An analysis in 1996 showed the impact of the work of female outreach workers to be large and growing. Researchers found that when contraceptive prevalence was relatively low, the main determinant of whether women continued using contraception was client motivation and, as the underlying cause of that, the clients' demographic characteristics (level of income, urban residence, level of education, and so forth). As the proportion of women trying contraception grew as a result of the government's major efforts to change attitudes and make services available, the main determinant of whether women sustained use of contraception was whether they had ongoing contact and support—that is, whether they were visited at home by a young woman from the family planning program. According to Hossain and Phillips,[11] "Household outreach substitutes for client motivation, providing an incentive for practicing contraception that would not otherwise arise. As time progresses, the effect of outreach in sustaining use gains in importance."

Not all observers have been impressed by the quality of services offered through the outreach workers, however, and suggest that the strategy may have run its course now that demand for contraception is higher. Janowitz and colleagues found that the home visits were very short—often shorter than five minutes—and that women did not tend to depend on the home visitors for information. "The vast majority of clients view the fieldworker program as a convenience and not as an important source of information."[13] Still others have questioned the value of the door-to-door approach because of gender considerations: The approach "often fails to provide adequate information and support to contraceptive users and may actually reinforce women's isolation and powerlessness by accommodating existing gender norms."[14]

contraceptive options, increasing the use of contraception, and decreasing fertility rates.

By 1991, when a contraceptive prevalence survey was conducted, almost all Bangladeshi women had some knowledge of modern contraception. Between 1975 and 1997, the proportion of married women who had ever used contraception increased fivefold, from about 14% to nearly 70%.[16] The current use of contraception (also known as the contraceptive prevalence rate, or CPR) increased by more than six times, from around 8% to 49% (see Figure 13-1). In relative terms, the use of modern methods increased and traditional methods decreased. With the wider availability of a range of methods, the use of sterilization and other long-acting methods declined, while the use of oral contraceptives and other temporary methods increased.[9]

The provision of a wide range of contraceptive methods was shown to be an important influence on the increase in overall use of contraceptives. The experience of the Matlab evaluation showed that when a full range of methods was made available, 80% of women continued using contraception for more than one year, while when only condoms and oral contraceptives were available, only 40% of women sustained use.

Most important, fertility declined—from 6.3 births per woman in the early 1970s to about 3 births per woman in 2004.[17] The greatest decline in fertility rates was observed among women aged 35 years and older.[16] With this change, Bangladesh became one of few poor countries to achieve major fertility declines without draconian measures, such as China's one-child policy.

Of course, the family planning program alone can take only partial credit for the increase in demand for and use of contraceptives. During the same 30-year period, life in Bangladesh was improving in many ways, particularly for women, and some of those changes directly affected the likelihood that couples would choose smaller families. Between 1973 and 1996, for example, primary school enrollment increased by 1.8 times for boys and almost tripled for girls. Enrollment in secondary school increased by about 2.5 times for boys and by more than five times for girls.[19] Correspondingly, employment opportunities for women have increased, and traditional cultural practices have eroded somewhat in the face of global communication and mass media.

Although these factors are important in fostering greater contraceptive use, they do not overwhelm the independent effect of the availability of family planning services. Khuda et al used multiple regression analysis to disentangle the effects of changes in women's status and economic conditions from the independent effects of the family planning program.[9] Their research found that six factors primarily account for the reproductive change in Bangladesh: communication between husbands and wives about family planning, desire for children, women's education, women's employment status, access to mass media, and the effects of the family planning program, including availability of contraceptives. In addition, it is likely that program efforts have influenced several of the other factors, including communication about family planning between husbands and wives.

BOX 13-3 Use of Social Marketing Methods

The early messages of the family planning campaign—"a small family is a happy family"—were not hitting the mark, so market researchers were asked to look at the problem. They found that almost all Bangladeshi women were in favor of family planning but for cultural reasons could not use contraception if their husbands objected. It was the men's attitudes, rather than the women's, that were the obstacle. Recognizing this, a mass media campaign was designed with minidramas for radio, television, movies, and mobile vans to appeal to male audiences. Within one year, male attitudes showed a change, with a much larger share of men doing what they were urged to do in the media campaign: talk with their wives about contraceptive options. Mass media also were used to solve a problem the program faced: harassment of the female outreach workers. In the program's early days, before family planning was widely accepted, many outreach workers faced the threat of violence from irate villagers, primarily men. Thus, two of the country's most renowned writers were asked to create a storyline that would show the value of the outreach workers' efforts, in both urban and rural environments. A compelling soap opera heroine named Laila was created; in the drama, she eventually took a job as a family planning outreach worker. This gave an entertaining platform to convey messages both about family planning and about the importance of respecting the outreach workers.

The effect was swift and positive. In its first year, the program received 10,000 letters, many telling about how the program had changed husbands' attitudes about the family planning program. The success of this use of media was so great, in fact, that it inspired similar initiatives in Kenya, Tanzania, Brazil, Mexico, India, and other countries.[18]

FIGURE 13-1 Trends in current use of family planning methods among currently married women aged 15–49 years in Bangladesh, 1975–2004.

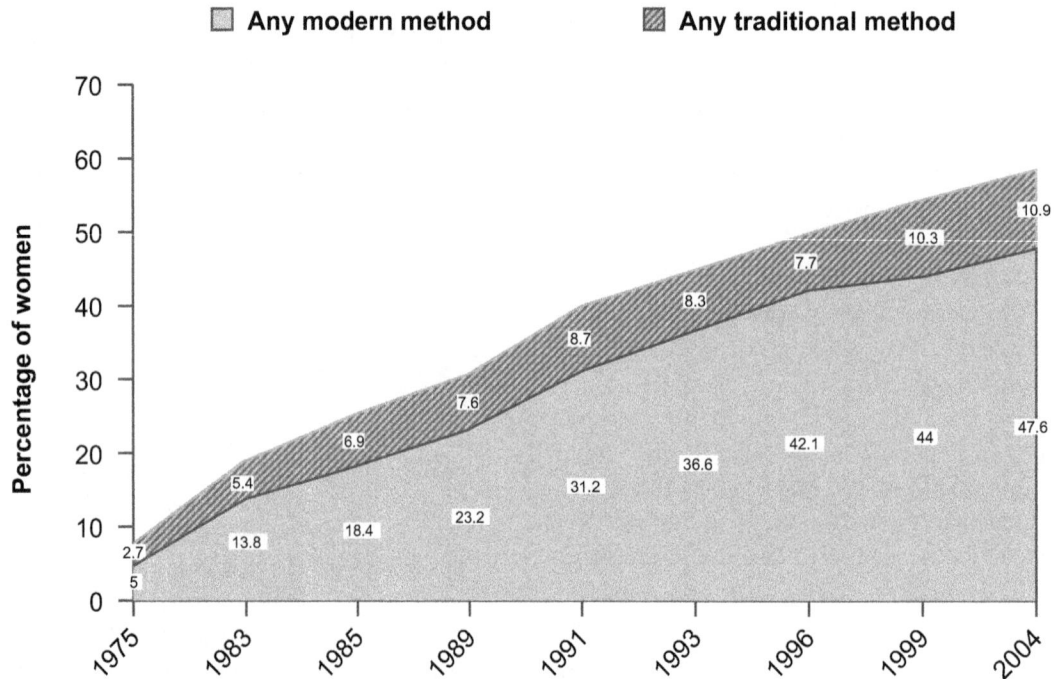

Source: National Institute of Population Research and Training (NIPORT), Mitra and Associates, and ORC Macro. *Bangladesh Demographic and Health Survey 2004.* Dhaka, Bangladesh, and Calverton, Maryland [USA]: National Institute of Population Research and Training, Mitra and Associates, and ORC Macro; 2005.

BALANCING AIMS

The Bangladesh family planning program is far from perfect. Since about 1995, declines in fertility have slowed. Many observers have noted opportunities to increase the program's efficiency, to respond more effectively to women's needs, and to better link family planning and health. The question of the optimal outreach strategy remains unanswered.

One of the changes introduced into the program, the expansion to provide a broader set of reproductive health services, is clearly a positive development. Some data suggest that during the years when the focus was exclusively on the use of contraception, the death rate during pregnancy and delivery increased slightly because of inattention to services such as antenatal care and skilled attendance at birth.

However, the expansion in the mandate of the program brings with it difficulties and may be partially responsible for the plateauing of family planning uptake in recent years.

The current challenges, significant though they are, do not erase the fact that Bangladesh has done something few other countries at its level of social and economic development have been able to accomplish: It has complemented efforts to change attitudes about family size with the provision of family planning services to bring about a sustained and dramatic decrease in fertility. Although the original motivation for the program was to attain demographic aims, the government was able to learn the lessons of history and create a program that rejected coercive approaches and responded to couples' needs.

REFERENCES

1. United Nations. *World Population Prospects 1950–2050: The 2002 Revision*. New York, NY: United Nations, Department of Economic and Social Affairs, Population Division; 2003.

2. United Nations Fund for Population Activities. *State of the World's Population*. New York, NY: United Nations Fund for Population Activities; 2002.

3. DaVanzo J, Adamson DM. Family planning in developing countries: an unfinished success story. Population Matters Issue Paper. RAND Corporation. Available at: http://www.rand.org/publications/IP/IP176/. Accessed December 13, 2006.

4. Ross JA, Winfrey WL. Unmet need for contraception in the developing world and the former Soviet Union: an updated estimate. *Int Fam Plann Perspect*. 2002;28(3):138–143.

5. Levine R, Langer A, Birdsall N, Matheny G, Wright M, Bayer A. Contraception. In: Jamison DT, Breman JG, Measham AR, et al, eds. *Disease Control Priorities in Developing Countries*. 2nd ed. New York, NY: Oxford University Press; 2006:1075–1090.

6. Bayer A. Unmet need for contraception in the 21st century. Population Resource Center. Available at: http://www.prcdc.org/summaries/unmetneed/ unmetneed.html. Accessed December 13, 2006.

7. Economic and Social Commission for Asia and the Pacific. *Population Data Sheet*. Bangkok, Thailand: United Nations; 1999.

8. United Nations Development Program. *Human Development Report 1994*. New York, NY: Oxford University Press; 1994.

9. Khuda B-e-, Roy NC, Rahman DM. Family planning and fertility in Bangladesh. *Asia-Pacific Popul J*. 2000;15(1):41–54.

10. Khuda B-e-, Helali J. Agriculture development in Bangladesh: a macro study on sustainability considerations. Dhaka, Bangladesh: University Research Corporation; 1991.

11. Hossain MB, Phillips JF. The impact of outreach on the continuity of contraceptive use in rural Bangladesh. *Studies in Fam Plann*. 1996;27(2):98–106.

12. Rob U, Cernada G. Fertility and family planning in Bangladesh. *J Fam Plann*. 1992;38(4):53–64.

13. Janowitz B, Holtman M, Johnson L, Trottier D. The importance of field workers in Bangladesh's family planning programme. *Asia-Pacific Popul J*. 1999;14(2):23–36.

14. Schuler SR, Hashemi SM, Jenkins AH. Bangladesh's family planning success story: a gender perspective. *Int Fam Plann Perspect*. 1995;21(4):132–137.

15. Routh S, Khuda B-e-. An economic appraisal of alternative strategies for the delivery of MCH-FP services in urban Dhaka, Bangladesh. *Int J Health Plann Manage*. 2000;15:115–132.

16. Mitra SN, Al-Sabir A, Cross AR, Jamil K. *Bangladesh Demographic and Health Survey 1996–1997*. Dhaka, Bangladesh: National Institute for Population Research and Training; 1997.

17. National Institute of Population Research and Training (NIPORT), Mitra and Associates, and ORC Macro. *Bangladesh Demographic and Health Survey 2004*. Dhaka, Bangladesh and Calverton, Maryland [USA]: National Institute of Population Research and Training, Mitra and Associates, and ORC Macro; 2005.

18. Manoff R. Getting your message out with social marketing. *Am J Trop Med Hyg*. 1997;57(3):260–265.

19. Khuda B-e-, Mabud MA, Duza MB, et al. *Population Report of the Task Force on Bangladesh Development Strategies for the 1990s: Policies for Development*. Vol. 1. Dhaka, Bangladesh: University Press Ltd; 1991:117–139.

Curbing Tobacco Use in Poland[*]

[*] Case drafted by Molly Kinder.

ABSTRACT

Geographic area: Poland

Health condition: In the 1980s, Poland had the highest rate of smoking in the world. Nearly three quarters of Polish men aged 20 to 60 smoked every day. In 1990, the probability that a 15-year-old boy born in Poland would reach his 60th birthday was lower than in most countries, and middle-aged Polish men had one of the highest rates of lung cancer in the world.

Global importance of health condition today: Tobacco is the second deadliest threat to adult health in the world and causes 1 in every 10 adult deaths. It is estimated that 500 million people alive today will die prematurely because of tobacco consumption. More than three quarters of the world's 1.2 billion smokers live in low- and middle-income countries, where smoking is on the rise. By 2030, it is estimated that smoking-related deaths will have doubled, accounting for the deaths of 6 in 10 people.

Intervention or program: In 1995, the Polish parliament passed groundbreaking tobacco-control legislation, which included the requirement of the largest health warnings on cigarette packs in the world, a ban on smoking in health centers and enclosed workspaces, a ban on electronic media advertising, and a ban on tobacco sales to minors. Health education campaigns and the "Great Polish Smoke-Out" have also raised awareness about the dangers of smoking and have encouraged Poles to quit.

Impact: Cigarette consumption dropped 10% between 1990 and 1998, and the number of smokers declined from 14 million in the 1980s to under 10 million at the end of the 1990s. The reduction in smoking led to 10,000 fewer deaths each year, a 30% decline in lung cancer among men aged 20 to 44, a nearly 7% decline in cardiovascular disease, and a reduction in low birth weight.

Only two major causes of death are growing worldwide: AIDS and tobacco. While the course of the AIDS epidemic is uncertain, one can be more sure that current smoking patterns will kill about 1 billion people this century, 10 times more than the deaths from tobacco in the 20th century.[1] Much of this burden will fall on poor countries and the poorest people living there. While smoking rates have fallen in rich countries over the past two decades, smoking is on the rise in developing countries.[2] Currently, more than three quarters of the world's 1.2 billion smokers live in low- and middle-income countries, and smoking-related deaths are estimated to double in number by 2030.

As Poland's story shows, there is reason to hope that concerted efforts to tackle the growing smoking problem in low- and middle-income countries can succeed. In many instances, this will likely take a very high level of political commitment—enough to counter the significant economic influence of the tobacco industry—as well as state-of-the-art communication strategies to induce major shifts in attitudes toward smoking.

LIGHTING UP: DANGERS OF TOBACCO

Smoking causes an astonishingly long list of diseases, leading to premature death in half of all smokers. Tobacco is implicated in numerous cancers including bladder, kidney, larynx, mouth, pancreas, and stomach. Lung cancer is the most common disease caused by smoking, and overall, smoking is responsible for about one half of all cancer deaths.[3] Smoking is also a major cause of cardiovascular diseases, including strokes and heart attacks, and of respiratory diseases such as emphysema. Additional health threats are emerging as research advances. A recent study in India found that smoking accounts for about half of the country's tuberculosis deaths and may well be increasing the spread of infectious tuberculosis.[4]

Cigarette smoking takes a heavy toll not only on smokers but also on those around them, particularly young children. Passive smoking (inhaling smoke in the surrounding air) contributes to respiratory illnesses among children including ear infections, asthma attacks, sinus infections, and throat inflammations. Tobacco use in and around pregnant women can contribute to sudden infant death syndrome, low birth weight, and intrauterine growth retardation.[5]

Smoking places an economic burden on individuals, families, and societies chiefly because of its massive death and disability toll and also because of the high cost of treatment, the value of lost wages, and the diversion of income from other basic needs such as children's food.[6] Because the poor are more likely to smoke than their rich neighbors, the economic and health impact of smoking disproportionately burdens the poor. In Poland, most of the gap in risk of dying early between uneducated and educated men is due to smoking.[7] Furthermore, because cigarettes claim the lives of half of their users, often during their prime years, smoking robs countries of valuable labor and strains health systems.

CURBING TOBACCO USE

Compared with controlling other health scourges, stopping the deadly effects of smoking requires changing personal behavior rather than undergoing complex medical procedures. Preventing smoking-related cancer and respiratory disease simply requires that smokers quit smoking and that fewer people light up their first cigarette. Because most

tobacco deaths over the next few decades will occur among today's smokers, getting adults to quit is a special priority.[2,8]

However, despite the clear health and economic benefits, quitting is extremely difficult. In addition to having to combat the addictive nature of nicotine, those seeking to reduce cigarette consumption are stymied by the fact that smoking is an ingrained social norm whose popularity is sustained through billions of dollars worth of cigarette advertising (which in the United States alone totaled over $11 billion in 2001).[9] Moreover, many smokers in developing countries are unaware of the link between smoking and health—just as was the case in the United States and other industrialized countries before the mid-1960s. In China, for example, a survey discovered that more than half of Chinese smokers and nonsmokers thought that smoking did "little or no harm."[10]

Although changing the behavior of smokers is daunting, it can be done—and it has been done. Governments and civil society can implement proven and highly cost-effective interventions to control tobacco use. Governments have at their disposal a range of legislative measures that can limit the supply of cigarettes and promote nonsmoking behavior, including increasing taxes on tobacco products; limiting tobacco advertising and promotion; limiting the harmful ingredients in tobacco products; requiring health warnings on products and advertisements; and establishing "nonsmoking" areas.[2,8,10] Both the government and civil society can work to educate the public about the negative health effects of smoking.

Implementation of such interventions requires high levels of political commitment, as well as the determination and energy of civil society and antitobacco advocates to counter commercial interests. Tobacco companies are well financed and have played a key role in thwarting progress in tobacco control internationally.[11]

POLAND: HIGHEST CIGARETTE CONSUMPTION IN THE WORLD

Before the fall of the Berlin Wall in 1989, Poland had the highest cigarette consumption in the world. In the late 1970s, the average Pole smoked more than 3,500 cigarettes each year. Nearly three quarters of Polish men aged 20 to 60 smoked every day, and by 1982, 30% of adult women smoked regularly.[12,13]

The impact on the health of Poles was staggering. In 1990, the probability that a 15-year-old boy born in Poland would reach his 60th birthday was lower than most countries in the world—even India and China. Half of these early deaths were attributable to tobacco consumption.[12] Middle-aged Polish men had one of the highest rates of lung cancer in the world—

higher than every European country except for Hungary—and other smoking-related illnesses, such as laryngeal and oral cancer, were at all-time high levels. It is estimated that 42% of cardiovascular deaths and 71% of respiratory disease in middle-aged men were due to smoking.

Few Poles were quitting, largely because of the political and social climate of the time. Because the state-run tobacco production was a significant source of revenue, the government—which controlled information—did not fully disclose the negative consequences of smoking. As a result, Polish smokers were less informed about the dangers of smoking than most of their European neighbors. In addition, tobacco-control laws were rarely enforced, and stronger tobacco-control legislation introduced in the early 1980s was rejected by the government because it was seen as a threat to government revenue during an economic downturn.

The dramatic social, economic, and political changes ushered into Poland after the fall of communism initially exacerbated Poland's addiction to tobacco. When a market economy replaced the state-run system in 1988 and 1989, the tobacco industry was one of the first to be privatized—opening the country to the powerful influence of multinational corporations. In less than a decade, multinationals had taken over more than 90% of Poland's lucrative tobacco industry. Suddenly, cigarettes in Poland were available in abundant supply and in more tempting variety. International brands flooded the market, along with popular new domestic brands like Solidarnosc and Lady Di. Adding to their appeal, cigarettes were also cheap, less than the price of a loaf of bread—thanks to deals made between the corporations and the Polish government that kept prices down during the first half of the 1990s.

At the same time, democratic changes sweeping the country brought with them a potent force: savvy and state-of-the-art marketing. Tobacco companies poured more than $100 million into Poland, making the tobacco industry the largest advertiser in the country. The industry aggressively set out to increase consumption by 10% a year. As a result, smoking rates in the early 1990s climbed steadily, particularly among children aged 11 to 15.[17]

ROOTS OF THE TOBACCO-CONTROL MOVEMENT

As the tobacco epidemic was escalating in the early 1990s, historic changes in Poland set in motion powerful influences that helped amplify antitobacco voices.

Poland's scientific community laid the foundation of the antitobacco movement when they first established the in-country scientific evidence illustrating the devastating health impact of smoking. Research conducted in the 1980s by

the Marie Sklodowska-Curie Memorial Cancer Centre and Institute of Oncology contributed to the first Polish report on the health impact of smoking, highlighting in particular the link between smoking and the escalating cancer outbreak in Poland. The body of evidence about the harmful effects of smoking and the need for tobacco-control legislation were further strengthened through a series of international workshops and scientific conferences held in Poland.

With solid evidence now in hand, Poland's budding civil society took up the call for tobacco-control measures. Health advocates in Poland were first brought together around the antismoking cause in the 1980s as civil society was experiencing a renewal. During this time, antitobacco groups such as the Polish Anti-Tobacco Society formed and began to interact with the WHO, the International Union Against Cancer, and other international groups.

Later in the new political milieu, when nongovernmental organizations (NGOs) could freely form, Poland's civil society had an even stronger voice. In 1990, Poland hosted "A Tobacco-Free New Europe" conference of western and eastern European health advocates, which resulted in a set of policy recommendations that would later prove instrumental in shaping Poland's own antitobacco laws. Finally, the Health Promotion Foundation was established to lead health promotion and antitobacco education efforts.

The free media was essential to the success of the advocates' movement to control tobacco use. In the new democratic era, the Polish press could cover health issues, including the reporting of scientific studies illustrating the health consequences of smoking. The dissemination of this information raised awareness about the dangers of smoking and shaped public opinion about tobacco-control legislation. It also provided a venue for health advocates to broadcast special advertisements with health messages, such as how to take the steps to quit smoking.

Finally, democracy provided a window for the most powerful tool in the fight against smoking: tobacco-control legislation.

THE SMOKE CLEARS: IMPLEMENTING TOBACCO-CONTROL MEASURES

In 1991, legislation was brought to the Polish Senate, which introduced a comprehensive set of tobacco-control measures based on the recommendations from the 1990 international conference and the WHO. The motion faced intense opposition from tobacco companies, sparking a heated public debate that lasted several years. Advocates consistently defended the bill by reiterating the scientific evidence of the public health threat of smoking, while the powerful tobacco lobbies countered by emphasizing their right to advertise freely and the potential threat to Poland's economy. The tobacco lobbies poured an unprecedented amount of money into fighting the legislation, wielding a force as a special interest never before seen in Poland. Media coverage of the debates helped shape public opinion, which eventually swayed toward the health advocates—the "David" against the "Goliath" tobacco lobby.

In November 1995, the Polish parliament passed the "Law for the Protection of Public Health Against the Effects of Tobacco Use" with a huge majority of 90% of the votes. The groundbreaking legislation included:

- A ban on smoking and the sale of cigarettes in health care centers, schools, and enclosed workspaces
- A ban on the sale of tobacco products to minors under 18 years of age
- A ban on the production and marketing of smokeless tobacco
- A ban on electronic media advertising (including radio and television) and restrictions on other media
- The printing of health warnings on all cigarette packs to occupy 30% of at least two of the largest sides of the packs—the largest health warnings on cigarette packs in the world at that time
- Free provision of treatment for smoking dependence

The sweeping legislation has served as a model for other countries. The European Union followed the Polish precedent in 2003 and required similar health warnings on all cigarette packs. In 1999 and 2000, the tax on cigarettes increased 30% each year, and a total ban on advertising was passed in 1999. [†] In just a few years, Poland had transformed from one of the *least* favorable climates in Europe for tobacco controls to one of the *most* favorable.

According to legislation, Poland is required to dedicate 0.5% of all tobacco taxes to funding prevention programs. In practice, the tobacco-control movement has not received the full 0.5% allocation and continues to lobby the government for increased funds for prevention programs. However, one recipient of tobacco tax revenue, the Health Promotion Foundation, has led health education and consumer awareness efforts with a profound impact on smoking patterns in Poland. Since the early 1990s, the foundation has launched an annual campaign each November called the "Great Polish Smoke-Out" to encourage smokers to quit. For a time, the smoke-out, the largest public health campaign in Poland, included a competition that invites Poles who have quit smoking in the past year to send a postcard for the chance to win a week-long stay in Rome and a private audience with the Polish-born Pope John Paul II. The campaign attracted extensive media attention and uses television, radio, and print media to spread the core messages of how and why to quit. Throughout the year, health education promoted by schools, the Catholic Church, and local civic groups has reinforced the campaign's messages.

The campaign is popular, and 80% to 90% of Poles have heard of it. Each year, between 200,000 and 400,000 Poles credit the campaign with their successful quitting. Since the first smoke-out in 1991, more than 2.5 million Poles have permanently snuffed their cigarettes because of the campaign.

Because raising tobacco taxes has long been recognized as one of the most effective tobacco-control policy interventions, health promotion foundations like the one in Poland are becoming more common around the globe. Increasing the price of cigarettes not only keeps many from starting to smoke, but tobacco taxes can also be a source of sustained funding for tobacco control and other health promotion activities. Health promotion foundations financed by these taxes are not limited to supporting tobacco control: funds can also be used to subsidize treatment for HIV/AIDS, tuberculosis, or malaria; to conduct wider disease prevention and information campaigns; and to provide opportunities for training or other capacity building for health professionals that are otherwise unavailable.

TOBACCO CONSUMPTION AND CANCER RATES PLUMMET

Because of the extensive tobacco controls and the health education efforts, far fewer Poles now smoke. Cigarette consumption dropped 10% between 1990 and 1998. In the 1970s and 1980s, Poland had an estimated 14 million smokers, including 62% of adult men and 30% of adult women. By the end of the 1990s, this figure had dropped to less than 10 million Polish smokers, with 40% of adult men and 20% of adult women smoking.

The decline in tobacco use has led to a corresponding improvement of health in Poland. The total mortality rate in Poland, taking into account all causes of death, fell by 10% during the 1990s. The decline in smoking is credited for 30% of this reduction in deaths, translating into 10,000 fewer deaths each year. At the end of the 1990s, lung cancer rates in men aged 20 to 44 had dropped 30% from their peak levels just a decade earlier and fell 19% in middle-aged men between 45 and 64 years (see Figure 14-1). Decreased smoking rates have contributed to one third of the 20% decline in cardiovascular diseases since 1991. Infant mortality has fallen as well, and the percentage of babies born with low

---

† The impact of these additional measures is not captured in this chapter.

FIGURE 14-1 Standardized mortality rates among Polish males, 1959–1999.

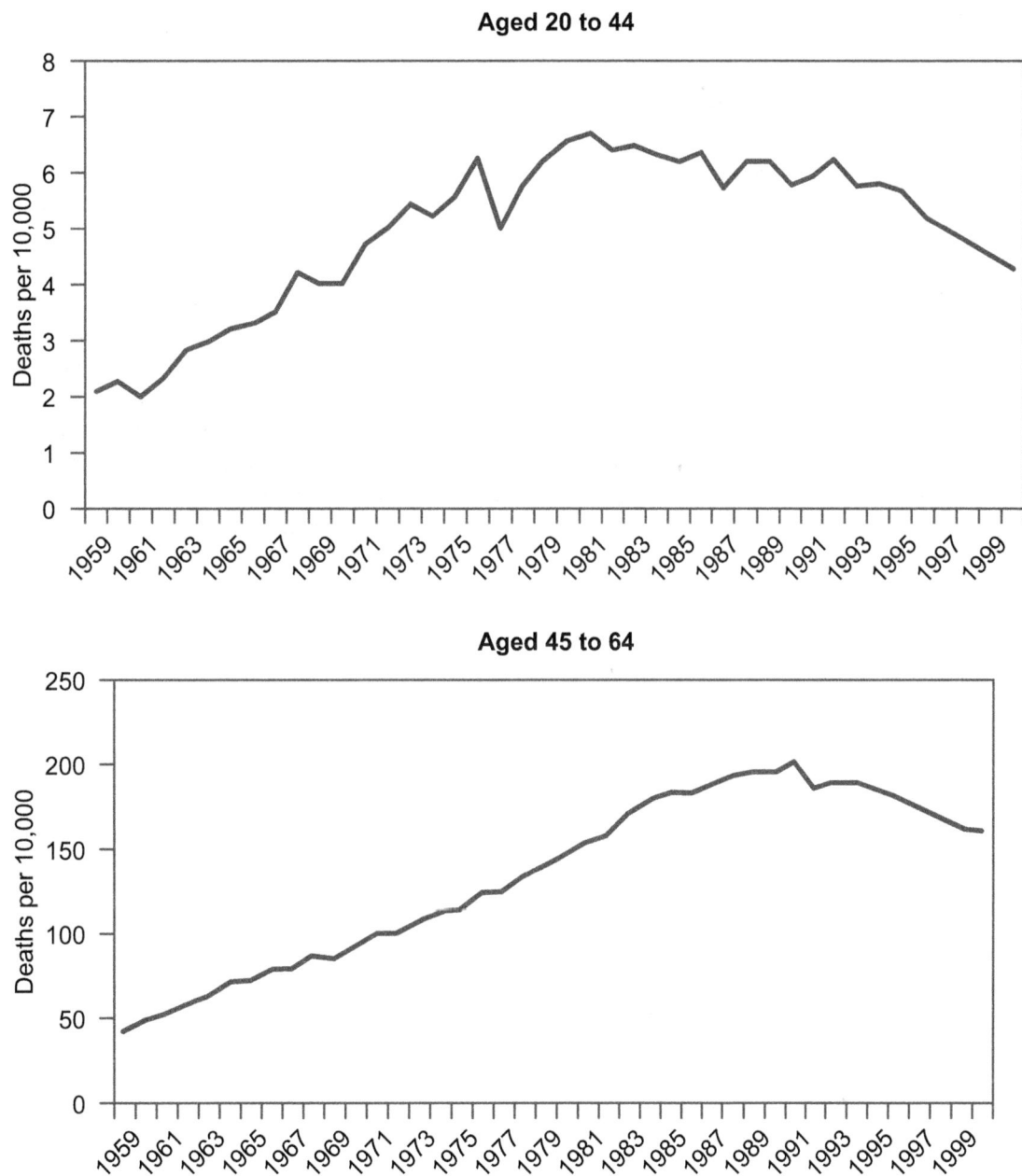

Aged 20 to 44

Aged 45 to 64

Source: Personal communication, Zatonski W, July 2, 2004.

birth weight has dropped from over 8% in 1980 to less than 6% a decade later. About one third of this reduced risk stems from decreased smoking among pregnant women. In total, life expectancy during the 1990s in Poland increased by four years for men and more than three years for women.[13]

Comparing the path of Poland with its neighbor Hungary, a country that did not implement tobacco-control measures, further illustrates the dramatic impact of Poland's efforts. In the 1980s, before Poland initiated controls and health awareness campaigns, lung cancer rates in the two countries were roughly equivalent. Throughout the 1990s, lung cancer rates in Hungary continued to climb, at the same time that they were falling by one third in Poland; today rates in Hungary have peaked at their highest levels ever for young and middle-aged residents.

STRENGTHENING TOBACCO CONTROLS WORLDWIDE

Both South Africa (Box 14-1) and Poland share a common lesson in battling tobacco. Once smoking is seen for what it is—the leading cause of preventable deaths among adults worldwide—then governments do act. They do so with a set of tools that are powerful, cost-effective, and save millions of lives.

Importantly, the national experiences of Poland and South Africa have not remained confined to the two countries. The leadership created in South Africa about tobacco control was strengthened into global leadership during five years of negotiations, which led to the world's first treaty for public health, the Framework Convention on Tobacco Control. The South African negotiating team played a decisive role in ensuring that the most effective text was accepted first by African countries—and that no watering down could be tolerated—and later by all 192 governments that adopted it in May 2003.

In May 2003, all of WHO's member states unanimously adopted the convention, indicating their commitment to stronger efforts to reduce tobacco use through many of the same interventions that proved successful in Poland and South Africa: health education, tobacco-control legislation, cigarette taxes, warnings on cigarette packs, restrictions on smoking in public places, and bans on all cigarette advertising and promotion. By the end of 2006, more than 130 countries had ratified the treaty and were beginning to implement it. Although still in its early days, the treaty has played an important role in changing the way that most governments approach tobacco use.

BOX 14-1 South Africa's Story

Until the 1990s, South Africa's tobacco industry—controlled almost entirely by one company—exerted immense power and operated virtually untouched by government restrictions or taxes. The tobacco industry was seen as a major source of government revenue, taxes, jobs, and advertising dollars. The dominant tobacco company, Rembrandt, was established in 1948, when the National Party came to power, and was seen as a symbol of Afrikaaner success in business—and therefore beyond question in policy debates about tobacco. With strong ties to the media and the apartheid government, nothing stood in its way.

When the African National Congress came to power in 1994, the antismoking movement gained a valuable ally in incoming President Nelson Mandela. Mandela had made his strong antismoking stance known during World Tobacco Day in 1992 and through his call for a "world free of tobacco." Unlike the previous Afrikaaner government, Mandela's African National Congress party had no ties to the tobacco industry and placed a much higher priority on healthcare for all. The first health minister of the new government, Nkosazana Zuma, was an ardent supporter of the tobacco-control cause and fearlessly pursued the tobacco control that her predecessor Rita Venter had begun, despite intense opposition from the industry. Even before assuming office as the minister of health in 1994, she committed the African National Congress to take a leadership role when she addressed the first All-Africa Tobacco Control Conference in Harare in 1993.

Despite the influence of the tobacco industry, public health researchers worked tirelessly to bring attention to the dangers of smoking: Professor Harry Sefterl's work from the 1970s stimulated many to recognize that unless action was taken, South Africa faced pending chronic disease epidemics. Derek Yach, a researcher who had established evidence on the economic and health impacts of smoking, collaborated in the mid-1980s with local civic groups such as the Tobacco Action Group and international partners to promote tobacco-control efforts.

The first major victory for the antitobacco movement occurred in 1995 with the passage of the Tobacco Products Control Act. The act introduced health warnings, banned smoking on public transportation, and established restrictions on youth under 16 purchasing cigarettes. Although relatively mild in reach, the legislation was an important milestone because it was the first schism between the government and the tobacco industry.

The tobacco-control policies implemented in the second half of the 1990s were bolstered by research at the University of Cape Town, which established the rationale and evidence base for increased taxes on smoking, considered by the group's researchers to be the most cost-effective and powerful way of rapidly reducing smoking. Studies demonstrated that because of the sensitivity of demand for cigarettes to changes in prices, an increase in prices would cause a decline in consumption and at the same time increase tax revenue. Health advocates argued that a tax increase of 50%—in their view necessary because the real value of taxes had fallen 70% between 1970 and 1990—would lead to 400,000 fewer smokers and an increase in tax revenue of approximately $92 million.[14,15]

In 1997, taxes on cigarettes were increased by 52%, to reach 50% of the value of the retail price of cigarettes. Between 1993 and 2001, the real value of cigarette taxes increased by 215%. In 1999, the Tobacco Products Control Amendment Bill was passed, outlawing smoking in enclosed public places, banning tobacco advertising and sponsorship, and requiring explicit health warnings on all cigarette packs.

The results of the price increases and control measures have been striking. Cigarette consumption fell from 1.9 billion packs in 1991 to 1.3 billion in 2002—a decline of more than 30%, peaking after the 1997 tax increases. The sharpest drops have been among youth and the poor, two groups that are most sensitive to changes in price. Smoking prevalence among the youth has dropped from 24% in 1993 to 19% in 2000. At the same time that consumption dropped, tax revenues in South Africa doubled since 1994.

Yach has credited the mix of basic science and political commitment with the passage of one of the world's most far-reaching tobacco-control policies. "You need the right combination of science, evidence, and politics to succeed," he explained. "If you have one without the other, you don't see action."[16]

REFERENCES

1. Peto R, Lopez AD. The future worldwide health effects of current smoking patterns. In: Koop EC, Pearson CE, Schwarz RM, eds. *Global Health in the 21st Century*. New York, NY: Jossey-Bass; 2000.

2. Jha P, Chaloupka F. The economics of global tobacco control. *BMJ*. 2000;321:358–361.

3. Peto R, Lopez A, Boreham J, Thun M, Heath C Jr. Mortality from tobacco in developed countries: indirect estimates from national vital statistics. *Lancet*. 1992;339:1268–1278.

4. Gajalakshmi V, Peto R, Kanaka TS, Jha P. Smoking mortality from tuberculosis and other diseases in India: retrospective study of 43,000 adult male deaths and 35,000 controls. *Lancet*. 2003;363:507–515.

5. Gajalakshmi CK, Jha P, Ranson L, Nguyen S. Global patterns of smoking and smoking-attributable mortality patterns. In: Jha P, Chaloupka FJ, eds. *Tobacco Control in Developing Countries*. Oxford, England: Oxford University Press; 2000.

6. Bonu S, Rani M, Nguyen S, Jha P. Household tobacco and alcohol consumption and child health in India. *Health Policy*. In press.

7. Bobak M, Jha P, Nguyen S. Poverty and smoking. In: Jha P, Chaloupka FJ, eds. *Tobacco Control in Developing Countries*. Oxford, England: Oxford University Press; 2000.

8. Jha P, Chaloupka F. *Curbing the Epidemic: Governments and the Economics of Tobacco Control*. Washington, DC: World Bank; 1999.

9. Federal Trade Commission. *Cigarette Report for 2001*. Washington, DC: Federal Trade Commission; 2003.

10. Jha P, Chaloupka F, eds. *Tobacco Control in Developing Countries*. Oxford, England: Oxford University Press; 2000.

11. Yach D, Hawkes C, Gould L, Hofman K. The global burden of chronic diseases: overcoming impediments to prevention and control. *JAMA*. 2004;291:2616–2622.

12. Zatonski W. *Evolution of Health in Poland Since 1988*. Warsaw, Poland: Marie Sklodowska-Curie Memorial Cancer Center and Institute of Oncology, Department of Epidemiology and Cancer Prevention; 1998.

13. Zatonski W, Harville E. Tobacco control in Poland. *Eurohealth*. 2000;6(2):13–15.

14. Abedian I, van der Merwe R, Wilkins N, Jha P, eds. *The Economics of Tobacco Control: Towards an Optimal Policy Mix*. Cape Town, South Africa: University of Cape Town; 1998.

15. Van Walbeek C. The tobacco epidemic can be reversed: tobacco control in South Africa during the 1990s. Available at: http://archive.idrc.ca/ritc///////SA-finalreport.pdf.. Accessed January 12, 2007.

16. Malan M, Leaver R. Political change in South Africa: new tobacco control and public health policies. In: de Beyer J, Brigden LW, eds. *Tobacco Control Policy: Strategy, Success, and Setbacks*. Washington, DC: World Bank and International Development Research Center; 2003.

Preventing Iodine-Deficiency Disease in China*

* The first draft of this case was prepared by Gail Vines.

ABSTRACT

Geographic area: China

Health condition: China bears the heaviest burden of iodine deficiency in the world. In 1995, 20% of children aged 8 to 10 showed signs of goiter. Overall, some 400 million people in China were estimated to be at risk of iodine-deficiency disorders, constituting 40% of the global total.

Global importance of the health condition today: Iodine deficiency—a range of disorders including goiter (enlarged thyroids), stillbirths, stunted growth, thyroid deficiency, and mental defects—affects 13% of the world's population, or 740 million people. Iodine deficiency is the leading cause of preventable intellectual impairment in the world and may forfeit as much as 15% of a person's intellectual potential.

Intervention or program: In 1993, China launched the National Iodine Deficiency Disorders Elimination Program to eliminate iodine deficiency, with technical and financial assistance provided through the donor-funded Iodine Deficiency Disorders Control Project. Both the programs have raised awareness of the health impact of iodine deficiency, strengthened the capacity of the salt industry to iodize and package salt, monitored and enforced the quality of the salt, and promoted compliance among the salt industry through enforcement of licensing regulations and legislation banning noniodized salt.

Cost and cost-effectiveness: Fortifying salt with iodine costs approximately 2 to 7 cents per kilogram, or less than 5% of the retail price of salt in most countries. The Chinese government invested approximately $152 million.

Impact: By 1999, iodized salt was reaching 94% of the country, up from 80% in 1995—and salt quality had improved markedly. As a result, iodine deficiency has been reduced dramatically. Total goiter rates for children aged 8 to 10 have fallen from 20.4% in 1995 to 8.8% in 1999.

Many classic public health programs affect whole communities by reducing the risk of diseases—for example, by improving water supplies or reducing exposure to environmental hazards. In such programs, individuals do not have to take action and in many instances are unaware that the program is in place while they benefit from it. Because benefits are spread out over a vast population, these programs tend to be very inexpensive on a per capita basis. A special kind of population-based program is the fortification of foods with nutrients that all need for good health.

The story of how China introduced iodized salt to prevent the multiple disabling disorders associated with iodine deficiencies represents one such program. [Others include salt fluoridation in Jamaica (Case 18) and fortification of wheat with folic acid in Chile (Case 16).] The success derives from the appropriateness of the technology and the political and financial support for start-up.

TINY AMOUNTS OF IODINE TO OFFSET HUGE HEALTH RISKS

A teaspoon of iodine, spread over a lifetime, is all that is needed to prevent a host of debilitating health problems collectively known as iodine-deficiency disorders. Although the human body needs just a minute quantity of iodine in the diet (100 to 150 micrograms each day), iodine deficiency is common throughout the world. Thirteen percent of the world's population, or 740 million people, are afflicted with iodine deficiency and suffer from a range of health problems associated with the disorder, including goiter (enlarged thyroids), stillbirths, miscarriages, neonatal and thyroid deficiency, mental defects, stunted growth, spastic weakness, and cretinism (a condition of mental retardation, deaf mutism, and short stature).[1] Furthermore, iodine deficiency is the leading cause of preventable intellectual impairment in the world, causing some 50 million people to suffer brain damage.

Iodine is essential for the proper functioning of the thyroid and for cell replication. A shortage of this micronutrient disrupts the action of the thyroid, the source of hormones that regulate body metabolism, growth, and development. Overcompensating thyroid glands become enlarged and create the visibly swollen necks known as goiter. Goiter is so frequent in many iodine-deficient countries that it has come to be regarded as normal.

During pregnancy, a severe shortage of iodine can result in stillbirths and miscarriages or babies born with spastic weakness, physical deformities, and irreversible mental retardation. After birth, iodine remains vital for optimum brain development during infancy and early childhood, and iodine-deficient people may forfeit as many as 15 IQ points—a loss of 15% of a person's intellectual potential.[2,3] Studies have also shown there is a generalized loss of IQ points among the whole population in areas with mild to moderate iodine deficiency.[4]

Iodine, an element found naturally in soil and water in many parts of the world, is scarce in many inland or mountainous regions. Many parts of the world, ranging from the Himalayas and the Andes to Central Africa, are notoriously deficient in iodine, where heavy rainfall, floods, or glacier melts have leached iodine-rich compounds out of the soil.

Fortunately, a simple technology exists to eliminate iodine deficiency: fortifying a commonly eaten food. Salt is the vehicle of choice in most parts of the world. Universally consumed daily in small but consistent amounts, salt can reach everyone, including the poorest members of the community. Moreover, mixing salt with an iodine-compound produces no discernable change in the product and is relatively cheap to produce. Although the technology of salt iodization is simple, implementation on a national scale requires a coordinated effort of political, administrative, legal, technical, and sociocultural changes.

Since the 1990s, the percentage of households in developing countries that use iodized salt has skyrocketed, climbing from less than 20% to 70% in 2000.[5] China's experience with iodine deficiency control is emblematic of this success, and the achievements in reducing the prevalence of iodine deficiency and goiter in China represent a tremendous public health success story.

CHINA: 40% OF THE WORLD'S BURDEN OF IODINE-DEFICIENCY DISORDERS

China bears the heaviest burden of iodine deficiency in the world. Studies in 1995 found that 20% of schoolchildren between the ages of 8 and 10 years had enlarged thyroid glands. Overall, some 400 million people in China were estimated to be at risk of iodine-deficiency disorders, constituting 40% of the global total.

The Chinese government spearheaded efforts in the early 1990s to address the burgeoning public health problem. The Minister of Health and other high-ranking officials became strongly committed to taking action when research showed that even mild to moderate iodine deficiencies could intellectually compromise children—posing a perceived threat to the one-child-per-family policy. In 1993, the Chinese government launched the National Iodine Deficiency Disorders Elimination Program. At the time, awareness of the dangers of iodine deficiency was weak, particularly in many regions of China at highest risk, where goiter was regarded as normal. Furthermore, people living in salt-producing regions or on salt hills did not buy salt because they did not want to pay for it. Ensuring a nationwide supply of commercially marketed iodized salt and promoting universal compliance were thus tremendous challenges.

To help China achieve its goal of eliminating iodine deficiency, the World Bank, the United Nations Children's Fund (UNICEF), the World Health Organization (WHO), and other agencies provided financial and technical assistance through the Iodine Deficiency Disorders Control Project from 1995 to 2000. The donor-funded project focused on supporting the development of technological infrastructure necessary to produce, package, and distribute iodized salt throughout the country. The Chinese government's national program as a whole entailed legal regulation, monitoring, enforcement, and public awareness campaigns.

NATIONAL EFFORT

An important first step was informing the public about the seriousness of iodine deficiency and the need to buy only iodized salt. In some communities, goiter was so commonplace that even health workers did not realize the gravity of the problem. High-level political commitment of provincial governors boosted the nationwide public health campaign, which used posters on buses, newspaper editorials, and television documentaries to inform consumers and create a demand for fortified salt. Yet consumer demand on its own could not solve the problem. Public awareness of iodine-deficiency disorders was a vital first step but just as important were measures to ensure a reliable supply of the salt.

Judicious interventions in the salt production industry have helped ensure access to iodized salt (see Box 15-1). The China National Salt Industry Corporation controls the production of edible iodized salt in each province through the licensing of salt producers (factories) and of monopoly provincial salt companies that carry out wholesale and retail packaging. The variation in organizational structures between provinces has complicated reform. Some salt factories are owned by county-level governments, as in Guansu and Liaoning, and may have limited resources. By contrast, those that are owned and run by provincial salt companies, such as Guangxi Salt Company, generally have better access to financial resources, technology, and management, thanks to profits from their control over retail packaging and distribution.

During this initiative, 55 existing salt iodation factories were upgraded to increase their production, and 112 new iodation centers were established. Some 29 new bulk packaging systems complemented 147 new retail packaging centers, with carton packaging technology installed at two locations, which enabled consumers to easily recognize iodized salt. The technology for manufacturing modern packing machines was transferred from Europe to a local machinery-manufacturing firm. The domestic firm can now make the machinery required to meet future demands within China and will be in a position to compete in the international market, given its cost advantages.

The central and provincial governments in China have taken an active role in promoting compliance in the salt industry through the enforcement of licensing regulations and through legislation banning the sale of edible noniodized salt. Both government persuasion and direct assistance were necessary to motivate the salt industry to comply with iodation. As a first step, the central government made provincial governors aware of the seriousness of the problem, stimulating prompt action that reached even remote villages. The government also provided technological assistance that enabled licensed salt producers to readily adopt iodation.

Effective monitoring and enforcement, in addition to adequate incentives for industry compliance, are needed for the enforcement of quality control. First, production must be monitored because the amount of iodine added to salt matters: too little, and the treated salt is ineffective; too much, and it could be deleterious. Furthermore, distribution and retail sales must be monitored. Consumers cannot detect fraud, and because iodine in salt dissipates easily, the packaging, storage, and shelf life of the salt must be monitored to ensure adequate iodine levels. Hence, enforcement of quality controls is of paramount importance to the long-term success of salt iodation.

In China, the ability to hold producers accountable is strong, thanks to the concentration of production and distribution in a nationally controlled network. Provincial salt companies that produce iodized salt cooperate with local police to expose dealers of illegal salt operations, who accounted for about 10% of the Chinese salt market in 1998. In Wuxi and many other cities, salt inspectors patrol each day to sample salt in retail stores, restaurants, hotels, and households. The crackdown has been successful, and many illegal salt dealers have been apprehended. In any case, more than half of the "illegal salt" is itself iodized, having been smuggled out of the factories.

The more dangerous illicit commodity—noniodized salt—is either industrial salt fraudulently passed off as edible salt or raw salt consumed by local people living near salt hills or by the sea. In provinces such as Fujian, Guangdong, and Liaoning, where sea salt is traditionally produced, the China National Salt Industry Corporation encouraged selling this raw salt to refinement centers for iodation. Such interventions support small producers while at the same time reducing the amount of noniodized salt on the market. Pricing strategies are also important; smuggling of noniodized salt between provinces is inadvertently encouraged because quality salt is more costly in some provinces compared with others.

MAJOR HEALTH IMPACT

By the end of 2000, substantial progress had been made toward achieving universal salt iodation, and as a result the virtual elimination of iodine-deficiency disorders in China. By 1999, iodized salt was reaching 94% of the country, compared with 80% in 1995. Moreover, as a result of the government's program the quality of iodized salt has improved. Salt samples with an iodine content of 20 to 60 parts per million—considered high quality— increased from 30% in 1995 to 81% in 1999.

BOX 15-1 Salt Iodation in Madagascar

Iodine deficiency is also being tackled successfully in Madagascar, in a strikingly different social and industrial setting. In 1995, when salt iodation began, iodine deficiency was widespread, especially among the poorest communities living in the highlands. Nationwide, goiter rates among primary schoolchildren stood at 45%. The Nutrition Services of Madagascar's Ministry of Health and the United Nations Children's Fund designed a national iodine deficiency control program in Madagascar with World Bank assistance worth $1 million between 1993 and 1998.

Iodized salt was first introduced in Madagascar in 1995. In just four years, the proportion of households with iodized salt rose from zero to more than 98%. Over the same period, goiter rates among primary schoolchildren fell from 45% to 7%. Iodine levels in children's urine have also been monitored, with levels above 100 micrograms per liter a sign of adequate intake. In 1992, none of the children tested reached this level, while in 1998 an encouraging 91% did.

The program's success in increasing coverage with iodized salt stems from the primarily voluntary compliance of the large and medium-sized salt companies on the island. A handful of producers dominate the salt industry in Madagascar: One very large company, partially owned by the government, produces more than 40% of the country's salt. Four medium-sized companies manufacture another 35%, and a number of small companies produce the remaining 25%.

All the producers were targeted by the program and offered training and educational workshops, potassium iodate solution at no cost (until 2000), and leased iodating equipment. Since medium-sized producers have incentives to produce iodized salt to protect their market share in a competitive environment, they voluntarily complied. Furthermore, monitoring the five largest producers was also made easier by their small number. The Ministry of Health and Ministry of Commerce participate in monitoring and enforcement, publicizing their "check-and-seize" operations.

The program has had less success at enforcing compliance and quality control among small producers. Most of these small producers, scattered across the vast southwest coastal region, do not produce salt regularly, and when they do it is often wet, dirty, and noniodized. They sell their salt at a much lower price to distributors and have no incentives to use or repair their communal iodating equipment. Much of this poor quality salt is sold in the highland regions, where goiter is a common affliction. One solution may be for the authorities to consider shifting their focus from noncomplying small salt producers to distributors. "Small salt producers are numerous, elusive, and uncontrollable, whereas distributors are few and more manageable," reports Chor-ching Goh, a World Bank economist. "Authorities can provide disincentives—confiscation or fines—to discourage wholesale distributors from purchasing noniodized salt."[1] If distributors universally demand iodized salt, in time, virtually every salt producer should be motivated to iodize.

The health impact has been striking: Surveys of schoolchildren in 1995, 1997, and 1999 showed dramatic reductions in iodine deficiency. Across the country, far fewer children now show signs of goiter. Total goiter rates for schoolchildren aged between 8 and 10 have fallen, from 20.4% in 1995 to 8.8% in 1999 (see Table 15-1).

ECONOMIC IMPACT

In 1993, the World Bank's *World Development Report* estimated that a comprehensive and sustainable approach to address micronutrient deficiencies would cost less that 0.3% of GNP a year. Yet these deficiencies continue to have a substantial economic impact throughout much of the developing world; as much as 5% of GNP of many countries may be lost to deaths, disability, lower educational attainment, and decreased productivity. For China, this amounts to a loss of approximately $50 billion from micronutrient deficiencies, including iodine deficiency.[6]

The total cost of the salt iodation program in China is difficult to estimate, not least because costs are distributed across many government agencies, and practices vary across the country. In Hunan and Tianjin, for instance, provincial governments reimburse their health bureaus for carrying out tests on salt samples, while in other provinces salt testing is financed by the salt industry itself or shared between the industry and the health sector.

Costs of iodation itself are low, once the technology is in place—normally in the range of 2 to 7 cents per kilogram, which is less than 5% of the retail price of salt in most countries. But the industry must also provide laboratory monitoring to ensure quality control backed by a team of inspectors in the marketplace. Some estimates place the government's investment at approximately $152 million. To help finance

TABLE 15-1 Main Indicators of Iodine Status in China, 1995, 1997, and 1999

INDICATOR	1995	1997	1999
Iodized salt			
National mean coverage (percent)	80.2	90.2	93.9
Percentage of qualified iodated salt samples with:			
Iodine level > 20 ppm	39.9	81.1	88.9
Iodine level 20 to 60 ppm	29.7	69.0	80.6
Urinary iodine content among schoolchildren aged 8 to 10			
Median household iodine level (parts per million)	16.2	37.0	42.3
Average (µg/L)	164.8	330.2	306.0
Percentage with iodine content < 50 µg/L	13.3	3.5	3.3
Number of provinces with median iodine < 100 µg/L	5.0	1.0	1.0
Total goiter rates among schoolchildren aged 8 to 10 (percent)			
Tested by palpation	20.4	10.9	8.8
Tested with B-ultrasound	—	9.6	8.0
Grade 2 goiter	2.1	0.5	0.3

Source: Chor-ching (2002).[†]

† Reprinted with permission from the UNU *Food and Nutrition Bulletin* 2002;23:280–291.

this investment, the Chinese government set a new higher price for quality iodized salt; this price increase was estimated to represent less than 1% of the household budget and therefore affordable for most families. The World Bank deemed the project—financed with approximately $20 million from the Bank—extremely cost-effective, costing between 4 and 5 cents per beneficiary in external funding. Its success in saving lives and dollars has made China's iodation experience a model for other fortification interventions (see Box 15-2).

COMMITMENT AND REMAINING CHALLENGES

China's program to eliminate iodine-deficiency disorders continues, and a very high commitment to enforcing regulation on universal salt iodization in China remains. The country maintained a high national mean coverage—95% in 2002—for adequate iodized salt. Schoolchildren are regularly monitored for urinary iodine, and in 2002 the average urinary iodine (µg/L) was 241. It is estimated that only 16% of the population has low levels of urinary iodine (less than 100 µg/L) (Rae Galloway, personal communication, May 12, 2006).

The central government has pledged to retain control of the salt industry over at least the next decade, and in October 2003 China hosted an international conference to renew its commitment to eliminating iodine deficiency. To ensure success, the adequacy of iodine in salt must continue to be monitored and incentives must be modified as needed to increase compliance rates in the salt industry. Because national coverage of iodized salt reached over 90% in 2001, central and local governments concentrate on targeting resources where consumption of iodized salt is still low: the poor and remote mountainous areas in western China where fewer than half the people consume iodized salt and instead use cheaper, locally produced raw salt.

In China, local authorities in several provinces, including Guangxi, Hebei, and Shandong, have convinced residents in remote mountainous regions to buy iodized salt delivered directly to their villages. However, in provinces where local officials were not committed to the program, wholesalers were not paid and deliveries ceased. Similar problems arise in regions where inhabitants have easy access to salt hills, dehydrated salt lakes (as in Xinjian), or sea salt (as in Jiangsu) and are reluctant to pay for salt.

In such situations, careful research will be needed to find out why local people are not consuming iodized salt,

BOX 15-2 Untapped Potential? DEC-Salt Fortification to Prevent Lymphatic Filariasis

Just as one of the most common substances on earth, salt, was used as the vehicle to carry iodine to communities with evidence of iodine deficiency, so it has been tested to treat or prevent other diseases. Experiences in China and several other countries have shown that fortifying salt with a compound called diethylcarbamazine (DEC) can help eliminate lymphatic filariasis, a mosquito-transmitted parasitic disease. Causing painful genital enlargement and elephantiasis, lymphatic filariasis is responsible for the loss of approximately 4.6 million DALYs per year.[7] Along with the physical discomfort caused by the disease, those infected with the disease often fall victim to social isolation and poverty.

Distribution of DEC tablets to individuals poses logistical challenges, and early experiences suggest that DEC salt is an attractive option for controlling the disease in endemic areas. In the 1970s, the approximately 13,000 inhabitants of Taiwan's Quemoy Islands were treated with DEC-fortified salt for six months as a final step in eliminating the disease. Follow-up surveys until 1982 showed that people who had consumed the fortified salt had no microfilaria in their blood, and thus could not transmit the disease.[8]

A larger experience in China demonstrates that DEC-fortified salt can be extremely effective as a complement to mass drug distribution. Despite its vast population and high prevalence rates of lymphatic filariasis in many provinces, this combination of approaches was successful in eliminating this infection in China, which has had no evidence of new cases or of transmission for over five years.[9]

As in the case of iodization in China, fortifying salt with DEC can be extremely cost-effective. Compared with administration of DEC in tablet form, which can cost between $4.40 to $8.10 per DALY averted, DEC-fortified salt is estimated to cost $1.10 to $3.62.[7]

and alternative remedies adopted. If price is a deterrent, subsidies may be the solution. In some cases, increasing public awareness may be sufficient to ensure compliance, but other ways of providing iodine—through well or irrigation water, for instance—may be more effective. Alternatively, the old-fashioned way of distributing iodine, in capsules containing iodized oil or via long-lasting injections, may particularly suit nomads living in remote regions. Through a variety of approaches, China is fast approaching the day when iodine deficiency will be unknown throughout its population.

A CLASSIC PUBLIC HEALTH SUCCESS

The success of the fortified salt program in China in reducing iodine-deficiency disorders offers lessons to future public health campaigns targeting other micronutrient deficiencies such as iron and vitamin A. The Chinese government aligned social goals with the salt industry, and the health sector successfully built a commitment to eliminate iodine deficiency. Concurrently, the salt industry seized the opportunity of the investment in iodine deficiency elimination to restructure and modernize the industry, which put it on a firmer technical and commercial footing. Donor coordination was strong and effective, managed by the Chinese government and the donors themselves, and the major players offered mutual support across all activities. In addition, the financing strategy was clearly defined first. Most important, the Chinese government, on all levels, made a firm and long-standing commitment to eliminating iodine deficiency, allowing all sectors across the country to work together to achieve impressive results.

REFERENCES

1. Chor-ching G. Combating iodine deficiency: lessons from China, Indonesia, and Madagascar. *Food Nutr Bull.* 2002;23(3):280–290.

2. World Health Organization. *Nutrition—Micronutrient Deficiencies: Iodine Deficiency Disorders.* Available at: http://www.who.int/nutrition/topics/idd/en/. Accessed January 12, 2007.

3. Bleichrodt N, Borni M. A meta-analysis of research on iodine and its relationship to cognitive development. In: Stanbury JB, ed. *The Damaged Brain of Iodine Deficiency.* Elmsford, NY: Cognizant Communication; 1994.

4. Ma T, Wang D, Chen ZP. Mental retardation other than typical cretinism in IDD endemias in China. In: Stanbury JB, ed. *The Damaged Brain of Iodine Deficiency.* Elmsford, NY: Cognizant Communication; 1994.

5. United Nations Children's Fund. Iodine deficiency still leaves millions of children at risk of mental retardation. Press release, October 15, Beijing. Available at: http://www.unicef.org/media/media_14979.html. Accessed January 12, 2007.

6. World Bank. *World Development Indicators 2002.* New York, NY: World Bank Publishing; 2002.

7. Remme JHF, Feenstra P, Lever PR, et al. Tropical diseases targeted for elimination: Chagas disease, lymphatic filariasis, onchocerciasis, and leprosy. In: Jamison DT, Breman JG, Measham AR, et al, eds. *Disease Control Priorities in Developing Countries.* 2nd ed. New York, NY: Oxford University Press; 2006:433–450.

8. Fan PC. Filariasis eradication on Kinmen Proper, Kinmen (Quemoy) Islands, Republic of China. *Acta Tropica.* 1990;47(3):161–169.

9. Editorial Board of Control of Lymphatic Filariasis in China. Control of lymphatic filariasis in China. Manilla, Philippines: World Health Organization, Western Pacific Region; 2003.

CASE **16**

Preventing Neural-Tube Defects in Chile*

*Case drafted by Jessica Gottlieb.

ABSTRACT

Geographic area: Chile

Health condition: Neural-tube defects (NTDs), the second most common congenital malformation after congenital heart disease, affected about 400 babies in Chile per year in the years before the fortification intervention. The NTD rate of 17.2 per 10,000 live births had been unchanged from 1967 to 1999.

Global importance of the health condition today: Each year, neural-tube defects affect more than 300,000 newborns worldwide. Anencephaly and spina bifida, the two most common NTDs, are important contributors to infant and fetal mortality: All infants with anencephaly are stillborn or die shortly after birth, and those born with spina bifida suffer lifelong disabilities and require extensive medical care.

Intervention or program: Aware of the effect of folic acid on the prevention of neural-tube defects and encouraged by public health experts, the Chilean Ministry of Health introduced new legislation in early 2000 stipulating that all domestically produced wheat flour must be fortified with folic acid. Flour mills began producing, distributing, and marketing wheat flour in compliance with the new legislation, and the government helped to regulate and monitor the quality of fortified flour.

Cost and cost-effectiveness: With existing technologies, the cost of adding folic acid to the premix for fortified flour is approximately 15 cents per ton of wheat flour, making the cost of fortification only 16 cents per woman of reproductive age receiving the target amount of folic acid. With the total cost of rehabilitation for a child affected with spina bifida averaging $100,000, Chile's health system saved an estimated $11 million per year (based on 110 cases in one year).

Impact: Shortly after the fortification legislation was passed, 91% of wheat bread was being produced with fortified flour. A year later, blood folate levels in women of reproductive age increased three- to fourfold. Chile's fortification intervention produced a dramatic decrease of the NTD rate—a reduction of approximately 51% for spina bifida and 46% for anencephaly.

Chile, a country credited for its rapid social and economic progress relative to its Latin American neighbors, again asserted its leadership in public health when in the year 2000 the government successfully implemented the cost-saving fortification of wheat flour with folic acid to prevent neural-tube defects, a congenital malformation. Like other micronutrient programs, the low cost of inputs and the large scale of reach and impact add up to unbeatable cost-effectiveness. In this case, Chile's evidence-based approach to identifying promising interventions, and rapid rollout, resulted in both better health of children and savings to the health system through the prevention of one common type of birth defect, neural-tube defects.

DISABILITIES AS A HEALTH PRIORITY

Birth defects, along with learning, physical, and developmental disabilities of many types, are estimated to affect 10% to 20% of children and are increasingly recognized as an important public policy concern in low- and middle-income countries such as Chile, which has the second highest rate of disability prevalence in the region next to Brazil.[1] Recent decades have seen major advances addressing infectious diseases, but few programs focused on prevention of long-term disabilities. Governments are increasingly seeking ways to provide (often high-cost) support to those children and families affected and, when possible, to prevent the disabilities in the first place. The fortification of pregnant women's staple foods with folic acid has been identified as one of the most viable and cost-effective interventions in low- and middle-income countries to prevent congenital anomalies.[2]

Folic acid fortification has proven successful in countries such as the United States and Canada. Since 1995, the US Centers for Disease Control and Prevention (CDC) has recommended that women of childbearing age consume 400 micrograms of folic acid daily before conception and continuing into pregnancy. Because the synthetic folic acid added to fortified foods is more "bioavailable" or about twice as effective as naturally occurring folate, fortified foods and supplements are preferred to changes in diet. Since 1998, the US Food and Drug Administration (FDA) has mandated that certain foods such as cereals, breads, and pastas be "enriched" or fortified with 140 micrograms of folic acid per 100 grams of grain.[3] A study in 2001 estimated that the folic acid fortification program in the United States contributed to a 19% decline in birth prevalence of neural-tube defects.[4]

NEURAL-TUBE DEFECTS

Each year, neural-tube defects (NTDs), the second most common congenital malformation after congenital heart disease, affect more than 300,000 newborns worldwide.[5] NTDs generally occur in the first 28 days of pregnancy when the fetus' neural tube or spine fails to close properly. This results in the incomplete development of the brain, spinal cord, or their protective coverings. Anencephaly and spina bifida are the two most common NTDs and are important contributors to infant and fetal mortality. All infants with anencephaly are stillborn or die shortly

after birth. Those born with spina bifida have a chance at surviving, but only with extensive medical care. If infants with spina bifida do survive, they are likely to have severe, lifelong disabilities.

Few known measures can treat problems resulting from the failure of the neural tube to close, and dealing with the problem on a population level requires preventive interventions. As demonstrated in the United States and Canada, consumption of the B vitamin folic acid before conception and during early pregnancy can significantly reduce the number of NTDs occurring in newborns. Large-scale interventions have been found to reduce the prevalence of NTDs by as much as 50%.

AN OUNCE OF PREVENTION

In Chile, one quarter to one third of all health care costs for catastrophic events occur in the neonatal period and represent the single largest demand on health care.[6] Catastrophic health conditions such as congenital malformations not only are a burden on the nation's health care system, but also represent a substantial proportion of the household's income and are rarely covered sufficiently by insurance plans. At very low cost, Chile's decision to fortify wheat flour to prevent children from being born with neural-tube defects relieved a tragic and expensive burden on families and on the Chilean health care system.

In spite of recent declines in Chile's infant mortality rate, the rate of congenital malformations went unchanged in the years prior to the fortification intervention. About 400 babies affected with NTDs were born in Chile each year, and the NTD rate of 17.2 per 10,000 live births was unchanged from 1967 to 1999.[7]

NTD rates in the United States before its fortification interventions were significantly lower than those in Chile. This difference can be attributed, in part, to low consumption in Chile of the vegetables and fresh fruits containing naturally occurring folate, as well as cooking habits.[8] In addition, families in the United States and other countries may choose to terminate pregnancies upon prenatal diagnosis of NTDs, but termination of pregnancies for any reason is forbidden by law in Chile.

High prevalence of NTDs implies not only high mortality, particularly for anencephaly, but also extremely high costs of clinical care and management for complications of spina bifida. In addition to the physical and emotional tolls upon the family, surgery, clinical care, and rehabilitation for each spina bifida patient is estimated to cost about US$120,000 in Chile from birth to 18 years of age.

THE DEVELOPMENT OF AN NTD PREVENTION STRATEGY

In Chile, where folate supplements and fortified breakfast cereals and other commercial products are out of reach for most income groups, it was necessary to develop a new method of reaching pregnant women with folic acid. "Aware of the effect of folic acid on the prevention of neural-tube defects, in 1997 a group of academics from Chile's Institute of Nutrition and Food Technology convinced authorities from the Ministry of Health to convene a working group to evaluate the feasibility of implementing folic acid fortification to prevent NTDs," says Eva Hertrampf, one of the leading academics from the institute, known as INTA. The working group, composed of academics (pediatricians, nutritionists, geneticists, food technologists), industry representatives (millers, premix vendors, pharmacists), and professionals from the Ministry of Health (representatives from the nutrition unit, monitoring, and primary child care programs) recommended that Chile adopt the fortification of wheat flour with folic acid to prevent NTDs. As later happened in Mexico with milk fortification (see Text Box 16-1), strong evidence was marshaled by the research community to support the government's decision to introduce an important nutrition intervention.

Wheat flour fortification appeared to be the best option for a number of reasons. First, wheat flour is a staple food in Chile; 90% of it is consumed as bread. It is estimated that Chileans eat about 160 g of wheat flour per day, the equivalent of eight slices of wheat bread.[7] Second, Chilean mills have been fortifying wheat flour with micronutrients since the 1950s and even before that with baking aids and whiteners.[10] These early experiences with fortification were important for both economic and technical reasons. Because the mills were already equipped with the requisite equipment, it was much less costly to introduce folic acid to the premix for flour at the time the new fortification intervention was introduced. The Ministry of Health also had quality controls in place since 1967 when it became mandatory to fortify flour with iron. A national laboratory controls quality by randomly sampling wheat flour for analysis on a regular basis.

In January 2000, the Chilean Ministry of Health introduced new legislation stipulating that folic acid must be added to the premix. The level of mandated folic acid, 2.2 mg/kg, was tailored to the target group for the intervention. If women of childbearing age consumed the estimated average amount of fortified wheat flour, they would receive the 400 µg/day of folic acid recommended for the prevention of NTDs.

The government, the food industry, and the mills each

BOX 16-1 The Influence Potential of Evidence: Milk Fortification in Mexico

As with wheat flour fortification, Chile was a regional leader in milk fortification. In the 1980s, Chile began fortifying milk with iron and distributing it to infants with the result of significant reductions in anemia.[10] This experience was one of the influences behind a recent decision in Mexico to fortify milk with micronutrients to address observed problems in child malnutrition.

In 1999, the results of a national nutrition survey in Mexico signaled a serious problem: Despite significant investments in health and nutrition throughout the 1990s, a large share of Mexican children, especially those in rural and primarily indigenous areas, still suffered from malnutrition. One in four children suffered from anemia, and up to half of children exhibited signs of other micronutrient deficiencies.

These research findings helped influence decision making by government leaders. When presented with the poor nutrition findings, the Ministry of Health decided to coordinate with the Ministry of Social Development, which was responsible for many poverty reduction programs that had nutrition components. Knowing of successful milk fortification programs, public health researchers seized this opportunity to recommend that the Social Development Ministry take advantage of an existing milk distribution program and fortify the milk with micronutrients.

For 30 years, the Community Milk Supply Program (Programa de Abasto Social de Leche), implemented by the Liconsa company, had provided subsidized milk to as many as 4.6 million Mexican children. As a result of the collaboration between the public health researchers and the two government ministries, a fortification component was added to the Liconsa milk distribution program in late 2002. The new program, *Liconsa fortificada*, distributed fortified milk with appropriate amounts of iron, zinc, vitamin C, and folic acid to compensate for the deficiency of these micronutrients in children's diets. Beneficiaries of the program were chosen according to socioeconomic and demographic studies that focused on geographic zones with a high prevalence of malnutrition. Early results of the program indicate a decrease in the prevalence of anemia from 27% to 17% and the prevalence of iron deficiency from 20% to 4% among children aged 12–24 months who consumed the fortified milk.[11]

played a part in the rollout of the legislative mandate. The mills had the most immediate role in implementing folic acid fortification. Thanks to their early involvement in the decision to fortify wheat flour and the small size of the milling community, little advocacy by the health authorities was required to turn the legislative mandate into action. The food industry was responsible for producing, distributing, and marketing wheat flour in compliance with the regulations of the government. To ensure the effectiveness of the fortification intervention and to continually inform program design, the government was charged with the responsibility of regulating and monitoring the quality of fortified flour.

EVALUATING THE IMPACT OF THE FORTIFICATION PROGRAM

With much of the current impact data on folic acid fortification derived from the United States and Canada, the Chilean intervention offered an opportunity to measure program impact in a middle-income country. The evaluation of Chile's experience was important not only to Chilean authorities, but also to neighboring Latin American countries that could utilize the results to pursue similar fortification programs.[13]

Researchers at the University of Chile's Institute of Nutrition and Food Technology collaborated with the University of Florida to undertake an impact evaluation with support from the Pan-American Health Organization, the March of Dimes, the US CDC, and the Chilean Ministry of Health. The researchers considered two outcomes—bread folate content and folate status in women of childbearing age—and one type of impact—the frequency of NTD in the population. Bread folate content was measured by testing the folic acid content of bread at 50 randomly selected bakeries in the capital, Santiago, three and six months after the mandate to fortify with folic acid. Through folate extraction methods, the researchers determined that shortly after the 2000 mandate by the Ministry of Health, 91% of bread sampled was produced with fortified flour.

Ten months after the fortification mandate, a study was conducted on the folate status of 605 women of reproductive age in Santiago. Researchers discovered a three- to fourfold increase in blood folate levels in these women, demonstrating that consumption of a food staple fortified with folic acid effectively improves folate status. As expected, the women in the study indicated that they did not consume other foods fortified with folic acid or supplements because they were culturally unacceptable, scarce, and economically infeasible. The increases in folate levels can thus be attributed to the introduction of folic acid in the wheat flour they regularly

consume (see Figure 16-1). Nearly half of women of reproductive age were at risk of folate deficiency before the fortification intervention, but very few neared these levels after the intervention.

In spite of encouraging results from these intermediate outcomes, the real impact of the folic acid fortification program was determined by measuring the prevalence of neural-tube defects in the Chilean population. A surveillance system for congenital malformations had been in place in Chile for more than 30 years and was able to provide data on some births, but not enough. In 1999, the CDC helped finance a hospital-based surveillance system in nine public hospitals to register NTDs. Because nearly all deliveries occur in institutional settings, this new system was able to account for 25% of all births in Chile. Evidence from both surveillance sources indicated that NTD rates were at 17 per 10,000 live births before fortification. After wheat flour fortification with folic acid was mandated in 2000, the surveillance demonstrated a dramatic decrease of the NTD rate in Chile to 10 per 10,000 live births—an approximate 51% decrease for spina bifida and 46% decrease for anencephaly.[†]

To determine whether this observed decrease could be attributed to the folic acid fortification program or a preexisting trend, a group of Brazilian researchers who have conducted a congenital malformation surveillance study since the 1980s in Latin America analyzed their findings. Based on a population survey from two prefortification periods (1982–1989 and 1990–2000), the researchers determined that NTD prevalence rates were not decreasing in Chile before the mandate to fortify wheat flour with folic acid. In addition, the rates of decrease after fortification are comparable to decreases in prevalence in other countries with folic acid fortification programs such as Canada and the United States.[13]

AT ALMOST NO COST

Thanks to existing technologies, the cost of adding folic acid to the premix for fortified flour is very low, approximately 15 cents per ton of wheat flour. The cost of fortification was only 16 cents per woman of reproductive age receiving the target amount of folic acid. This implies that two cases of NTDs prevented per year would recover the annual fortification cost.[14] With NTDs being cut by more than 40% per year, the fortification intervention more than paid for itself.

---

† Rates included the prevalence of the main three types of NTD: anencephaly, encephalocele, and spina bifida. Encephalocele decreased by only 26%, which explains the greater decreases in anencephaly and spina bifida.

Adding an average of less than 0.5% to the retail price of wheat flour, this cost was easily absorbed by the milling industry. Because the mills already had most of the machinery and quality controls in place, relatively little overhead cost was associated with the addition of folic acid to the other micronutrients already used in fortification processes. The considerable cost of research, data collection, and information-sharing needed to support Chile's fortification intervention was made possible by contributions from donor agencies and benefited many beyond Chile's borders. With the milling industry taking on the minor costs of fortification and the total cost of rehabilitation for a child affected with spina bifida averaging $100,000, Chile's health system saved an estimated $11 million per year (based on 110 cases in one year).[15]

A SUCCESS BUILT ON PARTNERSHIP

Key to Chile's success in its folic acid fortification program was a strong alliance among partners in the public and private sectors. This exemplary public-private partnership was fostered by a clear understanding of roles and responsibilities as well as a strong sense of the imperative to collaborate to achieve effective planning, implementation, and sustainability of the program.

The government provided the enabling legislation and the regulatory apparatus to support micronutrient fortification in the public and private sectors. Academics at the national level contributed to the success through advocacy, monitoring, and impact evaluation efforts. And the milling industry enabled fortification through advanced technological capacity. Collaboration between partners was positively influenced by existing linkages between the research community and public health agencies in Chile. The private sector also has a long history of supporting research and development and interacting with legislators.

Chile's success has been contagious. "The long tradition of fortification in Chile inspired ALIM," says Hertrampf, referring to the Latin American Association of Industrial Millers, established in 1982 to harmonize quality procedures and combat unfair competitive practices. Spurred by advocates within PAHO, the US Agency for Inernational Development (USAID), the World Bank, and UNICEF, ALIM advanced the fortification agenda in 1997 when its association millers agreed to support the mandatory fortification of wheat flour.

Chile's recent success with folic acid fortification continues to inspire. In 2001, Argentina adopted mandatory fortifica-

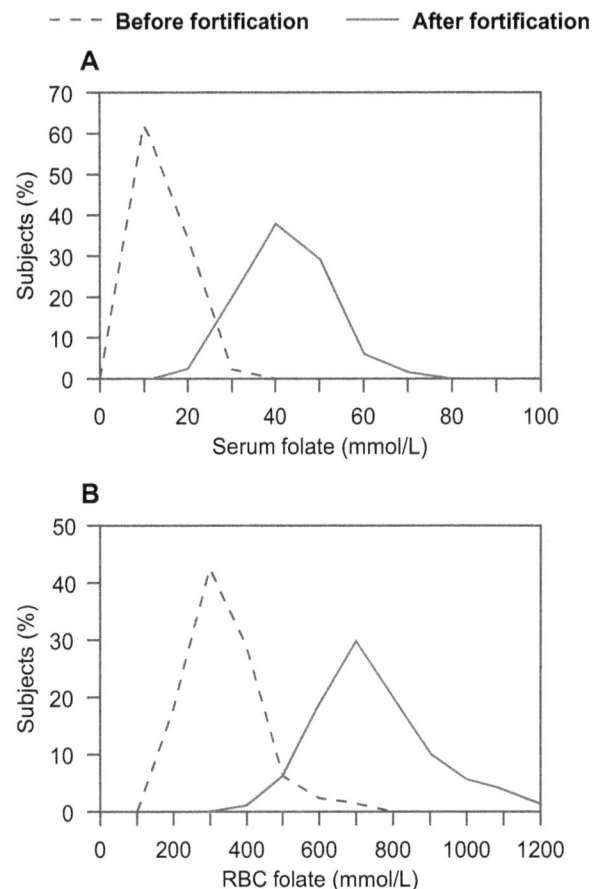

FIGURE 16-1 Serum (A) and red blood cell folate (B) levels in women of reproductive age before and after folic acid fortification, Santiago, Chile, 1999–2001.[13]

tion of wheat flour with folic acid. And in October 2003, Chile's Institute of Human Nutrition and Food Technology cosponsored a conference with PAHO and the CDC to standardize and strengthen similar programs in neighboring countries. Since then, almost every Latin American country has implemented a regulation to fortify wheat flour with folic acid.

REFERENCES

1. Inter-American Development Bank. Data on disability. Available at: http://www.iadb.org/sds/SOC/site_6215_e.htm. Accessed January 12, 2007.

2. Durkin M, Schneider H, Pathania VS, et al. Learning and developmental disabilities. In: Jamison DT, Breman JG, Measham AR, et al, eds. *Disease Control Priorities in Developing Countries.* 2nd ed. New York: Oxford University Press; 2006:933–952.

3. March of Dimes. Increased use of folic acid could cut brain and spinal cord birth defects by as much as 70 percent. Available at: http://www.marchofdimes.com/aboutus/14458_18069.asp Accessed January 12, 2007.

4. Honein MA, Paulozzi LJ, Mathews TJ, Erickson JD, and Wong LY. Impact of folic acid fortification of the US food supply on the occurrence of neural-tube defects. *JAMA.* 2001;285(23):2981–2986.

5. Botto LD, Moore CA, Khoury MJ, Erickson JD. Medical progress: neural-tube defects. *N Engl J Med.* 1999;341(20):1509–1519.

6. World Bank, Human and Social Development Group: Argentina, Chile, and Uruguay Country Management Unit. *Chile Health Insurance Issues: Old Age and Catastrophic Health Costs.* Washington, DC: World Bank; 2000. Report 19940.

7. Pan American Health Organization. Flour fortification with iron, folic acid and vitamin B12. Regional meeting report; October 9–10, 2003; Santiago, Chile. Washington, DC: Pan American Health Organization.

8. Allen LH. Folate and vitamin B12 status in the Americas. *Nutr Rev.* 2004;62(6):S29–S33.

9. Darnton-Hill I, Mora JO, Weinstein H, Wilbur S, Nalubola PR. Iron and folate fortification in the Americas to prevent and control micronutrient malnutrition: an analysis. *Nutr Rev.* 1999;57(1):25–31.

10. Stekel A, Olivares M, Cayazzo M, Chadud P, Llaguno S, and Pizarro F. Prevention of iron deficiency by milk fortification. II. A field trial with a full-fat acidified milk. *Am J Clin Nutr.* 1988;2:265–269.

11. Rivera J. Improving nutrition in Mexico: the use of research for decision making in nutrition policies and programs. In: Freire WB, ed. *Nutrition and an Active Life: From Knowledge to Action.* Washington, DC: Pan American Health Organization; 2005. Scientific and Technical Publication, No. 216;183–204.

12. Hertrampf E, Cortes F, Erickson JD, et al. Consumption of folic acid-fortified bread improves folate status in women of reproductive age in Chile. *J Nutr.* 2003;133(10):3166–3169.

13. López-Camelo JS, Orioli IM, da Graca Dutra M, et al. Reduction of birth prevalence rates of neural-tube defects after folic acid fortification in Chile. *Am J Med Genetics.* 2005;135A:120–125.

14. Hertrampf E, Cortés F. Folic acid fortification of wheat flour: Chile. *Nutr Rev.* 2004;62(6):S44–S48.

15. Hertrampf E. Folic acid fortification of wheat flour and the prevention of neural-tube defects in Chile: a successful experience. In: Freire WB, ed. *Nutrition and an Active Life: From Knowledge to Action.* Washington, DC: Pan-American Health Organization; 2005. Scientific and Technical Publication, No. 216;93–105.

Eliminating Measles in Southern Africa*

* The first draft of this case was prepared by Phyllida Brown.

ABSTRACT

Geographic area: Seven countries in southern Africa: Botswana, Lesotho, Malawi, Namibia, South Africa, Swaziland, and Zimbabwe

Health condition: In 1996, the seven countries of southern Africa reported a total of 60,000 measles cases and 166 measles deaths.

Global importance of the health condition today: Measles, one of the most contagious infections known in humans, ranks among the top four childhood killers worldwide. Despite the existence of a safe and effective vaccine, an estimated 30 million to 40 million cases of the disease and some 454,000 deaths occurred in 2004. Just under half of these deaths were in sub-Saharan Africa, where measles kills more children than HIV/AIDS.

Intervention or program: In 1996, the seven southern African countries agreed on a plan to eliminate measles. The strategy consisted of routine immunization for babies at nine months, a nationwide catch-up campaign to provide a second opportunity for immunization to all children aged nine months to 14 years, and follow-up campaigns in young children every three to four years. In addition, the countries organized surveillance for cases of measles and improved laboratory facilities so that suspect cases could be confirmed.

Cost and cost-effectiveness: The majority of the funding for the measles initiative came from national budgets. An estimate of the total cost of the program is $26.4 million, with the average cost per immunized child at $1.10. The cost of increasing routine coverage from 50% to 80% has been estimated at about $2.50 per year of healthy life gained, making measles immunization an extremely cost-effective intervention.

Impact: Between 1996 and 2000, the number of measles cases across southern Africa fell from 60,000 to 117. The number of reported measles deaths fell from 166 to zero.

Measles is one of the most contagious human infections. Along with acute respiratory infections, diarrheal disease, and malaria, it ranks among the top four childhood killers worldwide. Nearly 9 out of 10 measles deaths claim the lives of children under the age of five. Malnutrition, especially vitamin A deficiency, strongly increases the risk of death from measles. Of an estimated 454,000 deaths from measles in 2004, more than 216,000 were in sub-Saharan Africa.[1] South Asia had the second largest number of measles deaths, with 202,000 in 2004.

With a pennies-per-dose vaccine, reducing child mortality from measles through high levels of vaccination should be affordable in the developing world, making measles as rare a disease in the poorest countries as it is in the richest. As the story of seven countries in southern Africa demonstrates, a concerted effort to immunize children against measles can work—as long as the organization, political leadership, and funding are there.

IMPACT ON CHILD HEALTH

The measles virus spreads through the air, attacking vulnerable surfaces in the body, such as the lungs, the lining of the intestines, and the cornea. The infection results in a wide range of symptoms including pneumonia and diarrhea. The most visible signs include fever, cough, runny nose, red lips, red rims to the eyes, rash, peeling skin, and difficulty breathing.

In developing countries, the chance that a child infected with the measles virus will die of the disease ranges from about 5% to 15%, but the proportion can be higher in overcrowded conditions or during outbreaks.[2] Among those who survive measles, a substantial number suffer serious complications, including blindness, loss of hearing, and nerve damage.

Since the vaccine was added to the Expanded Programme on Immunization in the 1980s, making it routine in most parts of the world, measles mortality worldwide has fallen by more than 80% compared with the prevaccine era.[3] In large areas of the world, including the Americas, Mongolia, and the Philippines, measles transmission has been interrupted or controlled at very low levels. Yet in most of Africa and parts of South Asia, the death toll from the disease has stayed stubbornly high. This is largely because vaccination has not reached as many children as it should. Overall in sub-Saharan Africa, coverage in the past decade stayed well below the levels of other basic children's vaccines such as diphtheria, tetanus, and pertussis. During the 1990s, coverage reached an average of 60% across the continent;[4] in 15 African countries, fewer than half of all 1-year-olds were immunized against the disease.[5]

High coverage matters for measles, more than for almost any other vaccine-preventable disease. Measles is so contagious that the proportion of the population vaccinated must be above 90% to stop the spread of the virus. At lower coverage levels, enough susceptible individuals will remain to create a "pool" within which the virus can spread. With coverage above 90%, the population achieves what epidemiologists call "herd immunity"—a condition created when immunization levels are so high that even the small minority not immune are still protected from the disease.

At just 26 cents per dose,[5] including the safe injection equipment, the cost of measles immunization is not the problem. Instead, practical issues have kept coverage low. First, the vaccine must be given after 9 months of age—about six months later than the other basic vaccines—because

before that age an infant still carries the mother's antibodies. These antibodies "passively" protect the baby so the vaccine fails to trigger an active immune response. Unfortunately, though, it is much harder to reach 9-month-olds than newborns: Mothers may be working outside the home nine months after delivery, or pregnant again. If the clinic is many miles from home—as is often the case in sub-Saharan Africa—families may be unable to make the trip. Many babies simply miss their routine measles vaccination. Adding to the difficulty of reaching older babies is the fact that in about 15% of the children vaccinated at the recommended age, their immune systems fail to make protective antibodies unless they receive a second booster dose.[6]

AGGRESSIVE POLICY TO CUT MEASLES MORTALITY

In Latin America and the Caribbean in the 1990s, researchers and immunization teams showed that they could overcome most of the difficulties in reaching and effectively immunizing older babies by using a strategy known as "catch up, keep up, and follow up."[7] This strategy, designed by Dr. Ciro de Quadros and recommended by the Pan American Health Organization (PAHO), consists of the following three components:

- A single nationwide "catch-up" campaign in which mobile teams vaccinate all children in a particular age group, usually between 9 months and 14 years, within just a few days. This approach reaches children who missed their routine measles immunization and also provides a second dose for any child in whom the first dose failed. If coverage reaches 90% or above, the chances of the virus spreading anywhere within this age group are sharply reduced, and the health impact is dramatic and immediate.
- Sustained routine coverage ("keep up") at levels of at least 80%
- Regular "follow-up" campaigns every three to four years to prevent the number of susceptible cases in the population rising to the critical mass required for transmission.

Applying this strategy, the countries in Latin America and the Caribbean worked together to bring down the annual number of measles cases from around 250,000 in 1990 to 537 in 2001.[5]

ACTION IN SOUTHERN AFRICA

While immunization teams across Latin America and the Caribbean were pursuing this approach, some health officials in southern Africa had also begun to act. One key player was

Dr. Robin Biellik, an epidemiologist and team leader for the Expanded Programme on Immunization in southern Africa at the WHO Regional Office for Africa in Harare, Zimbabwe. Before arriving in southern Africa, Biellik had worked with de Quadros at PAHO in Brazil in the 1980s, focusing on polio eradication (see Case 5). When Biellik arrived in southern Africa, immunization teams there were also concentrating on polio eradication. In fact, the success of the polio campaigns, which significantly reduced the number of cases, led to an intensified interest in measles elimination. Measles cases and deaths also were declining, but the disease remained a much greater health threat than polio. "The decision makers were saying, 'What we're really interested in is the thing that is killing our kids,'" recalls Biellik.

Dr. Adelaide Shearley, former immunization program manager for Zimbabwe and then WHO immunization adviser for Namibia, explains that health officials had observed the success of measles elimination strategies in Latin America and the Caribbean and believed that the same success could be achieved in southern Africa. By 1996, seven nations—Botswana, Lesotho, Malawi, Namibia, South Africa, Swaziland, and Zimbabwe—had agreed on plans to eliminate measles.

POLITICAL AND POPULAR SUPPORT, AND FAVORABLE STARTING CONDITIONS

Before these countries embarked on the elimination strategy, many already had relatively strong and effective immunization services compared with many other African nations (see Box 17-1 for a description of how another country raised the coverage of immunization from a low level). Since the mid-1980s these other countries had achieved average routine coverage of about 80% against measles, although in some countries and in some years the figure was lower.[4,8] This helped lay the foundation for the initiative.

Despite the good starting conditions, however, politicians in some countries had to be convinced that the investment was worthwhile, says Shearley. Measles campaigns—intensive efforts outside of routine immunization services—cost up to $1.10 per vaccinated child, depending on transport costs. However, says Shearley, the decision makers understood the potential benefits to public health and the potential savings from greatly reducing the incidence of a disabling and often deadly disease. Parents, too, needed persuasion, particularly about the need for a second dose. But the appearance of measles cases in some older children helped health workers make the case that 15% of children need a booster dose. Because no one can tell who those children are second doses are recommended for all.

In Zimbabwe, where some parents refused to allow their children to be immunized on religious grounds, the immunization program hired a private-sector marketing company to use road shows to communicate the benefits of the measles vaccine. Three countries—Zimbabwe, Botswana, and South Africa—introduced public health statutes to discourage the religious refusal of vaccination.[8]

CATCH UP, KEEP UP, FOLLOW UP

In each country, the ministry of health planned and implemented the strategy, with technical support from WHO in Harare. Reflecting distinct needs and resources, each of the seven countries followed slightly different pathways but used common principles. All countries began with a national catch-up campaign. South Africa used its ongoing series of polio national immunization days to deliver measles vaccine to all children aged between 9 months and 14 years during 1996–1997. Botswana divided the campaign into two geographic areas, one in 1996 and the other in 1997. Swaziland and Lesotho immunized children in two age groups, one in 1998–1999, the other in 1999–2000; Swaziland, like South Africa, combined measles immunization with polio national immunization days. Malawi, Namibia, and Zimbabwe did their catch-up campaigns in a single year. In Lesotho, Malawi, and Namibia, health workers gave children vitamin A supplements along with the measles vaccine.

Because of the importance of monitoring the impact of the campaigns, countries also increased their surveillance od measles cases. The WHO trained surveillance staff at national and provincial levels, who in turn developed guidelines tailored to their country's needs. Those guidelines were used to train national medical and public health staff at the provincial and district levels. To provide the laboratory structure to investigate all suspected measles cases by testing samples for antibodies to the measles virus, the WHO worked with national staff to train technicians and designated the National Institute of Virology in Johannesburg as a regional reference laboratory.

Between 1996 and 2000 the campaigns reached almost 24 million children, and the reported coverage of these campaigns averaged 91% across the seven countries. Some, such as Botswana and Malawi, reported universal coverage. Routine immunization continued throughout each country. All seven countries also did follow-up campaigns between 2001 and 2003, up to four years after completing their catch-up campaigns.[8]

BOX 17-1 Against All Odds: DTP Immunizations in the Democratic Republic of Congo

A smaller immunization success story has emerged in the war-torn country of Democratic Republic of Congo (DRC), which has suffered 10 years of conflict. Despite ongoing violence, political instability, and economic hardship caused by the war, the DRC was able to garner support from the international community, national leaders, and local community members to triple DTP3* coverage within a period of six years.

In the early 1990s, DTP3 immunization coverage plummeted from what had been a stable 40% to about 20%, as a result not only of the severe national instability but also of an abrupt break of bilateral and multilateral cooperation.[9] Coverage rates remained at around 20% for nearly a decade until a new infusion of funds and external support led to an upward trend in coverage, which in 2004 was around 64%.[10]

This three-fold increase in coverage rates of DTP3 can be attributed to a better planning process, greater community involvement, multisector partnerships and coordination interventions, and social mobilization. Initially focused on polio eradication, an interagency coordinating committee was organized in 1995 to improve coordination among partners in their planning, technical, and financial activities. This partnership between the Ministry of Health, World Health Organization, UNICEF, bilateral aid agencies, nongovernmental organizations, and missionary groups proved successful in addressing the nation's severe polio outbreak and was soon expanded to include routine immunization services.

But improving immunization coverage within a conflict zone takes special efforts.[11] In 1999, UN Security Council Resolution 1234 documented "the commitment by the parties to the conflict in the Democratic Republic of the Congo to stop fighting in order to allow an immunization campaign."[12]

In following years, warring DRC factions observed a truce and supported national immunization days (NIDs) during which children received their annual dose of life-saving vaccinations. Financial and material support was provided at the national level to produce public information materials such as posters, radio and television programs, and megaphones. On a local level, commercial activities were suspended during NIDs to ensure that parents could take their children to be immunized. Community members went to church authorities to inform their congregations of the dates and locations of immunizations, and volunteers used alternative transportation such as bikes and motorboats to administer immunizations.

The dynamic and comprehensive strategy helped boost immunization coverage so that thousands of children are now receiving all three doses of the DTP vaccine.[13] Although the DRC still has a long way to go before reaching the goal of 80% DTP3 coverage set by the Global Alliance for Vaccines and Immunizations, the commitment of immunization program officials and partners to increasing immunization coverage over the last decade has resulted in remarkable progress.

---

* DTP3 signifies the three doses of diphtheria toxoid, tetanus toxoid, and pertussis vaccine needed for full protection from these diseases.

RESULTS: A 100% DROP IN MORTALITY

By 2000, six of the seven countries (all but Lesotho) had completed their catch-up campaigns. For these six, surveillance data could therefore be analyzed. In 1996, they had reported a total of 60,000 measles cases; by 2000, the number of confirmed cases was just 117, a reduction of close to 100%. The number of reported measles deaths had been 166 in 1996; in 2000, it was zero.[8] Lesotho's campaign was completed in 2001. There were no measles deaths there during that year.[4]

Other data also show how measles virtually disappeared from southern Africa over the five years. In two provinces in South Africa, hospitals compared the number of children admitted with measles before and after the catch-up cam-

paign. They recorded a 96% reduction in cases and a 100% reduction in deaths. In Malawi, hospital wards were reportedly closed following a sharp fall in the number of admissions for measles.[14] Between the start of the southern African initiative in 1996 and 2002, an estimated 170,000 measles deaths were averted because of the actions of the governments of the seven countries, their international partners, and the health care workers who implemented the campaigns. (See Box 17-2 on extending this success further in Africa.)

NATIONAL GOVERNMENTS FINANCED THE EFFORT

The majority of funding for the measles initiative came from national government budgets. The South African government funded its own activities in full; other countries received

BOX 17-2 Extending Success in Africa: The Measles Initiative

The striking success of the southern African countries' strategy demonstrates that careful and sustained immunization can effectively control measles. The success leads to a question: Can the strategy also work in other African countries where the burden of measles has long been greater? For example, during those five years, the southern African initiative prevented the deaths of an estimated 170,000 children. But in the rest of sub-Saharan Africa, some 2.5 million children died of the disease during the same period.[4] Many of the countries with the highest burdens are dealing with conflict or its aftermath, extreme poverty, and multiple competing health problems, making nationwide vaccination coverage much more daunting.

To tackle this situation head on, a major initiative was launched across sub-Saharan Africa in 2001. Governments of all measles-endemic countries in the region are working with the Measles Initiative, an alliance of the American Red Cross, the International Federation of Red Cross and Red Crescent Societies, the Centers for Disease Control and Prevention, the United Nations Foundation, the WHO, and UNICEF to implement accelerated disease control activities across the continent.

The basic model that has been successful elsewhere—"catch up, keep up, follow up"—is being applied. A particular emphasis has been placed on a WHO- and UNICEF-endorsed guideline of providing a second opportunity for vaccination, in addition to the first dose at nine months, to ensure that those children who did not receive a first dose or who did not respond to their first dose are ultimately immunized.

To generate local demand for vaccinations, the initiative has employed community-based mobilization. Volunteers are recruited from the community and trained to educate caretakers—mostly mothers—about the importance of routine immunization. Volunteers are organized to reach families through door-to-door visits to document eligible children.

Children are mobilized as well: "measles songs" are taught in school, and children march through the streets in parades, brandishing posters and banners extolling the importance of immunization. To further improve primary health care services in the region, the initiative also delivers additional child survival interventions such as vitamin A supplementation, insecticide-treated bed nets for malaria prevention, integrated management of childhood diseases, polio vaccines, and deworming medication.

The initiative's success has been striking: between 2001 and the start of 2006, more than 213 million children have been immunized in 40 sub-Saharan African countries. Measles cases and deaths have been slashed 60% across the continent since 1999, saving an estimated 1.2 million lives.[1] The original objective of halving the death toll of measles by 2005 compared with 2000 levels has nearly been achieved. The program has now set even more ambitious goals of reducing global measles death by 90% by the year 2010, compared to 2000 levels. To achieve these targets, the initiative faces the challenge of extending their success in the large countries with the highest measles burdens, including Nigeria, India, and Pakistan. Efforts also must be sustained to strengthen case management and disease surveillance and to ensure that at least 90% of infants are vaccinated against measles before their first birthday.

modest external support from sources such as UNICEF, the US Centers for Disease Control and Prevention, and the UK Department for International Development. These funds supplemented the resources from each country's ministry of health budgets. The total expenditure for each country has not been published, but a very rough estimate of expenditure by all countries combined, based on a cost of $1.10 per immunized child and 24 million children vaccinated, is $26.4 million.

Governments were convinced to support the strategy, and to continue to support it, in part because measles vaccination is highly cost-effective. The cost of increasing routine coverage from 50% to 80% has been estimated at around $2.50 per year of healthy life gained.[15] To put this in context, interventions that cost less than gross national income (GNI)

per capita for each year of healthy life gained are considered to be cost-effective.[16] The seven southern African nations involved in the elimination strategy have generally higher incomes than in much of Africa, although political instability and AIDS have seriously affected several of their economies. While Malawi is notably very poor, with GNI of just $160 per capita, Namibia, South Africa, and Swaziland all have GNIs in excess of $1,000 per capita. In stark contrast, the Democratic Republic of the Congo, to the north, has a GNI of $90 per capita.[17]

However, the added cost of the measles campaigns, on top of routine services, must also be taken into account. In estimates from a set of African countries where catch-up campaigns have been pursued in 2001, Dr. Mark Grabowsky and colleagues suggest that the average cost per death prevented is

$319 in the first year, and $104 over three years, figures they consider "extraordinarily cost-effective."[18] Dr. Nigel Gay of the Communicable Disease Surveillance Centre of the Health Protection Agency, Colindale, United Kingdom, has estimated the cost-effectiveness of the combined intervention of improving routine coverage to 80% and doing catch-up campaigns. Depending on the age group covered by the campaign, the incremental cost per death averted could range from $20 to around $800.[19]

SLIPPING ROUTINE COVERAGE—AND THE FIRST DEATHS FOR SEVERAL YEARS

Overall, measles transmission and deaths have remained at extremely low levels in the group of seven southern African countries since 2000. However, as in Latin America, the elimination strategy has occasionally proved "leaky," allowing a few clusters of measles cases to break through. In most instances, those affected have not been vaccinated, including children whose parents refuse immunization on religious grounds and those from families whose private doctors had wrongly advised them that they did not need to participate in the catch-up campaign.

In Gauteng province in South Africa, three hospital-based outbreaks occurred in 1999 among infants younger than nine months who were born to HIV-positive mothers. Two babies died. The hospitals began a policy of immunizing all infants aged six months or over who were admitted, and measles transmission was halted.[8]

However, in 2002 and 2003 more serious outbreaks occurred. Cases believed to have been imported across the border from neighboring Angola triggered one outbreak in Engela in northern Namibia and, it is thought, another outbreak in the capital, Windhoek. The outbreak in Namibia continued for 18 months between 2002 and 2003, resulting in 1,218 reported cases and 13 deaths.[20] Transmission was subsequently interrupted following a major vaccination campaign in June 2003. In Zimbabwe an outbreak started in September 2003, primarily among children whose parents refused vaccination on religious grounds, causing 80 cases and 20 reported deaths.[20] Another outbreak was detected in Johannesburg and was traced to an immigrant community.

If routine coverage were sufficiently high in these areas, imported infections could not have spread to others. But they did, suggesting that the main problem is inadequate routine coverage.[21] In Namibia, national coverage may have slipped to around 60%, and among those who refused vaccination in Mutare district in Zimbabwe, coverage was 75%.[22] As a result, the weighted average of routine measles coverage in the seven southern African countries fell from 87% in 2000 to 72% in 2001 and 73% in 2002. "If we want to maintain the elimination phase we have to raise our coverage to more than 80% and do follow-up campaigns," says Shearley. In 2003, this goal was accomplished with reported coverage stabilizing at 81%.[20]

MAINTAINING THE SUCCESS

Tackling diseases such as measles is hardly a one-time effort. It requires steady, conscientious effort by public health workers, backed by committed governments in the seven countries. Virtually all the impressive gains could be eroded unless the routine immunization system keeps up, the surveillance system identifies suspected measles cases in a timely manner, and confirmed cases are thoroughly investigated to prevent secondary spread. Like other campaigns, the intense effort against measles succeeds only within a functioning public health architecture.

REFERENCES

1. World Health Organization. *Weekly Epidemiol Record.* 2006;10:81;89–96.

2. Birmingham M, Stein C. The burden of vaccine preventable diseases. In: Bloom B, Lambert P-H, eds. *The Vaccine Book.* San Diego, Calif: Elsevier Science; 2002.

3. World Health Organization. *Measles Mortality Reduction and Regional Elimination Strategic Plan 2001–2005.* Geneva, Switzerland: WHO, UNICEF; 2001. WHO V&B/01/13/Rev.1.

4. Otten MW Jr, Okwo-Bele J-M, Kezaala R, Biellik R, Eggers R, Nshimirimana D. Impact of alternative approaches to accelerated measles control: experience in the African region, 1996–2002. *J Infect Dis.* 2003;187(suppl 1):S36–S43.

5. World Health Organization. *State of the World's Vaccines and Immunization.* Geneva, Switzerland: World Health Organization; 2002.

6. World Health Organization. *The World Health Report.* Geneva, Switzerland: World Health Organization; 2002.

7. Hersh BS, Tambini G, Nogueira AC, Carrasco P, de Quadros C. Review of regional measles surveillance data in the Americas, 1996–99. *Lancet.* 2000;355:1943–1948.

8. Biellik R, Madema S, Taloe A, et al. First five years of measles elimination in southern Africa: 1996–2000. *Lancet.* 2002;359:1564–1568.

9. Ministry of Health, DRC. *Financial Sustainability Plan of the Expanded Progamme on Immunization Submitted to GAVI and the Global Vaccine Fund.* Brazzaville, DRC: Ministry of Health; 2005.

10. World Health Organization, UNICEF. *Review of National Immunization Coverage 1980–2004: Democratic Republic of Congo.* Geneva, Switzerland: WHO/UNICEF; 2005.

11. Nelson D, Shimp L. *The Immunization Interagency Coordination Committee Model: Example from DR Congo.* Arlington, Va: BASICS II; 2002.

12. United Nations Security Council. S/RES/1234. April 9, 1999.

13. BASICS, WHO, UNICEF. *Communication for Immunization and Polio Eradication in the Democratic Republic of the Congo: A Joint Case Study by BASICS, WHO, and UNICEF.* November 1999. http://www.changeproject.org/pubs/lessonslearneddrc.pdf. Accessed January 12, 2007. Arlington, VA: BASICS.

14. World Health Organization Regional Office for Africa. Measles wards close in Malawi. *WHO/AFRO/EPI Bull.* 2000;1:1.

15. Edmunds W, et al. *The Cost-Effectiveness of Haemophilus influenzae type b (Hib), Hepatitis B (HBV) and Measles Vaccination in Developing Countries.* London, England: City University and Public Health Laboratory Service Communicable Disease Surveillance Centre; 2000.

16. World Bank. *World Development Report: Investing in Health.* Washington, DC: World Bank; 1993.

17. World Bank. Gross national income statistics. Available at: http://www.worldbank.org/data/countrydata. Accessed January 12, 2007.

18. Grabowsky M, Strebel P, Gay A, Hoekstra E, Kezaala R. Measles elimination in southern Africa [letter]. *Lancet.* 2002;360:716.

19. Gay N. Effectiveness and cost-effectiveness of measles strategies. Available at: http://www.afro.who.int/ddc/vpd/2000tfi/measlescontrol/costeffectiveness.pdf. Accessed January 12, 2007.

20. Otten M, Kezaala R, Fall A, et al. Public-health impact of accelerated measles control in the WHO African region 2000–2003. *Lancet.* 2005;366:832–839.

21. World Health Organization Regional Office for Africa. *Measles Control Activities in Namibia in 2003.* Harare, Zimbabwe: World Health Organization African Regional Office; 2003.

22. World Health Organization Regional Office for Africa. Report on Measles Outbreak in Manicaland Province, Zimbabwe. Harare, Zimbabwe: World Health Organization African Regional Office; 2003.

CASE 18

Preventing Dental Caries in Jamaica*

* The first draft of this case was prepared by Phyllida Brown.

ABSTRACT

Geographic area: Jamaica

Health condition: In the early 1980s, dental caries in Jamaica was widespread. On average, children had 6.7 decayed, missing, or filled teeth, and fewer than three in every 100 children were free of caries.

Global importance of health condition today: Dental caries, or tooth decay, is one of the most common chronic health problems of children. Untreated caries is painful and may affect diet, school attendance, and sleep. Tooth decay can have significant negative health and social consequences in later life.

Intervention or program: In 1987, at the encouragement of a dentist from the country's Ministry of Health, Jamaica's only salt producer began producing and selling fluoridated salt. The Ministry of Health and the Jamaican Parliament completed the necessary legal and regulatory framework, and the government provided biological and chemical monitoring of the salt.

Cost and cost-effectiveness: Salt fluoridation costs only 6 cents per person annually. Cost savings from the program are extraordinary: For each $1 spent on salt fluoridation, $250 will be saved in reducing the need for future dental treatment.

Impact: By 1995, the health of children's teeth in Jamaica had improved dramatically. In both 6-year-olds and 12-year-olds, the index of the severity of caries had fallen by more than 80%.

Some public health programs attract wide financial and political support because the health conditions they address are seen as severe, even life threatening. Others are out of the public view because they tackle smaller problems, albeit concerns that may profoundly affect quality of life. Donors rarely line up to fund such programs, and politicians make little effort to lead the charge. However, such modest initiatives—exemplified by Jamaica's successful effort to reduce the incidence and severity of dental problems among children—can demonstrate how small amounts of money,

applied intelligently, can quietly and steadily raise the health status of populations.

PROBLEM OF DENTAL CARIES

Dental caries is the progressive loss of tooth mineral and the invasion of the demineralized tooth by bacteria. It develops when bacteria stick to the surface of the tooth, forming plaque. When a person eats food containing simple sugars, the bacteria use the sugars for their own metabolic needs and produce acids as by-products.

Caries is common among children worldwide, and, though declining, remains a persistent problem in many regions.[1] Poor oral health can add significantly to the disadvantages a child faces, in terms of both personal health and life chances. Untreated caries is painful and may affect diet, school attendance, and sleep. Unresolved oral health problems can affect a child's speech and language, as well as appearance, self-image, and even social functioning.

Poor oral health can be lifelong and span many generations. Impaired eating habits and persistent oral infections can continue into adulthood and contribute to overall health. Biomedical and epidemiologic research has found that pregnant women with long-standing gum disease significantly increase their risk of having a premature birth and other adverse outcomes. In fact, one study found that pregnant women with periodontal disease are seven times more likely to deliver a preterm or low birth weight baby, controlling for other factors.[2] In short, although dental caries rarely makes it to the top of the health priority list, it merits attention as an important determinant of both child and adult health.

In many populations, a disadvantaged minority of children suffer a much higher burden of caries than their more affluent peers and also are less likely to have received treatment. In the United States, for example, almost 37% of children aged 2 to 9 years living below the poverty level have at least one untreated carious tooth, compared with 17.3% of nonpoor children in this age group. A similar pattern is evident in other countries.[1]

PREVENTION OF DENTAL CARIES WITH FLUORIDE

Dental treatment is expensive, and the costs of treating caries mount with the progression of the disease. In many developing countries, treatment is unavailable because of a shortage of dentists.[1] It is in such settings where prevention can make the biggest difference.

Since the mid-20th century, researchers have known that much dental caries can be prevented. In countries and areas where fluoridated water, toothpaste, or salt has been made available, the prevalence of caries has fallen sharply, despite the fact that people continue to consume large amounts of sugar.

In 1945, the town of Grand Rapids, Michigan, became the first to deliberately add fluoride to its water. The levels of caries in the town's children were then compared over a period of years with those of children in a "control" town, Muskegon, where water was not fluoridated. In Grand Rapids, dental caries declined significantly. Several other studies in other cities followed, each showing similar results. In a review of 95 studies conducted between 1945 and 1978,[3] Murray et al reported that water fluoridation reduced caries by around 40% to 50% in primary teeth and 50% to 60% in permanent teeth.[4] Since that time, parts of the developing world in which dental caries poses a serious problem for both children and adults have sought to adapt the approach of fluoridation to local circumstances.

JAMAICA'S INTERVENTION TAKES SHAPE

In the early 1980s, Dr. Rosalie Warpeha, a Catholic nun trained as a dentist who had lived for many years in Jamaica and worked with the Jamaican Ministry of Health, surveyed Jamaican children's teeth and found that severe caries was widespread. By age 12, fewer than 3 in every 100 children were free of caries, and on average children had 6.7 decayed, missing, or filled teeth.[5] Characterized by an inquiring mind and dogged commitment to finding solutions to vexing problems, Warpeha sought ways to introduce fluoridation to reduce the prevalence of this problem; she identified salt, rather than water, as the vehicle. Regulated water distribution systems are largely unavailable outside the capital, Kingston, and many people use rainwater.[6]

Jamaica's circumstances were highly favorable for introducing fluoridated salt, says Dr. Saskia Estupiñán-Day, regional adviser on oral health for the Pan American Health Organization (PAHO). All of the island's water supply naturally contains very low levels of fluoride, so fluoridated salt could be used everywhere. Equally important, the island has one sole salt producer, Alkali Limited, so the intervention could be achieved fairly simply.

In 1984, Warpeha visited Alkali Limited. Trevor Milner, a chemical engineer there, was interested in what she had to say. "She sold us the idea of salt fluoridation," he says. Warpeha also told Milner and his colleagues the results of Colombian community trials (see Box 18-1). She knew that Alkali Limited already iodized its salt. "Why not add fluoride too?" she asked. "We said, yes, this looks like something we could do," says Milner.

There were questions to answer first, however, says Milner. Which fluoride chemical should be used? At what levels? Would the fluoride interact with other compounds in the salt? For answers, Milner and other chemical engineers from salt manufacturers in Latin America and the Caribbean traveled to Switzerland, with support from PAHO, to learn about salt fluoridation. After this visit, Alkali Limited installed the necessary equipment at a cost of about $3,000, which the company recovered with a slight increase in the price of salt. In 1985 and 1986 the Ministry of Health and the Jamaican Parliament completed the necessary legal and regulatory framework for salt fluoridation. A major advertising campaign informed Jamaicans of the fluoridation program, and in 1987, fluoridated salt went on sale. The salt contained 250 mg per kilogram of potassium fluoride, a concentration used for domestic salt in Switzerland and France.

The Ministry of Health provided biological and chemical monitoring of the salt, while the company performed its own quality control tests daily. The Jamaican Bureau of Standards monitored the fluoride concentration of the salt.

MAJOR IMPROVEMENTS IN ORAL HEALTH

In 1995, Warpeha and Estupiñán-Day and their colleagues again surveyed children's teeth. They found a dramatic improvement. The index of the severity of caries had fallen by more than 80% in both 6-year-olds and 12-year-olds.[7] The risks appeared to be minimal: fewer than 1% of children examined showed any evidence of excess exposure to fluoride, and even in these cases the problem was mild.

These striking results delighted the researchers. "We were surprised and very happy," says Estupiñán-Day. "It was almost too good to be true." Independent scientists confirmed the findings and, in a separate line of evidence, the island's dentists reported that the incidence of dental caries was rapidly diminishing.

ARE THERE OTHER EXPLANATIONS?

Because the introduction of fluoridated salt in Jamaica was a national-level community intervention, it is impossible to be certain that the fluoridated salt alone achieved the reduction in dental caries. Communities elsewhere in the world without access to fluoridated water or salt have also seen some modest reduction in dental caries in recent decades, usually attributed to the introduction of fluoride-containing toothpastes.[4] In Jamaica, fluoridated toothpaste had been available for 12 years before the 1984 survey and may have already reduced caries levels somewhat by that date. However, in the absence of data on the proportion of children using fluoride toothpastes in 1984 or 1995, it is impossible to judge what part these toothpastes may have played in improving children's teeth during the decade. During the 1980s and early 1990s children in Jamaica rarely had access to dental health education in school, and school dental services were very limited. (See Box 18-2 for information about a new, lower-cost approach to treatment.) Estupiñán-Day and her colleagues concluded that although a combination of factors may have been responsible for the improvement in children's teeth, salt fluoridation is "the likeliest factor."

The program has continued to be implemented successfully since 1995, thanks, in part to passage of legislation to protect the fluoridation program; fluoridated salt is also being exported from Jamaica to neighboring countries. (Warpeha continued to conduct research about dental health in Jamaica up until the time of her death in 2006.)

COST-EFFECTIVENESS OF SALT FLUORIDATION

The cost of the chemicals is low, at about 1 cent per person per year. Taking into account the entire cost of the fluoridation program, including equipment, running costs, and monitoring, salt fluoridation in Jamaica costs around 6 cents per person annually. This is an even lower cost than water fluoridation, which may cost up to 90 cents per person per year, depending on the size of the community.[4]

In treatment costs alone, the return on investment in salt fluoridation is substantial, leaving aside any less easily measured benefits such as reduced absence from school or improved health in later life. It is estimated that for each $1 spent on salt fluoridation in Latin America and the Caribbean, about $250 will be saved in reducing the need for future dental treatment.[7] "This makes fluoridation of salt one of the most cost-effective interventions known to modern public health," says Estupiñán-Day.

A LASTING LEGACY

Through its impact on the health and well-being of children from low-income households, and the demonstration effect that influenced other countries in the region, the Jamaican salt fluoridation program shows how much can be achieved with focused attention and creative problem solving.

BOX 18-1
Water or Salt?

Water fluoridation is effective only if the water supply system is regulated and the majority of inhabitants have access to the piped water system. In the 1960s and early 1970s, a community trial of salt fluoridation was conducted in Colombia, supported by PAHO and the US National Institutes of Health. Two communities receiving fluoridated salt—fluoridated at the rate of 200 mg of fluoride per kilogram—experienced reductions of nearly 50% percent in dental caries, compared with no reduction in a third community that served as a control, and compared with a 60% reduction in a fourth community that received fluoridated water.[8] Thus, while slightly less efficient than water fluoridation, salt fluoridation was shown to be highly beneficial.

BOX 18-2 Filling the Gap

Even with salt fluoridation, some children will get cavities. Once they do, the integrity of the teeth must be restored quickly and well to avoid extensive damage, as well as the pain and poor nutrition that go along with erosion of teeth. The traditional approach, for those with access to dental care, is to have the cavities filled with amalgam, using electric drilling equipment. While this type of restoration can be very functional and long lasting, it is also relatively costly and often unavailable to low-income populations.

Recognizing this gap, PAHO's oral health team sought an alternative. Exploring ways to expand access, Estupiñán-Day and colleagues saw promise in simple technologies known as atraumatic restorative treatment (ART), which uses hand instruments and inexpensive adhesive filling. Clinical studies in the early 1990s suggested that ART could give good results, but questions existed about its cost-effectiveness and large-scale implementation under field conditions.

In a recent study involving more than 2,000 children in three countries (Ecuador, Panama, and Uruguay), and with support of the Inter-American Development Bank, PAHO and its research collaborators compared three different approaches: traditional fillings using amalgam, applied by a qualified dentist; ART, applied by a qualified dentist after undergoing 40 hours of training; and ART, applied by a dental auxiliary with 40 hours of training. Children were randomly assigned to one of the three treatments, and then followed up at intervals of 12, 24, and 36 months.

The results, published in 2006, were very encouraging. Across a range of real-world conditions, the restoration of teeth using ART was excellent—precisely as good as the restoration using amalgam, and equally satisfactory whether performed by a dentist or an auxiliary. Even at the two-year mark, ART restorations held up very well.

Importantly, the costs were much lower. In Ecuador, for example, the average cost for an amalgam procedure was $7.77, while for an ART procedure it was $3.64 or $1.48, depending on whether a dentist or auxiliary performed the service. In Uruguay, the differential was even larger: it cost an average of $33.64 for a dentist to restore a tooth with amalgam, and only one tenth that amount for an auxiliary to use ART for the same purpose—with both types of treatment achieving excellent results.

This important study paves the way for widespread adoption of ART in government health services, particularly in low-income communities where dental services are scarce. It represents one more step toward improved oral health in the region of the Americas.

REFERENCES

1. World Health Organization. *WHO Oral Health Country/Area Profile Programme.* Geneva, Switzerland: WHO Collaborating Centre on Oral Health, University of Malmö, Sweden; 2003.

2. Offenbacher S, Katz V, Fertik G, et al. Periodontal infection as a possible risk factor for preterm low birth weight. *J Periodontol.* 1996;67:1103–1113.

3. Murray JJ, Rugg-Gunn AJ, Jenkins GN, Rugg-Gunn AJ, Jenkins GN. *Fluorides in Caries Prevention.* 3rd ed. Oxford, England: Butterworth-Heineman;1991.

4. US Department of Health and Human Services. *Oral Health in America: A Report of the Surgeon General.* Rockville, MD: National Institute of Dental and Craniofacial Research; 2000.

5. Warpeha RA. Dental caries and salt fluoridation. *Jamaican Pract.* 1985;5:6–8.

6. Estupiñan-Day S. *Salt Fluoridation in Caries Prevention.* Washington, DC: Pan American Health Organization; 2004.

7. Estupiñan-Day S, Baez R, Horowitz H, Warpeha R, Sutherland B, Thamer M. Salt fluoridation and dental caries in Jamaica. *Community Dent Oral Epidemiol.* 2001;29:247–252.

8. Mejía R. Experience with salt fluoridation in Colombia. First International Symposium on Salt Fluoridation, Pan American Health Organization. Washington, DC: Scientific Publication No. 501; 1986:54–66.

Treating Cataracts in India

ABSTRACT

Geographic area: India

Health condition: In India in the early 1990s, it was estimated that more than 80% of blind people, or more than 10 million individuals, suffered from bilateral cataract, and another 10 million individuals had cataract in one eye.

Global importance of the health condition today: The leading cause of global blindness, cataract is present in more than half of all cases. Cataract is an age-related condition in which the lens of the eye becomes clouded, blurring vision. In 1998, it was estimated that some 20 million people were blind due to cataract, and at least 100 million eyes have very poor vision as a result of cataract.

Intervention or program: In 1994, recognizing both the tremendous problem of adult blindness in India, and the short-comings in the existing cataract treatment program, the Cataract Blindness Control Program was begun in seven states in India where the need was most concentrated. The program consisted of introducing a new, more effective surgical technique; shifting from a strategy of providing treatment in mass camps to one in which fixed sites were used; partnering with Aravind Eye Hospital and other nongovernmental organizations for delivery of services; and improving management and training at all levels.

Cost and cost-effectiveness: The total cost of the project was about US$136 million, with close to 90% coming from the World Bank and the remainder from the government of India. In some settings, costs were as low as $10 per cataract operation, due to the efficiencies of high patient volume and the local production of high-quality artificial lenses. Overall, the cost-effectiveness of surgery in the South Asia region has been estimated at about $60 per disability-adjusted life year.

Impact: A cumulative total of 15.35 million cataract operations were performed within the seven years of the program, which was successful in improving the quality of care. Surgeries using the recommended technique increased from 3% before 1994 to about 42% (cumulative) between 1999 and 2002. Based on an estimated 3.5 million cataract surgeries in India in the year 2000, 320,000 people were saved from blindness.

Achieving major public health impact requires that interventions reach a large share of those who need them and are effective and affordable. In many of the cases in this volume, the greatest challenge was to ensure access to a simple and cost-effective preventive technology or treatment that could be delivered or administered by basic health workers. In the case of treating millions of cataract sufferers in India, the task was to both reach those in need *and* to ensure that the surgical treatment offered was of adequate quality to solve the problem, without needless complications. This represents a vast challenge, given major limitations in both the reach and the quality of health care delivery in India, but one that the government, working with key partners and deploying low-cost technologies, has been able to accomplish to a remarkable degree.

The cataract program in India, in its several phases, demonstrates some of the key features of "scaling up": introducing better and affordable technologies when they become available, building demand for a service that was previously unavailable, and getting to low unit costs by serving large numbers of patients efficiently. Initially, the goal of a broad coverage of services to treat blindness and severe vision loss was achieved by public education to convince people that treatment was possible, and by the use of "eye camps" to bring screening and treatment services to remote and impoverished areas that had not previously been well served by either government or private providers. Services then needed to be reoriented and upgraded, focusing on quality as well as quantity. Achieving good outcomes from treatment required the systematic introduction of improved techniques, training and retraining, attention to monitoring, and partnership between government and a broad range of funding and service-provision organizations to achieve high-volume, low-cost surgery. Through those actions, more than 300,000 people have been saved from a lifetime of blindness each year.

THE DEVASTATION OF BLINDNESS

Blindness affects rich and poor, young and old—but it is the poor and the old who suffer the greatest burden. Blindness affects an estimated 45 million people around the world; another 135 million are visually impaired.[1] About 90% of people who are blind live in low- and middle-income countries, and several diseases of poverty—including trachoma, onchocerciasis, and vitamin A deficiency—account for large shares of that burden.[1] (See Cases 10, 7, and 4.) Of every 10 blind individuals, about 9 are adults, with the incidence of blindness and other vision problems rising steeply above age 50. In India, vision problems represent an enormous problem; about 45 million Indians experience visual impairment, and about 12 million are blind.

It is estimated that nearly one quarter of the world's blind live in India.[2,3] In addition to age-related factors, risks for eye problems include exposure to excessive sunlight, poor sanitation and other environmental hazards, infection, and poor nutrition. Because of environmental risks and limited access to care, women from low-income households are particularly affected by several blinding eye diseases, including trachoma and cataract.

The household and social costs of blindness are high. About 3.1% of deaths worldwide are directly or indirectly due to cataract, glaucoma, trachoma, and onchocerciasis.[4] Annual worldwide productivity loss associated with blindness is estimated at $168 billion (using 1993 data).[5]* In India, the economic burden of blindness was estimated in 1997 to be about $4.4 billion annually.[6]

Cataract as the Cause

Worldwide, the leading cause of blindness is cataract, present in more than half of all cases. Described simply, a cataract is a clouding of the lens of the eye, due to a clumping of the protein elements of the lens or a discoloration that occurs with age, excessive sunlight exposure, diabetes, undernutrition, and other risk factors. The normal lens, clear and transparent, sits behind the colored iris and pupil and helps focus light on the retina, which converts the light images to electrical and chemical signals that are carried to the brain. A cataract blurs the image on the retina, producing a visual effect that is like looking through a window that is frosted or fogged with steam.

Cataracts can affect one or both eyes. In addition to blurry vision and changes in color perception, symptoms can include glare and halo effects from lights and sun, failing night vision, and double vision. Cataract is detected by an eye exam that includes a visual acuity test and dilated eye exam.

In 1998, it was estimated that some 20 million people were blind due to cataract.[1] Globally, at least 100 million eyes have very poor vision (visual acuity < 6/60) as a result of cataract.[7]

The problem of cataract in India has been profound, given the country's huge population and an above average incidence of cataract. Few extended families are untouched by the problem. In India in the early 1990s, it was estimated that more than 80% of blind people, or more than 10 million individuals, suffered from bilateral cataract, and another 10 million individuals had cataract in one eye.

In India, the problem affects a broad swath of the population. Cataract hits people earlier in life than in most other parts of the world. Almost half (45%) of cataract cases in India occur before 60 years of age, and women appear to be particularly hard hit, in part because exposure to smoke from indoor cooking represents a significant risk factor.[8] Because of the relatively early onset, those affected with cataracts face many years of severe vision loss and/or blindness.

---

* This is likely to be a slight overestimate because it assumes that all sighted persons are fully productive and all blind persons are completely unproductive.

In short, addressing the widespread problem of blindness in India requires dealing with cataract—and dealing with cataract requires surgical intervention. Successful treatment of cataract can then have benefits over many years for individuals and their families.

Treatment for Cataract

Surgical treatment for cataract has been around since the mid-1700s, becoming more widely available, safer, and more effective through a series of major advances in technique. Age-related cataracts—by far the most common—can be treated well with a two-step surgery: all or part of the lens is removed, and then eyesight is corrected with eyeglasses or an intraocular corrective lens.

Two approaches have been developed to remove the lens: With intracapsular cataract extraction, known as ICCE, the lens and surrounding lens capsule are removed in one piece. A plastic lens (an intraocular lens implant) is then placed, and remains permanently in the eye. This surgery requires a large incision and places significant pressure on a part of the eye known as the vitreous body. Because of these features, it has a relatively high rate of complications. ICCE also almost always requires patients to wear strong spectacles to correct for remaining refractive distortions. Traditionally, ICCE has been the procedure used in low-income environments because it is a relatively simple and quick surgery.

The alternative, more technically sophisticated approach is called extracapsular cataract extraction, or ECCE. In ECCE, the lens is removed but the lens capsule is left partially intact; an intraocular lens is then implanted. In general, ECCE requires a very small incision, and the complication rate is quite low. In some cases, the correction is so good that patients do not require glasses or other corrective lenses.

Although ECCE requires somewhat more skill by practitioners than ICCE, the outcomes confirm that the extra effort is worth it. The difference in efficacy between ICCE and ECCE is dramatic: In a study of outcomes after cataract surgery in India, covering about 3,600 operated eyes, researchers found that patients who had ECCE surgery had a 2.8 times higher chance of obtaining a good outcome after surgery, compared to those who had undergone an ICCE procedure. Among those who had obtained ECCE surgery, some 71% had a good outcome (vision >= 6/18 in the operated eye).[9]

THE GOVERNMENT OF INDIA'S EARLY EFFORTS

The government of India's response to the problem of blindness, and cataract in particular, has been impressive in its breadth and duration. In 1963, India became one of the first countries in the world to organize a centrally sponsored national program to deal with eye disease. The program initially was aimed at controlling trachoma, an eye infection that is easily spread, also disproportionately affects women, and commonly results in blindness (see Case 10). Over the following decade, it was broadened to include treatment of all visual impairment, as well as prevention of blindness.

In 1976, in recognition of the tremendous burden associated with cataract, India's National Program for Control of Blindness was formed to address the problem. The program emerged at a time when the government was implementing various types of health care—from family planning to immunization—through mass campaigns. It took a similar approach to dealing with cataract treatment. This was an approach that partially overcame the unwillingness of trained health workers, and physicians in particular, to work in remote areas. Temporary camps were established for short periods to provide specific types of services, including mass ICCE surgeries, to populations in the surrounding areas. The centrally directed program's activities were heavily oriented toward the expansion of access to surgical treatment. In addition to the camps, the program included establishing regional institutions of ophthalmology, development of mobile eye units, recruitment of eye care professionals, and an increase in various ophthalmologic services.

Help came from outside. In 1978, the National Program accepted assistance from DANIDA, the Danish International Development Assistance organization. This support primarily focused on nationwide expansion of infrastructure (equipment and mobile units) and for training of paramedical ophthalmic assistants. Funds were later added for central monitoring and evaluation.

As the program expanded, the volume of surgeries in the camps was indeed impressive. The number of individuals screened in a day might be upward of 600 in a camp, and the number of surgeries undertaken in a typical camp was 100 or more per day. Patients spent a very brief time recovering from surgery, and then were sent home with relatives. Once the screening and treatment were completed in a particular area, the team would pack up and move to the next, leaving few opportunities for postsurgical follow-up.

Although the program's quantitative achievements were remarkable in those early years, the impact on health was disappointing; outcomes were relatively poor. According to at least one study of 24 villages, less than half of those operated had good visual outcomes.[10] The reasons for this underperformance were many: First, the ICCE surgery itself had a significant failure rate, even under the best circumstances. And the camps were in no way the best circumstances. Surgeons were serving a rural population that did not always understand instructions for postsurgical care at home; it was difficult (and often impossible) to maintain a sterile field during the operation; and local doctors were either not present or not able to provide follow-up monitoring and care. And, while the program was increasingly successful at stimulating a demand for surgeries, it was unable to keep up with that demand. A backlog of people asking for treatment led to long lines and increased pressure to work quickly and move on.

In part in response to the shortcomings of the public sector program, the private sector—and particularly nongovernmental organizations—sought to fill the void. Among those NGOs, the Aravind Eye Hospital, founded by a charismatic and committed leader, demonstrated a remarkable ability to reach poor communities with a range of quality eye care, including surgical treatment of cataract (see Box 19-1).

In 1992, Aravind fostered a major innovation: the local manufacture of the previously imported intraocular lens, making surgery far more affordable. With this breakthrough in 1992, the path to large-scale use of superior surgical methods became possible.

FROM QUANTITY TO QUALITY: THE WORLD BANK PROJECT

In 1994, recognizing the tremendous problem of adult blindness in India, the shortcomings in the existing government cataract treatment program, and the promising approach pioneered by Aravind, the World Bank–assisted Cataract Blindness Control Program (CBCP) was begun in seven states in India where the need was most concentrated: Andhra Pradesh, Madhya Pradesh, Maharashtra, Orissa, Rajasthan, Tamil Nadu, and Uttar Pradesh. These include regions that are home to very poor, marginalized populations, living at subsistence level with little contact with public services.

Specific program objectives of CBCP were designed to support and enhance the work of the existing national program in several ways. First, the program sought to improve the quality of cataract surgery and lessen the prevalence of blindness by reducing the backlog of cataract blindness in the participating states. To achieve these objectives, the seven states would perform more than 11 million sight restoration surgeries during the seven-year project period. A particular concern was to induce a change in the treatment protocol—away from the unsatisfactory ICCE approach and toward the more complicated but ultimately more effective ECCE technique. To make this transition, the existence of the locally produced intraocular lens was a critical ingredient.

Second, the CBCP aimed at a particular type of "scale-up" of services, strengthening India's capacity to provide high-volume, high-quality, and low-cost eye care by upgrading health and management skills for eye care personnel. Importantly, the program envisioned improving service delivery through nongovernmental and public sector collaboration by assigning geographic areas to NGOs and government hospitals to avoid duplication of effort and to help improve performance. Aravind was the leading partner, and ultimately provided a large share of the total services.

Third, the program undertook specific actions to increase the coverage of eye care delivery among the underprivileged population groups including women and those in tribal areas and in geographically inaccessible and remote terrain. These actions included identification of patients blind in both eyes, who were given preferential access to services, and preparation of village registries of blind residents.

MANAGEMENT SUPPORT FOR THE PROGRAM

As Dr. Alfred Sommer points out, "High-volume cataract surgery requires exquisite organization, provision of inexpensive equipment and supplies, and a constant stream of patients eager to benefit from the procedure."[11] In other words, to achieve its aims the CBCP program had to pay considerable attention to getting the support functions for service delivery fully functional.

In contrast to situations where a "greenfield" program is being established where none previously existed, this was a challenge of reeducation, reorientation, and changing entrenched practices of surgeons, support staff, and managers. The main management elements included training; generating demand through information, education, and communication; tracking the data; strengthening institutional capacity; and expanding the role of international NGOs.

Training

Training of eye care professionals was an imperative of CBCP. A 16-week train-the-trainer program was delivered through medical colleges across India, ultimately training 100 faculty in ophthalmic hospitals. This was followed by two months of instruction for eye surgeons on the latest surgical techniques, such as intraocular lens and sutureless surgeries. More than 800 eye surgeons received this training. Education programs also included health workers and teachers, covering issues such as types of eye disease, treatments, and advantages and disadvantages of available surgical methods.

BOX 19-1 Aravind Eye Hospital

The Aravind Eye Care System, an NGO with a 30-year history of providing very low-cost vision care, has been a leading partner to the government of India in its blindness program and a leading example of social entrepreneurship in the health sector. Among the NGOs providing cataract treatment in India, Aravind is by far the largest, conducting more than 1,000 screening camps and performing close to 1 million cataract surgeries each year. Within the context of the CBCP, Aravind's role was particularly significant in Tamil Nadu, where some 95% of the surgeries were performed under the organization's auspices.

Aravind had its start in 1976 when its founder, Dr. Govindappa Venkataswamy, after mandatory retirement from government service at age 58, opened a 12-bed hospital in the South Indian city of Madurai. Starting with little money but a strong sense of mission toward saving the vision of those in need—and inspired, serendipitously, by the large-scale success of the McDonald's fast-food marketing strategy—over time Dr. Venkataswamy established a network of specialty eye hospitals throughout India that uses a sustainable business model to provide high-quality patient care. He devoted himself to this effort until his death in 2006; his family continues his work.

Three key elements define the Aravind business model:

- Economies of scale—With excellent management and high patient volume, Aravind keeps productivity high, with surgeons performing 25–40 procedures daily; unit costs are maintained at the very low level of about $10 per cataract operation.
- Cross-subsidies—Aravind provides free or very low-priced care to two thirds of its patients with the revenue derived from the one third of patients who are able to pay moderate prices. The only difference in the treatment of those who do and don't pay is in the amenities, such as the air conditioning in the recovery room.
- Vertical integration—Recognizing that the imported intraocular lenses constituted a major component of the total surgical costs, Aravind obtained a transfer of technology through the US-based Seva Foundation, and additional support from the Combat Blindness Foundation, to permit it to manufacture these lenses at a fraction of the cost. The manufacturing activity scaled up quickly, from 35,000 in 1992–1993 to nearly 600,000 lenses today. Now, at the Aurolab subsidiary established for this purpose, a workforce of about 200 young women from rural backgrounds produces lenses to a global standard of quality that are used at Aravind, as well as at facilities throughout India. The affordably priced intraocular lenses are exported to some 85 countries around the world, providing another source of revenue for Aravind. The system of eye hospitals also is considered one of India's premier ophthalmic training institutions, providing a steady flow of well-prepared professionals and support staff.

Beyond the mechanics of the business model was the leadership of Dr. Venkataswamy—a surprising combination of marketing savvy and spirituality. "If Coca-Cola can sell billions of sodas and McDonald's can sell billions of burgers," Dr. Venkataswamy asked, "why can't Aravind sell millions of sight-restoring operations, and, eventually, the belief in human perfection? With sight, people could be freed from hunger, fear, and poverty. You could perfect the body, then perfect the mind and the soul, and raise people's level of thinking and acting."[12] With this approach, he attracted both financial and technical support from many organizations outside of India, from Lions Club to the World Health Organization to the Seva Foundation, and inspired a generation of health professionals in South Asia and beyond.

Generating Demand Through Information, Education, and Communication

The program included significant resources for the provision of information to the general population about the potential to cure cataracts through a relatively simple surgical procedure. Individuals affected by cataract and their families were informed through both public and NGO outreach that services were available and that full recovery of sight was possible. This aspect of the program built directly on the Aravind experiences, which had demonstrated that even very poor patients in rural areas valued effective treatment for cataracts. As researchers and clinicians from Aravind had found, "The magnitude of IOL [intraocular lens] acceptance among these patients has surpassed even our expectations and projections. Since this change seems to occur from within the community, there is every reason to expect the demand to increase in an exponential fashion. This clearly indicates that the rural patient is prepared to meet the cost of an IOL provided the visual results are convincing."[13]

Tracking the Data

A simple management information system was devised for use at the state, district, and central levels. Data from the cataract surgery records provided detailed information for every person operated on for cataract, as well as financial status for all districts. Funds were released based on information from this system. At a district level, the system could be used for evaluating the monthly performance of the District Blindness Control Society, the ophthalmic surgeon, and the civil surgeon (or chief medical officer) against a fixed target.

The data provided a good leading indicator of trends and needs. Tracking studies developed by the Indian Institute of Health Management Research and by the National Program for Control of Blindness were carefully designed to build a benchmark against which to measure progress with established survey elements for statistical analysis. A combination of measures attempted to capture both the number of individuals treated and the outcomes of the surgeries.

Strengthening Institutional Capacity

Based on the experiences of previous blindness control programs, the Cataract Blindness Control Project committed to the decentralization of eye care services in the seven participating states. Toward that end, district blindness control societies were established, each headed by a district program manager. Each district was assigned eye surgeons and paramedical ophthalmic assistants to diagnose patients, conduct surgeries, and perform follow-up care.

Expanding the Role of International NGOs

In addition to the many Indian NGOs participating in the CBCP, significant organizational, professional, and financial contributions have been made by the following international NGOs:

- Sight Savers International, based in the United Kingdom, is active in more than 50 countries worldwide. India is one of its oldest programs. Sight Savers supported (and continues to support) NGOs and eye hospitals throughout India. It funds training courses, such as the intraocular lens training course in the Aravind Eye Hospitals and programs for rehabilitation of incurably blind persons.
- Christoffel Blinden Mission (CBM), based in Germany, is the largest NGO working on blindness control and rehabilitation in 105 countries in Asia, Africa, Latin America, and Europe. The CBM total budget for 1994 was over US$100 million. Eventually, CBM has come to support 127 eye care projects in India; these are mainly Christian NGO eye hospitals in rural and underserved areas.
- Lions International SightFirst program activities have been implemented through local Lions Clubs all over India. SightFirst funds cataract surgeries performed by local NGOs. They have constructed eye hospitals and funded a training institute for community ophthalmology—Lions Aravind Institute for Community Ophthalmology at the Aravind Eye Hospital in Madurai.
- DANIDA supported the NPCB starting in 1978 and the CBCP through 1996, with emphasis on equipment and training including the development of local education programs such as school vision screening programs.

MAJOR ACHIEVEMENTS

Although the achievements of the program were not subject to a rigorous impact evaluation, there is little doubt that much was accomplished: many more people obtained surgical treatment; that treatment was, on average, much more effective than earlier methods; and the move from performing surgeries in the camps to fixed facilities greatly reduced the postsurgical risks. In short, better outcomes for more people.

At the most basic level, the program was successful in increasing access to services and improving the quality of care provided, and the health outcomes achieved. A rapid assessment conducted in 2001–2002 found that the program had expanded access—a cumulative total of 15.35 million cataract operations were performed within the seven years of the World Bank–funded program—and during that period 69% of those requiring cataract surgery received it. By the end of the program, which included a major communications effort, some 90% of the population the area included in the program was aware of the availability of a treatment for cataract blindness.

The appropriate surgeries are now being done: According to the rapid assessment, the number of surgeries using the recommended IOL technique increased from 3% before 1994 to about 42% (cumulative) in 1999–2002.

Although exceptions do exist, today eye surgeons have moved their operating theaters to safe and more sterile locations, away from the mobile camps. By 2001, only about 8% of conventional surgeries were taking place in camps. The remainder is done in fixed facilities, where better outcomes can be expected; 17% of those are in government facilities; 37% in NGOs; and about 38% in private facilities.[14] The camps have continued to play a crucial role as the locus for screening and follow-up care, as well as the provision of public information.

Surgical outcomes have improved with the introduction of improved procedures, well-equipped surgical facilities, and trained personnel: Postoperative visual acuity to an acceptable level (> 3/60) following surgery improved from 75% before 1994 to 82% in 1999–2002. Based on an estimated 3.5 million cataract surgeries each year in India (2000 figure), about 320,000 people were saved from blindness annually. Overall population prevalence of cataract blindness declined by 26%, from 1.5% at baseline to 1.1%, during the program period.[14]

COST AND COST-EFFECTIVENESS

The total cost of the World Bank–funded project was about US$136 million, with close to 90% coming from the World Bank and the remainder from the government of India. (Information on private contributions is unavailable.)

Cataract surgery, which can be performed at relatively low cost and can result in lasting reversal of vision loss, is among the most highly cost-effective interventions,[15] when the surgery done uses the appropriate method and among populations with relatively high prevalence, so that facilities and personnel are used efficiently. According to Baltussen et al, the cost-effectiveness of ECCE surgery is estimated at about $60 per disability-adjusted life year in the South and East Asia region (which includes India).[16] Interestingly, it is the model of care provided by NGOs through a combination of screening camps and then surgery at a base hospital providing high-volume services that has been demonstrated most cost-effective. The NGO public awareness campaigns are both motivating and educational; coupled with efficiencies of scale in serving the needy population and the ability to screen and select patients for cataract surgery, these facilities practice the most effective use of resources. More recent cost-effectiveness analyses by the Disease Control Priorities Project confirm that cataract surgery is one among several other surgical interventions, such as obstetric and abdominal operations, that can be made cost-effective in low-tech hospitals and other resource-poor settings.[17]

REMAINING CHALLENGES

Despite the achievements of the program in the participating states, major challenges remain. First, the states that did not participate in the program have much catching up to do. It is estimated that eliminating cataract blindness in the country would have required 9 million high-quality cataract surgeries annually during 2001–2005, and would require another 14 million during 2016–2020, given population growth and demographic change. This requires twice the current number of surgeries.

Second, because the program funded by the World Bank was focused entirely on reducing the prevalence of cataract blindness, no provisions were made to treat individuals who came to the screening camps with other types of eye problems. Thus, there has been a steady—and ever more obvious—neglect of other causes of blindness.

EFFECTIVE MANAGEMENT, USEFUL INFORMATION FOR PROVIDERS AND PATIENTS

Two central features of India's cataract program success provide key lessons for other efforts to scale up complex health programs to hard-to-reach populations. First, the program focused intensive attention on improving the management systems, from the organization of training programs, to the methods for identifying target populations and clients, to the organization of logistics and financing at the district level. Neither the expansion of services at relatively low cost nor the improvement in the quality of those services would have been possible without specific and constant attention to the management side of the program, including the recruitment of a strong management team at all levels.

Second, the program designers recognized from the inception that one of the core challenges was changing behavior—of providers (who needed to learn new approaches and methods) and the potential patients (who had to take action to obtain services to address a health problem that many thought was untreatable). Focused, sustained efforts were made to achieve these behavior changes. On the side of the providers, these efforts included training programs and sharing the results of research and monitoring to motivate improvements. On the side of the patients, massive communications efforts were undertaken, particularly by NGOs with close links to the community.

The experiences of Aravind and the government have had an impact far beyond India's borders. In fact, the success of the India program was a major motivating force behind the "VISION 2020: The Right to Sight" initiative of the WHO and the International Agency for the Prevention of Blindness. This international initiative is a multinational effort to generate and share accurate data on distribution and determinants of vision loss; the development and introduction of cost-effective ways to prevent and treat eye problems; and partnerships among governments, communities, and NGOs. With the advances in control of onchocerciasis and trachoma, prevention of xerophthalmia due to vitamin A deficiency, and treatment of cataract, the successes of those who work on eye care are among the most impressive in global health.

REFERENCES

1. World Health Organization. *Global Initiative for the Prevention of Avoidable Blindness.* Geneva, Switzerland: World Health Organization; 1997. WHO/PBL/97.61.

2. Frick K, and Foster A. The magnitude and cost of global blindness: a problem that can be alleviated. *Am J Ophthalmol.* 2003;135(4):471–476.

3. <Thomas st al 2005—

4. Murray CJL, Lopez AD. Global mortality, disability, and the contribution of risk factors: Global Burden of Disease Study. *Lancet.* 1997;349:1436–1442.

5. Smith AF, Smith JG. The economic burden of global blindness: a price too high! *Brit J Ophthalmol.* 1996;80:276–277.

6. Shamanna BR, Dandona L, Rao GN. Economic burden of blindness in India. *Indian J Ophthalmol.* 1998;46:169–172.

7. Foster A. Cataract—a global perspective: output, outcome and outlay. *Eye.* 1999;13:65–70.

8. Pokhrel AK, Smith KR, Khalakdina A, Deuja A, Bates MN. Case-control study of indoor cooking smoke exposure and cataract in Nepal and India. *Int J Epidemiol.* 2005;34(3):702–708.

9. Bachani D, Gupta SK, Murthy GVS, and Jose R. Visual outcomes after cataract surgery and cataract surgical coverage in India. *Int Ophthalmol* 1999;23(1):49–56.

10. Anand R, Gupta A, Ram J, Singh U, and Kumar R. Visual outcome following cataract surgery in rural punjab. *Indian J Opthalmol.* 2000;48(2):153–158.

11. Rubin H. The perfect vision of Dr. V. *Fast Company.* 2001;43:146. Available at: http://www.fastcompany.com/online/43/drv.html. Accessed January 12, 2007.

12. Sommer A. Toward affordable, sustainable eye care. *Int Ophthalmol.* 1994;18:287–292.

13. Venkatesh, PN and Raheem R. Changing trends in the intraocular lens acceptance in rural Tamil Nadu. *Indian J Opthalmol.* 1995;43(4):177–179.

14. World Bank. *Cataract Blindness Control Project Implementation Completion Report.* Washington, DC: World Bank; 2002.

15. Javitt J, Venkataswamy G, Sommer A. The economic and social aspect of restoring sight. In: Henkind P, ed. *ACTA: 24th International Congress of Ophthalmology.* New York, NY: JP Lippincott; 1983:1308–1312.

16. Baltussen R, Sylla M, Mariotti SP. Cataract surgery: a global and regional cost-effectiveness analysis. *Bull WHO.* 2004;82(5):338–344.

17. Debas HT, Gosselin R, McCord C, and Thind A. Surgery. In: Jamison DT, Breman JG, Measham AR, et al, eds. *Disease Control Priorities in Developing Countries.* 2nd ed. New York, NY: Oxford University Press; 2006:1245–1260.

Preventing Hib Disease in Chile and the Gambia*

* The first draft of this case was prepared by Phyllida Brown.

ABSTRACT

Geographic areas: Chile and the Gambia

Health condition: Researchers in Chile estimated that the incidence of *Haemophilus influenzae* type b (Hib) disease in Santiago during the late 1980s was 32 per 100,000 infants under 6 months of age, and 63 per 100,000 in infants aged 6 to 11 months. The proportion of children who died after contracting the disease was relatively high at 16%. In the Gambia, just over 200 children per 100,000 developed Hib meningitis in 1990.

Global importance of the health condition today: Worldwide, Hib disease is the leading cause of bacterial meningitis in children under 5 years of age and the second most common cause of bacterial pneumonia deaths in this age group. It kills an estimated 450,000 children every year and causes some 2 million cases of disease.

Intervention or program: Chile's Ministry of Health introduced the Hib vaccine into the routine immunization program for infants in 1996. The Gambia began administering the vaccine routinely as part of the national immunization program in 1997.

Cost and cost-effectiveness: The government of Chile has paid $3.39 million for the combined DTP-Hib vaccine, a figure that represents nearly 23% of the total immunization budget and 0.7% of the government health expenditure. In Chile, the price per dose is $3, and the government saves an estimated $78 for each case of Hib prevented. Aventis Pasteur's donation of the vaccines in the Gambia helped make the immunizations possible there, and financial support from the Global Alliance for Vaccines and Immunization will help sustain the program through 2008.

Impact: The incidence of Hib meningitis in Chile fell by 91% and that of pneumonia and other forms of Hib disease fell by 80% following an initial trial in 36 health centers in 1994. The number of children developing Hib meningitis in the Gambia dropped almost tenfold, from 200 per 100,000 to 21 per 100,000, in the 12-month period after the start of routine immunization. In the last two years of the study, there were just two cases.

Although it is a major cause of bacterial meningitis and pneumonia in young children worldwide,[1] the microbe *Haemophilus influenzae* type b (Hib) has avoided the notoriety of other major killers. Yet researchers have estimated that it is responsible for the deaths of some 450,000 people worldwide and at least 2 million cases of disease each year.[2,3] Hib menin-gitis is particularly lethal, killing 20–40% of the children who get it and leaving as many as half of the survivors with some lasting impairment, such as deafness or mental retardation.

In principle, most of this disease and suffering are avoid-able. Since the late 1980s, highly effective vaccines against Hib have been licensed (see Box 20-1). Their impact in the industrialized countries, where they are widely available, has been dramatic. For example, in the United States, within four years of the initial licensing of conjugate vaccines in December 1987, the number of young children diagnosed with Hib disease fell by 71%, with up to 16,000 cases of the disease prevented in 1991 alone.[4] Similarly, in the United Kingdom and Finland, Hib immunization resulted in as steep or even steeper declines in the incidence of the disease.[5,6]

For most low- and middle-income countries, the relatively high cost of Hib vaccines (up to $7.50 for three doses, compared with just a few cents for the basic vaccines such as diphtheria-tetanus-pertussis, or DTP) has kept them beyond reach (S. Jarrett, UNICEF supply division, personal communication, 2003). But, even with this cost, one study for the former Children's Vaccine Initiative estimated that the Hib vaccine could be delivered as part of routine immunization in sub-Saharan Africa for just $21 to $22 per life-year saved.[7] This makes it highly attractive to governments, given that anything costing less than $25 per life-year saved is considered an excellent "buy." However, governments of developing countries have been unable to take advantage of the potential, and because of this, one recent assessment concluded that Hib vaccines have merely dented the global burden of this disease, reducing the estimated number of cases per year by less than 40,000.[2]

BASICS OF HIB

The vast majority of Hib infections are in children under the age of 5 years of age. The age group at greatest risk of Hib meningitis globally is infants aged 6 to 11 months. In this group, the estimated annual incidence is 67 per 100,000.[1] After age 2, the risk of contracting Hib meningitis drops sharply. Overall, among children under 5 years, 23 per 100,000 develop Hib meningitis each year.

Infection patterns differ around the world; in sub-Saharan Africa the number of new cases in infants up to 11 months old is around 200 for every 100,000 infants, compared with some 60 per 100,000 in the Americas. Europe and Asia appear to have lower rates. Within each region, certain populations appear to have exceptionally high risks of Hib infection, including Navajo Indians and Alaskan Indians in the United States and Australian Aborigines.

On average, 14% of the children who develop Hib meningitis die, a measure known as the case fatality rate.[1] This is similar to the overall case fatality rate for severe acute respiratory syndrome (SARS), which the WHO (2002) estimates to be 15%. However, this global average for Hib meningitis masks sharp differences between wealthy and poor countries in children's chances of surviving the disease. In industrialized countries, the case fatality rate is just 3.2%, because virtually all children who develop meningitis have access to emergency and adequate medical treatment. In developing countries overall, the case fatality rate is more than five times greater, at about 17%. In sub-Saharan Africa, where a high proportion of children lack access to specialized medical treatment, more than one in four affected children die, a case fatality rate of about 28%.[1] For every child who develops Hib meningitis in a given year, researchers estimate, about five children develop Hib pneumonia, making it the most common reason for death among those infected with this microbe.

The long-term impact on survivors of the disease is rarely taken into account in assessments of the social and economic costs of Hib. In the Gambia, only 55% of meningitis survivors fully recover; the rest may experience learning disabilities, neurological problems, deafness, and other major health and social problems.[8] And treatment for Hib disease is becoming more complicated with the spread of antibiotic-resistant strains of the microbe.

All figures are approximate, because Hib pneumonia is relatively difficult to diagnose. Doctors typically do not establish exactly which microbes are responsible for a child's pneumonia before treating it. For this reason, also, case fatality rates for Hib pneumonia are more difficult to document than rates for Hib meningitis.

Researchers base their estimates of the incidence of Hib pneumonia on what proportion of *all* pneumonia cases are prevented when Hib vaccines are given. In both the Gambia and Chile, studies in the 1990s showed that mass Hib vac-

BOX 20-1
Conjugate Vaccines

Until the late 1980s the only available Hib vaccines were based on the polysaccharide, or sugary, capsule of the bacterium. These vaccines protected older children and adults but not young infants, who were at greatest risk of infection, because their immune systems did not respond well to the vaccines. The new generation of conjugate vaccines contains two components: the Hib polysaccharide capsule and, attached to it, a "carrier" protein antigen such as tetanus toxoid. This antigen stimulates a strong T-cell-related immune response from the infant immune system. Several Hib conjugate vaccines have been licensed, including combinations with DTP and DTP plus hepatitis B.

cination reduced the incidence of confirmed cases of pneumonia of all types by just over 20%,[9,10] leading researchers to conclude that Hib is responsible for about a fifth of all severe pneumonia in children under 5 years of age in these two countries.

CHILE: EVIDENCE OF NEED AND PUBLIC DEMAND

Chile has an average income per person of $5,220,[11] a figure that puts it among middle-income nations. Its infrastructure is largely modern, and immunization services are efficient, with more than 95% of infants receiving routine vaccines.

Chile's first step toward introducing Hib vaccine came in the late 1980s, when researchers at the Ministry of Health first estimated the incidence of Hib disease in the Santiago area and concluded that it was an important public health problem.[12] Until this point, there had been no information about the extent of the disease in Chile. The researchers analyzed clinical and laboratory records between 1985 and 1987 at all seven government hospitals in the Santiago area. They matched these data with census records to estimate the incidence of Hib in the Santiago population of children under 5 years, which was estimated at 500,000 at that time. During the study period they identified 343 cases of laboratory-confirmed Hib disease, including 242 cases of meningitis; the remainder were other forms of invasive Hib disease—that is, Hib pneumonia, Hib bacteremia, and other severe forms of the disease. The peak age for infection was between 6 and 11 months, with the risk rapidly reducing after infants passed their first birthday.

At first glance, the figures suggested that the incidence of Hib was only about half as high as in infants in the United States at the same time. However, there were strong reasons to believe that the figures underestimated the true extent of Hib disease in Chile. Dr. Rosanna Lagos, a pediatrician at the Center for Vaccine Development in Santiago and an expert in Hib, explains that the team found sharp variation between hospitals in the rates at which bacteria from patients' samples were successfully detected and cultured in the laboratory. The process of isolating and culturing bacteria is difficult and depends on the specialist skills and capacity of the laboratory and its staff. In the northern area of the city, where the local hospital had a specialist interested in Hib, the rate of detection was twice as high as in the rest of the city. The researchers assumed that the specialist's estimate was likely to be more accurate and on this basis estimated that the annual incidence of Hib meningitis in the Santiago area was 32 per 100,000 in infants aged 5 months and under, and 63 per 100,000 in infants aged 6 to 11 months.[12,13] These figures are comparable with those in other temperate industrialized countries where Hib was endemic before immunization.

In addition to indicating that Hib was a widespread problem in Chile, the study also revealed that the proportion of children who died after contracting Hib disease in Santiago was relatively high, at 16%. (In industrialized countries the case fatality rate is below 4%.) The researchers reasoned that outside the city, where access to hospital treatment would likely be less widespread, the chances of death would be equal or greater.

ASSESSING THE FEASIBILITY AND EFFECTIVENESS OF NATIONAL HIB IMMUNIZATION

Although two Hib conjugate vaccines were licensed in Chile in 1992, they were not initially introduced into the country's routine immunization system. Their licensure had been based on evidence of their *efficacy*—their biological protective effect—in controlled trials in the industrialized countries. In Chile, however, the Ministry of Health had not been convinced that the high costs of the vaccine would justify its routine use. Once the disease burden had been shown to be significant, however, the ministry agreed in 1994 that researchers should further explore the use of the Hib vaccine.[13] Rather than performing a randomized clinical trial of the vaccine's efficacy in controlled conditions, the researchers did what is known as an "intent-to-vaccinate" study. This observed the *effectiveness* of the vaccine—its impact on a large population of infants receiving it in the normal conditions of a routine immunization service. Thirty-six primary health centers in Santiago were enrolled for the study and administered the vaccine with other routine immunizations for a year. The researchers assumed that some children would fail to turn up for immunization and that some would receive only one or two of the three required doses. For a comparison group, they observed children in 35 additional centers in the city where Hib vaccine would not be offered.

To minimize the number of shots for children and to increase cost effectiveness, the researchers tested a combination of Hib conjugate vaccine and the established DTP antigens in the same syringe. In the 35 centers that did not receive Hib, children received only DTP as usual. The total number of children involved was more than 70,000. The vaccine for the large-scale study was donated by the manufacturer, Pasteur Mérieux Serums et Vaccins of France, now Sanofi Pasteur; additional external support for the studies came from the US National Institute of Allergy and Infectious Diseases.

HIB DISEASE FALLS 90% IN A YEAR

The results of the study were dramatic. Researchers compared the number of new cases of Hib meningitis and pneumonia diagnosed during the study period in the two groups of health centers. Among the children in the health centers where Hib vaccine was available, the number of meningitis cases was reduced by 91%, and the number of cases of pneumonia and other forms of Hib disease were reduced by 80%, compared with children in the DTP-only centers.[14]

The vaccine had won its case. Not only was it effective but also feasible and practical for health centers to combine DTP and Hib vaccines and deliver them within the routine system. "At this point, the Ministry of Health decided that it was a good moment to do it," says Lagos. The ministry introduced the vaccine into the routine immunization program for babies throughout Chile, starting in July 1996 (see Figure 20-1).

AFFORDABILITY, SUSTAINABILITY, AND PUBLIC DEMAND

Although the Chilean government's decision was based on the public health evidence, there was also a strong public demand for immunization against meningitis. The government faced a complex situation. Dr. Fernando Muñoz of the Ministry of Health explains that before the vaccine was introduced into the national immunization program, it was already being recommended and administered by private pediatricians to families who could afford to pay. "The national program was facing the need to solve this equity failure," he says.

An entirely different political problem had emerged at the same time. Chile had recently suffered from outbreaks of a different type of meningitis, meningococcus type B. A private laboratory producing a vaccine against meningococcus type B was lobbying for its product to be introduced, and the media picked up and ran with the campaign. However, the evidence for the vaccine's efficacy in infants and toddlers was not convincing, says Muñoz. "The ministry faced a dilemma." By introducing the Hib vaccine, the government managed to offer the public something that was useful, albeit against a different form of meningitis, instead of a vaccine of questionable efficacy. While Hib meningitis had a lower popular profile than meningococcal meningitis, its burden was now known to be substantial, and it did at least have a vaccine that had proved itself in rigorous trials. Demand for the vaccine against meningococcus type B gradually faded, says Muñoz.

National pride also played a part. The fact that Uruguay had introduced the Hib vaccine two years earlier spurred action in Chile. "The Chilean program of immunizations is seen in Chile as one of the great achievements of Chilean

public health," says Muñoz. "We have always seen ourselves as pioneers in the field, and it is hard to accept losing leadership in the region."

The cost of the vaccine was initially substantial, accounting for about half of the total immunization program, but the government funded it in full with public funds from general taxes. By 2003, that figure had fallen: The ministry was paying $3.39 million for the combined DTP-Hib vaccine, or 22.9% of the total immunization budget, which was approximately 0.7% of government health expenditure. The price per Hib dose dropped from around $15 in 1996 to around $3 in 2003 (personal communication, F. Muñoz, Chilean Ministry of Health, December 2, 2003). And in 1998, researchers concluded that the nation would save $78 for every case of Hib prevented, providing further evidence to support the public expenditure.[13] "Under Chilean regulations, EPI [Expanded Programme on Immunization] vaccines are considered as public goods and are provided free of charge to all the population," he says.

THE GAMBIA: AN INVESTMENT AGAINST POVERTY

The Gambia is among the poorest countries, with an average annual income of $280 per person.[11] It is starkly different from Chile, with a much less developed infrastructure. For example, the country has about seven telephone lines per 100 people compared with almost 60 in Chile.[15] However, the country's immunization coverage—the proportion of all children immunized with basic vaccines such as DTP—is relatively high, at 85%, compared with many sub-Saharan African countries,[8] and it spends a higher proportion of its gross domestic product on health, approximately 3%, than many other low-income countries.

Better primary healthcare has substantially reduced infant mortality, but it remains high at 90 per 1,000 live births, based on 2001 figures.[15] This is twice as high as in South Africa, although well below the levels of some other very poor African countries such as Niger (about 190 per 1,000 live births) or Mali (about 150 per 1,000 live births).

Although Gambians' access to health care has improved, many people still walk several kilometers to the nearest health facility, and 10% of the population lives more than 7.5 kilometers from any facility. There are only four doctors for every 100,000 people, compared with 15 in Nigeria and more than 150 in China.[15] The Gambian government also acknowledges disparities between its regions in access to healthcare, particularly in the eastern, upriver part of the country, and that "underfunding of the health sector persist[s] at all levels."[16]

FIGURE 20-1 Impact of Hib vaccination.

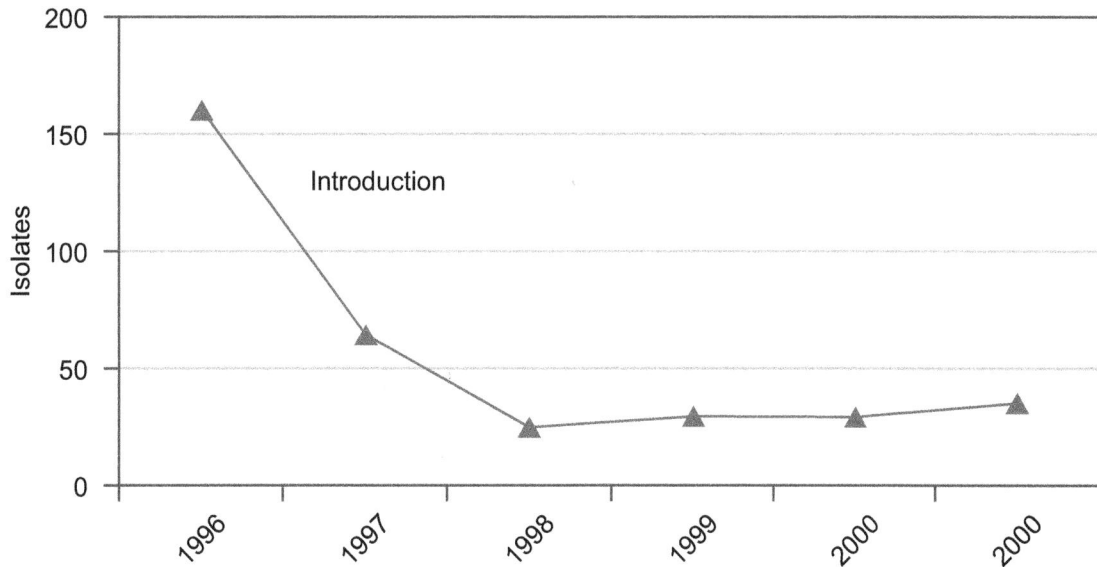

Source: Pan American Health Organization. "Monitoreo de las enfermedades causadas por Hib: Post-introducción de las vacunas." Presentation: XV Meeting of the Technical Advisory Group on Vaccine-preventable Diseases. Washington, DC: PAHO; 2002.

Many children are brought to clinics for immunization later than the recommended visits at 2, 3, and 4 months. "This is an important factor," says Dr. Richard Adegbola of the Medical Research Council Laboratories in Fajara, the Gambia. The age at which infants are most likely to become infected with Hib appears earlier in Africa than in higher-income settings such as the Americas; therefore, even slightly late vaccination puts children at very high risk of infection (personal communication, R. Adegbola, Medical Research Council Laboratories, June 2003).

Since 1990, the Gambia's health system has performed continuous surveillance of its infant population for Hib disease in the country's western region, where clinic, hospital, and laboratory facilities are adequate to effectively accomplish the task. In 1990, just over 200 children per 100,000 developed Hib meningitis each year.[9] Here, Hib struck younger, more seriously, and more frequently than in more developed countries: Less than half of patients make a full recovery from Hib disease in the Gambia, and a third of those that developed Hib meningitis died.[17]

New awareness of the scale of the Hib burden led the government and its international partners to take action. Between 1993 and 1995, researchers conducted a large, con-trolled trial of the Hib vaccine, involving 42,000 infants and requiring the participation of the three main hospitals and the health laboratories in the Gambia's western region. The trial used vaccine donated by its manufacturer Aventis Pasteur and was supported by a range of partners including the US Agency for International Development, World Health Organization (WHO), United Nations Children's Fund (UNICEF), the staff of the UK Medical Research Council, and others. Children were allocated at random to receive either DTP plus Hib vaccine or DTP alone. During the trial, and for up to 36 months afterward, all children with symptoms of invasive Hib disease (mainly meningitis and septicemia) were examined carefully with laboratory tests to culture bacteria, with lumbar punctures, blood tests, and chest X-rays as appropriate.

If any researchers expected the vaccine to produce a less dramatic effect in the Gambia than in an industrialized country, they were wrong. Compared with the children who received no Hib vaccine, the Hib-vaccinated group had 95% fewer cases of invasive Hib disease, confirming that the vaccine was as highly protective as in industrialized countries. The trial was also key in demonstrating the impact of the vaccine in reducing all types of pneumonia in Gambian infants by 21%, and a 60% protection against carriage in the child's second year.[17] As a result of the study, Dr. Kim Mulholland and his colleagues concluded that "the introduction of Hib vaccines into developing countries should substantially reduce childhood mortality from pneumonia and meningitis."[9]

FROM CLINICAL TRIAL TO MESSIER REALITY

The logical next step, then, was to introduce the vaccine into the national immunization program. However, cost was a major obstacle. Total expenditure on health in the Gambia is only $13 per person each year, with the government spending $6 per person and external funding and households contributing the remaining $7. And it costs $37 to fully immunize a child in the Gambia.[18,19] For at least the short- to medium-term, external support was needed to extend the benefits of the vaccine that the trial participants had enjoyed to the rest of the population—and to maintain those benefits for the participants' families.

A key question was whether the vaccine would work as well in real-life Gambian conditions as in a clinical trial. As in other low-income countries, health services in the Gambia struggle with interruptions in the vaccination supply chain, breakdown of refrigerators, and staff shortages, all of which can interfere with the delivery of immunization. Plus, the lack of coordination among funding sources can cause resources to be wasted; for some years, the program had in stock 14 ice-lined refrigerators, five refrigerators, six freezer-refrigerators, and one freezer—but none were in use.[19] Although the Gambia has invested considerable effort in improving its vaccine cold chain with the use of solar power and decentralizing vaccine storage and health care management to get vaccines where they are needed in a timely fashion,[16] the system is far from perfect. Researchers and health officials decided to perform a large-scale, long-range study of its effectiveness.

In 1997, an agreement was signed between the prime minister of the Gambia and Aventis Pasteur to carry out the study, involving the population of the country's western region, where about half the country's 1 million inhabitants live. Aventis Pasteur donated the vaccine for a five-year period. Between May 1997 and April 2002, the vaccine was administered routinely as part of the national (EPI), with continuous surveillance for cases of Hib disease. The study was conducted by Adegbola and others at the Medical Research Council Laboratories in Fajara, the Gambia, together with colleagues at the Gambian Ministry of Health, the Royal Victoria Hospital in Banjul, and the WHO. An interim report was published in 1999,[8] and the final results have now been reported to the WHO.[20]

SAVING LIVES

Adegbola and his colleagues have watched Hib virtually disappear. The number of children developing Hib meningitis dropped almost tenfold, from 200 per 100,000 to 21 per 100,000 in the 12-month period after the start of routine immunization. By the fifth year after routine immunization began, this incidence was reduced to zero.[17] Of the rapidly dwindling numbers of children who did develop the disease—fewer than 50—more than half had not been vaccinated, while all but two of the remainder had received incomplete immunization of just one or two doses. In the last two years of the study, there were just two cases; no cases have been reported in western Gambia since 2002.[17] Two doses of the vaccine demonstrated a 94% efficacy. The results demonstrate that this vaccine can be highly effective even in an impoverished country where the health system faces numerous logistic and financial challenges.

Equally important, says Adegbola, the vaccine appears to stop children from carrying Hib bacteria in their noses and throats and therefore reduces the transmission of the microbe from one person to another. Before the study, about 10% of children were Hib "carriers," but with the introduction of the vaccine this figure has dropped to less than 1% (personal communication, Adegbola, June 2003). This is particularly significant given the delays in immunizing some infants because the reduced transmission helps create herd immunity. "Even if children don't receive the vaccine at the time they are most susceptible, this [reduced carriage] tends to have an [additional] effect," says Adegbola.

Adegbola and colleagues note that the Gambia's success in virtually eliminating Hib disease was achieved even despite an irregular vaccine supply marked by periodic interruptions. Fewer than 70% of children completed the full schedule of immunizations and many of the vaccine doses were late. Thus, the country's experience provides encouraging evidence that Hib elimination can be achieved in other developing countries with strong but imperfect immunization delivery. With even modest immunization coverage and suboptimal conditions, all children can benefit.

ANOTHER FIVE YEARS

The agreement with Aventis Pasteur to provide free vaccine has now run its course. However, the Gambian government is able to continue providing Hib immunization to all children nationwide for at least five more years, starting in 2003. This is due to support from the Global Alliance for Vaccines and Immunization (GAVI), a partnership set up in 2000 between governments and their international partners, including

WHO, UNICEF, the World Bank, the Bill & Melinda Gates Foundation, and the vaccine industry. GAVI supports low-income countries to improve access to vaccines against major killers, including new and underused vaccines such as Hib and hepatitis B, by buying vaccines and investing in improved immunization services. In the longer term, the alliance seeks to enable governments to mobilize new resources for immunization from within their own budgets and from other sources, so that they can provide sustainable services.

OTHER LOW-INCOME COUNTRIES ADOPT HIB VACCINE

Other developing countries are now using the Hib vaccine. Most countries in Latin America and the Caribbean include the Hib vaccine as part of their routine EPI, thanks in part to the successful experiences of Chile and Uruguay, and the initial technical and financial support of the Pan American Health Organization in 1997 and 1998. Researchers concluded that the benefits of introducing Hib vaccine in the Cape Town area alone exceeded the costs of treating the disease by up to $500,000.[21] So, in 1999 South Africa started to include Hib immunization as part of its national program. With a major international effort and financial and techni-

cal support from the partners in GAVI, 10 additional low-income countries introduced Hib immunization in 2003 and 2004, providing protection for an additional 4 million children in total each year. Results are encouraging: A recent study demonstrated that three years after Kenya introduced Hib vaccine into its routine immunization program, rates of the disease were down 88%, preventing more than 3,000 hospitalizations per year.[22] By 2007, the vaccine will be introduced in several additional Asian countries, including Malaysia, Mongolia, and Sri Lanka, where the disease burden has recently shown to be higher than previously expected.[23]

The final chapter in the Hib story is not yet written. Whether large numbers of developing countries where Hib disease is a major problem will choose to introduce and sustain the use of the vaccine is not yet known. It depends in part on how and whether financing is made available—and how expensive the vaccine is over the medium term. The health impact in regions of the world where Hib vaccine has not yet been used on a large scale is also unknown, and researchers are following closely to see whether the positive experiences now being consolidated in Latin America and the Caribbean, and parts of Africa, will be shared elsewhere.

REFERENCES

1. Bennett JV, Platonov AE, Slack MPE, Mala P, Burton AH, Robertson SE. Haemophilus influenzae *type b (Hib) Meningitis in the Pre-Vaccine Era: A Global Review of Incidence, Age Distributions, and Case Fatality Rates*. Geneva, Switzerland: World Health Organization; 2002. WHO/V&B/02.18.

2. Peltola H. Worldwide *Haemophilus influenzae* type b disease at the beginning of the 21st century: global analysis of the disease burden 25 years after the use of the polysaccharide vaccine and a decade after the advent of conjugates. *Clin Microbiol Rev*. 2000;13(2):302–317.

3. World Health Organization. *The State of the World's Vaccines and Immunization*. Geneva, Switzerland: World Health Organization; 2002.

4. Adams WG, Deaver KA, Cochi SL, et al. Decline of childhood *Haemophilus influenzae* type b (Hib) disease in the Hib vaccine era. *JAMA*. 1993;269(2):221–226.

5. Slack M P, Azzopardi HJ, Hargreaves RM, Ramsay ME. Enhanced surveillance of invasive *Haemophilus influenzae* disease in England, 1990 to 1996: impact of conjugate vaccines. *Pediatr Infect Dis J*. 1998;17(suppl 9):S204–S207.

6. Peltola H, Kilpi T, Anttila M. Rapid disappearance of *Haemophilus influenzae* type b meningitis after routine childhood immunisation with conjugate vaccines. *Lancet*. 1992;340(8819):592–594.

7. Miller M, McCann L. Policy analysis of the use of hepatitis B, *Haemophilus influenzae* type b, *Streptococcus pneumonia*, and rotavirus vaccines in national immunization schedules. *Health Econ*. 2000;1:19–35.

8. Adegbola R, Usen SO, Weber M. *Haemophilus influenzae* type b meningitis in the Gambia after the introduction of a conjugate vaccine. *Lancet*. 1999;354(9184):1091–1092.

9. Mulholland K, Hilton S, Adegbola R, et al. Randomised trial of *Haemophilus influenzae* type b tetanus protein conjugate for prevention of pneumonia and meningitis in Gambian infants. *Lancet*. 1997;349:1191–1197.

10. Levine OS, Lagos R, Muñoz A. Defining the burden of pneumonia in children preventable by vaccination against *Haemophilus influenzae* type b. *Pediatr Infect Dis J*. 1999;18:1060–1064.

11. World Bank. *World Development Indicators*. Washington, DC: World Bank; 2004.

12. Ferreccio C, Ortiz E, Astroza L, Rivera C, Clemens J, Levine MM. A population-based retrospective assessment of the disease burden resulting from invasive *Haemophilus influenzae* in infants and young children in Santiago, Chile. *Pediatr Infect Dis J*. 1999;9(7):488–494.

13. Lagos R, Levine OS, Avendano A, Horwitz I, Levine MM. The introduction of routine *Haemophilus influenzae* type b conjugate vaccine in Chile: a framework for evaluating new vaccines in newly industrializing countries. *Pediatr Infect Dis J*. 1998;17(suppl 9):S139–S148.

14. Lagos R, Horwitz I, Toro J, Martin O, Bustamante PC. Large scale, post-licensure, selective vaccination of Chilean infants with PRP-T conjugate vaccine: practicality and effectiveness in preventing *Haemophilus influenzae* type b infections. *Pediatr Infect Dis J*. 1996;15:216–222.

15. United Nations Development Program. *Human Development Report*. New York, NY: United Nations Development Program; 2003.

16. Government of the Gambia. Proposal for support submitted to the Global Alliance for Vaccines and Immunization (GAVI) and the Vaccine Fund. August 2001. The Gambia Government EPI Review (quoted by Richard Adegbola, personal communication, May 8, 2003).

17. Adegbola RA, Secka O, Lahai G, et al. Elimination of *Haemophilus influenzae* type b (Hib) disease from the Gambia after the introduction of routine immunisation with a Hib conjugate vaccine: a prospective study. *Lancet*. 2005;366:144–150.

18. Department of State for Health and Social Welfare, the Gambia. Chapter 7—Health expenditures. Available at: http://www.dosh.gm/docs/general/per/PER _Chapter_7_Health_Expenditures.pdf. Accessed February 9, 2004.

19. Department of State for Health and Social Welfare, the Gambia. Details of Expenditure. Available at: http://www.dosh.gm/docs/budget. Accessed February 11, 2004.

20. Adegbola R. *Final Report: Introduction of* Haemophilus influenzae *type b Vaccination into the Gambia—An Effectiveness Study*. Geneva, Switzerland: World Health Organization; 2003.

21. Hussey GD, Lasser ML, Reekie WD. The costs and benefits of a vaccination programme for *Haemophilus influenzae* type b disease. *S Afr Med J*. 1995;85(1):20–25.

22. Cowgill KD, Ndiritu M, Nyiro J, et al. Effectiveness of *Haemophilus influenzae* type b conjugate vaccine introduction into routine childhood immunization in Kenya. *JAMA*. 2006;296:671–678.

23. Gessner BD, Sutanto A, Linehan M, et al. Incidence of vaccine-preventable *Haemophilus influenzae* type b pneumonia and meningitis in Indonesian children: hamlet-randomised vaccine-probe trial. *Lancet*. 2005;365:43–52.

APPENDIX A

Millions Saved Methods

The What Works Working Group was convened to answer the question "what works in global health?" by finding and documenting a set of large-scale international health interventions judged to be successful on the basis of objective criteria.

The Working Group, brought together under the auspices of the Center for Global Development's Global Health Policy Research Network, benefited from the participation of 16 experts in international health, development economics, public policy, and other relevant fields. Although members participated in their individual capacities, they came from a spectrum of institutional, disciplinary, and geographic homes and brought a range of perspectives to the table. The Working Group also benefited from a close working relationship with the Disease Control Priorities Project in Developing Countries (DCPP) of the Fogarty International Center at the US National Institutes of Health, which recruited many of the world's leading authorities to prepare state-of-the-art papers on specific health conditions and dimensions of health systems. This work was published as *Disease Control Priorities in Developing Countries,* 2nd edition (2006).

The Working Group followed a series of steps to select the cases represented in the book:

- Established the criteria for "success" and agreed upon what would constitute adequate evidence. The criteria were scale, importance, impact, duration, and cost-effectiveness.
- Solicited candidate cases from the experts recruited by the DCPP
- Based on the suggestions and background materials provided by the DCPP authors, as well as additional library research and consultation, determined which

cases best fit the criteria for success and had the strongest evidence base—supported by peer-reviewed journal articles and official project evaluations
- Prepared case texts based on documentary information and interviews with key informants, and asked technical experts knowledgeable about the intervention to review the texts to correct errors of fact

LIMITATIONS

As with every effort to capture and make sense of part of a complicated world, this project has limitations. In this case, there are limits to what we can infer because of our methods. To start with, we looked only at successes rather than at "failures" and thus can only make educated guesses about whether the elements we have identified are in fact specific to successful experiences.* Because we insisted on a clear causal chain between the program and a health outcome, the sample may be skewed toward more "disease- or condition-focused" experiences than if we had relaxed our standard of evidence. So, for example, we were unable to include management and financing reform cases because even those that document a change in utilization rarely if ever link that to a change in health status. We also primarily depended on English-language sources and likely missed important work available only in other languages.

Although we tried to understand the context within which the experience occurred, we viewed success through

---

* We considered examining "failures," but the lack of documentation about these experiences prevented any systematic effort.

an admittedly narrow frame and time period. We cannot claim that the cases in any way represent the optimal use of resources or left other important programs or populations better off or unaffected. It is indeed possible that the political attention, funding, and management effort that were instrumental in the successes documented here ended up making other initiatives within the health sector worse off—deprived of attention and resources—during the same period and after. This simply cannot be known from the data we have available. And while these programs were successful during the 5-year or longer period covered in the case texts, success is fragile. In fact, the future of several of these well-established public health successes is endangered because the health condition they address has slipped from public consciousness and political priorities, or because of conflict and social upheaval.

Discussion Questions

INTRODUCTION

1. *Human capital* is a term used to describe individuals' stock of health and education that is associated with their ability to be productive workers. What can you say about the differences in human capital in high-, middle- and low-income countries? And how is human capital related to the patterns of income and poverty? Consider how human capital leads to economic growth and poverty reduction. Consider how slow economic growth and poverty reduce the opportunities for increases in human capital.

2. What are the main ways in which economic development affects health? Consider both micro- (or household-) and macro- (or national-) level dimensions of this relationship: at the microlevel, the role of increased household income that results in better nutrition and access to health services; at the macrolevel, the ways in which a growing economy can permit the development of better delivery of health services. What is the correlation between infant mortality and per capita GDP? Prepare a graph and describe what you see; speculate about the reasons behind the patterns observed.

3. What could account for the improvements in health conditions in the developing world? Consider improvements in living conditions, nutrition, access to health services, and medical advances. What are ways in which economic development can have a negative impact on health, such as through the adoption of unhealthful behaviors, opening of markets to tobacco and low-nutrition foods, movement of people (and diseases) across borders, and other phenomena?

4. Which is more important, diseases that affect children, or diseases that affect working-age adults? Explore the meaning of *important*—important for social welfare, for economic growth, on moral or ethical grounds, and so on.

5. Do governments of rich countries have a responsibility to help poor countries achieve better health? Why or why not? How do you think national governments in wealthy countries act relative to the "right" approach. Are governments in high-income countries consistent in their policies? How have they responded to the AIDS crisis differently from other health problems in the developing world? Why?

6. Which regions of the developing world are the healthiest? Least healthy? What do you think explains this variation?

7. Why did the authors choose to look only at programs that operated at a national, regional, or global level? What are the challenges that programs face in "scaling up" pilot projects to a national scale?

8. The authors chose to examine programs that operated for at least five years, not necessarily those that are "financially sustainable." What is the difference between duration and sustainability? How would it be possible to identify financially sustainable programs?

9. What is cost-effectiveness? Why is this a criterion that policy makers and program planners care about?

10. How do the criteria affect the types of programs and/or interventions that are highlighted in the book?

CASE 1: ERADICATING SMALLPOX

1. Define eradication, extinction, elimination, and control.

2. Describe the characteristics of smallpox that made it an appropriate candidate for eradication.

3. Should a measles eradication program be initiated? Why or why not?

4. If polio is eradicated, should we destroy all poliovirus samples? Why or why not?

5. In 1965, why didn't the World Health Organization immediately undertake a full-scale eradication program after endorsement by the World Health Assembly?

CASE 2: PREVENTING HIV/AIDS AND SEXUALLY TRANSMITTED INFECTIONS IN THAILAND

1. What are the characteristics of the high-risk population that permitted this intervention to work? What are the implications of this for replication in other settings?

2. Is Thailand a model for programs in other countries? Why or why not?

3. A cost-effectiveness assessment was never done for this program. What should such an assessment have taken into account in terms of costs measured?

4. What current challenges face the Thailand AIDS program?

5. What are some of the other national experiences in AIDS prevention that have been cited in the popular press as "successes"? What evidence can you find in the scientific literature about the effectiveness of these programs?

CASE 3: CONTROLLING TUBERCULOSIS IN CHINA

1. What are some of the factors that contribute to the high burden of tuberculosis in China?

2. How might Russia and Eastern Europe benefit from the Chinese model?

3. What countries have the highest burden of multidrug-resistant TB? What do you think explains this pattern?

4. Is directly observed therapy coercive? Why or why not? Under what conditions does the state have the right to require individuals with communicable diseases to undergo treatment?

5. In addition to the implementation of the DOTS program, what else should the Chinese government be doing to reduce the burden of TB?

CASE 4: REDUCING CHILD MORTALITY THROUGH VITAMIN A IN NEPAL

1. What are the pros and cons of supplementation, dietary intake, and fortification?

2. What are incentives? How were they used in this case to motivate certain behaviors?

3. The use of female community health volunteers is an innovation in health service delivery. Discuss some of the social and political reasons that made them a success in Nepal.

4. Why do you think technical experts questioned the original observations about the impact of vitamin A on child mortality? Can you think of other instances in which the scale-up of a successful health intervention was delayed because of similar obstacles?

5. Can the vitamin A program in Nepal be replicated in other countries? What kinds of countries might see similar success? What countries might not?

CASE 5: ELIMINATING POLIO IN LATIN AMERICA AND THE CARIBBEAN

1. What were the starting conditions in the region of the Americas that facilitated the achievement of polio elimination?

2. Which societies and groups will benefit most from polio eradication?

3. Could or should interagency coordinating committees be established for general health programs?

4. In what ways did the polio elimination campaign strengthen the basic health system? How might you see polio eradication weakening the delivery of basic health services?

5. How might the polio eradication initiative contribute to the preparedness for and mitigation of avian influenza?

CASE 6: SAVING MOTHERS' LIVES IN SRI LANKA

1. What are the cultural and historical features of Sri Lanka that contributed to the success of the program?

2. If a country pursues a strategy of professionalizing midwifery as the "first line" support for prenatal care and delivery, what are the other elements of the health care delivery system that need to be in place?

3. How do you think conflict and civil unrest affect the health of women and families in Sri Lanka? What policy priorities would you pursue if you were the Health Minister? President?

4. Looking at countries that have a similar per capita GDP to Sri Lanka, what can you say about health status (e.g., maternal and infant mortality)? What are the main causes of maternal death in one or more of those countries? Are there strategies that Sri Lanka has employed that would address those causes of death?

5. In Sri Lanka, the government's ability to track trends in maternal deaths through the vital registration system was important to the implementation of their program. What are some of the difficulties that poor countries face in developing such systems? What alternatives to vital registration are used to measure maternal mortality? What are the pros and cons of alternative approaches?

CASE 7: CONTROLLING ONCHOCERCIASIS (RIVER BLINDNESS) IN SUB-SAHARAN AFRICA

1. How did the development of ivermectin improve the chances for success of this program? Does Merck have a sound "corporate conscience"? Why or why not?

2. What are the pros and cons of depending on drug donations for the implementation of a key health program? How were the challenges managed in this case?

3. What are the replicable characteristics of this public–private partnership in West Africa? What other diseases might be pursued by this type of regional program? What are the political requirements to make this type of regional program work?

4. Onchocerciasis control has had significant economic benefits by increasing the productivity of workers and making large rural areas habitable and arable. What are some other tropical diseases whose control could yield large economic benefits?

CASE 8: PREVENTING DIARRHEAL DEATHS IN EGYPT

1. How might we better address the cause of diarrheal disease? What might be done, for example, regarding clean water and sanitation?

2. How did the program change the attitudes and behavior of health professionals, and why was this important, given that ORT is a home-based treatment?

3. What are the cultural determinants of diarrheal disease in Egypt?

4. Are social marketing and public–private sector partnerships effective modes of intervention to decrease the incidence of and morbidity/mortality due to diarrheal disease? What other health interventions have used such methods?

5. In Bangladesh, a large nongovernmental organization implemented the ORT program. What are the potential advantages and disadvantages of NGO involvement in health service delivery?

CASE 9: IMPROVING THE HEALTH OF THE POOR IN MEXICO

1. Consider the compact of coresponsibility between the government and recipients. What is needed to make the compact work?

2. Why were the cash grants given to mothers? Do you think this was a good idea or a bad one? What might have been the positive and negative consequences of this choice?

3. Progresa established a type of entitlement program that now accounts for a relatively large share of the government's expenditures. What are the factors that designers should have taken into consideration regarding the sustainability of the program over time?

4. What are the preconditions for a successful conditional cash transfer program?

CASE 10: CONTROLLING TRACHOMA IN MOROCCO

1. What are the major causes of blindness in the developing world? What is the burden of blindness worldwide, and which regions are most affected? What are the economic and social consequences of blindness for developing nations?

2. Trachoma was eliminated in the United States before the advent of antibiotics to treat the disease. What are the factors that contributed to its decline in the United States? What does this tell us about the measures that should be taken in developing countries still affected by trachoma?

3. How might trachoma control in Morocco strengthen health service delivery for other diseases? In general?

4. Could this program be successfully implemented in Uganda or Ethiopia in your opinion? Why? Why not?

5. What do you think motivated Pfizer to donate antibiotics to treat trachoma? What are your views about the behavior of for-profit multinational pharmaceutical companies, and does this case alter your view?

CASE 11: REDUCING GUINEA WORM IN ASIA AND SUB-SAHARAN AFRICA

1. When will guinea worm disease be eradicated? What is hampering eradication efforts? Is control enough for guinea worm disease?

2. The fundamental intervention for guinea worm is behavior change. What does the guinea worm example tell us about the components of successful behavior change programs for other public health problems? Why did behavioral change work in guinea worm disease control? Can you think of another disease where behavior change can mitigate the public health impact so it is no longer a public health problem?

3. Why is it important in the guinea worm case—and for other similar parasitic diseases—to use DALYs instead of mortality as the indicator of severity of the problem? Consider the need to incorporate the toll of morbidity into the estimate of the burden of disease for ailments like guinea worm.

4. Conflict in sub-Saharan African countries has impeded progress of the guinea worm control campaign. What are some strategies that can or have been used to pursue public health goals in the face of civil strife?

5. What are the economic benefits of controlling parasitic disease? What evidence can you find in the literature that demonstrates the economic importance of parasites (hint: look at the historical experience of hookworm in the southeastern United States).

CASE 12: CONTROLLING CHAGAS DISEASE IN THE SOUTHERN CONE OF SOUTH AMERICA

1. Do you think the seven governments involved would have initiated the program in 1991 without PAHO? Beyond PAHO's influence, what aspects of this disease encouraged a regional effort?

2. Why was a regional approach so important in the control of Chagas disease? What other diseases can be controlled only with a regional effort?

3. The development of a new pesticide represented a turning point in the battle against Chagas. What were the benefits to the program of the new pesticide?

4. In what way does the Chagas case demonstrate the fragility of "success"? What are the technical, political, and financial inputs needed to maintain vigilance in control of a disease like Chagas?

5. Because the vector for Chagas thrives in traditional housing materials, it is a disease of poverty. Should the governments of the region have focused on poverty reduction in affected areas rather than the control of a specific disease? Why or why not?

CASE 13: REDUCING FERTILITY IN BANGLADESH

1. Is the reduction in fertility better or comparable to other population or reproductive health programs? How does the annual rate of fertility reduction for Bangladesh over the last 25 years compare to Kenya? India?

2. What do you think education has to do with fertility? Give examples.

3. What are five ways fertility affects development?

4. Will delay of age of marriage and/or birth spacing guarantee fertility reduction? Why? Why not?

5. What sorts of questions can be answered using longitudinal data collection such as is possible in the Matlab setting? Are there other ways to answer such questions? Consider the ability to answer questions about how specific outreach or other service delivery approaches affects demand for and use of services, long-term trends in family formation, fertility, women's labor market participation, and so forth.

CASE 14: CURBING TOBACCO USE IN POLAND

1. How might programs focus on youth and smoking in Poland? What social, behavioral, and epidemiologic trends should be monitored to track program impact over the long term?

2. How did advocates and scientists in Poland and South Africa take advantage of a political transition to advance their cause?

3. Do you think that the transition to democracy in both countries was necessary for the successful control efforts? What does this suggest about the relationship between democracy and health? Can you think of examples that contradict your answer? Consider successful health programs in nondemocratic countries, such as the two China cases or Cuba's successful health system.

4. What are the factors that account for the growing smoking problem in the developing world? What are the economic consequences of this phenomenon?

5. Describe and discuss the changes in smoking behavior in China and the potential health consequences. If you were an antitobacco advocate in China, what would you focus on?

CASE 15: PREVENTING IODINE DEFICIENCY DISEASE IN CHINA

1. The universality of salt makes iodine fortification effective. List three other candidates of "universal foods" that could be fortified with other micronutrients such as vitamin A, zinc, iron, and folic acid.

2. What factors are required to successfully deliver a micronutrient at a population level?

3. What are the economic consequences of a high prevalence of iodine deficiency? How do those compare to the costs of an effective intervention to prevent the disease?

4. If the fortified salt is produced by commercial suppliers, what is the role of the government in an iodized salt program? Consider the need for standard setting, regulation, enforcement, data collection, surveillance, and health education and health communications.

CASE 16: PREVENTING NEURAL-TUBE DEFECTS IN CHILE

1. Characterize the public–private partnership that was key to the success of Chile's fortification intervention.

2. Is Chile's fortification experience replicable in Africa? Why or why not?

3. Neural-tube defects affect a fairly small portion of the population compared to diseases like malaria and TB. What are some of the reasons a Minister of Health might choose to address NTDs? Can you think of other diseases with a similar profile?

4. There are different types of evaluation discussed in the chapter. Explain the differences between each, and the questions each are meant to address.

5. Chile's leadership in the region has influenced adoption of health interventions outside its borders. Can you identify other instances where the leadership of a country has inspired public health improvements in a region or around the world?

CASE 17: ELIMINATING MEASLES IN SOUTHERN AFRICA

1. In 2003, 610,000 children died from measles. Why? If a good vaccine exists, what are the factors that limit immunization in many countries in Africa and South Asia?

2. What measles immunization priorities should be considered in conflict and humanitarian emergency situations? What different priorities might be pursued in the emergency, recovery, and development stages?

3. Why does Nigeria have such high rates of measles mortality? Consider five to eight reasons.

4. What were the starting conditions in the seven countries that facilitated the success observed? Are these same conditions present throughout the sub-Saharan African region?

5. How did the polio eradication campaign stimulate progress on control of measles? Is measles a good candidate for eradication? Why or why not?

CASE 18: PREVENTING DENTAL CARIES IN JAMAICA

1. Are dental carries and dental health a global public health issue? Should dental health be a priority?

2. If you were health minister in Ethiopia, what proportion of your annual budget would you spend on dental health? What would you do?

3. What are the economic and social consequences of dental caries? Why might Jamaican children have particularly high prevalence of dental problems (before the salt fortification)?

4. Why was water fluoridation not the right approach in Jamaica, as it is in the United States? What would have been the consequences had the authorities chosen to fluoridate the water? Consider how improvements would have been seen only among children with access to publicly provided water—typically from wealthier families.

5. What are the arguments against community-level fortification interventions such as salt fluoridation? Do you agree or disagree with those arguments? What do you think it would take to convince those who believe that fluoridation of water or salt is a bad idea?

CASE 19: TREATING CATARACTS IN INDIA

1. Why were management and training such important parts of the cataract program in India?

2. What were three of the most important contributions of the Aravind Eye Hospital to the design and implementation of the cataract surgery program?

3. Are there other types of surgery that are "low-cost" and can be implemented at scale, the way cataract surgery is?

4. What do you think the World Bank provided in this program, beyond the financing?

5. What are the types of costs and benefits that should be taken into account for an economic analysis of the value of the cataract surgery program?

CASE 20: PREVENTING HIB DISEASE IN CHILE AND THE GAMBIA

1. If you were a minister of health, what would you need to know prior to making a decision to include Hib in your country's immunization schedule? Should Hib vaccine be added to the six routine childhood immunizations worldwide?

2. In Chile, why was it important that the technical personnel had the relevant data about the potential benefits of Hib vaccination at the time of the meningitis outbreak, even though the meningitis could not be prevented by the vaccine?

3. What were some of the real-world features of the Gambia that helped to make the case that delivery of Hib vaccine can be done in an African setting?

4. What are the immunization rates in Latin America? Which countries have the highest rates? Which countries have the lowest rates? What are some of the factors that account for the relatively good performance of the immunization program in Latin America, compared to the countries of South Asia and sub-Saharan Africa?

5. How widely has Hib been introduced in developing countries? What are some of the concerns that have been voiced about its introduction?

Glossary

Burden of disease.	An indicator that quantifies the loss of healthy life from disease and injury.
Child mortality.	The probability of dying between birth and age 5, expressed per 1,000 live births. The term *under-5 mortality* is also used.
Cold chain.	A transportation and storage system used to keep and distribute heat-sensitive vaccines at the correct temperature until they reach the users.
Cost-effectiveness.	Analysis of the net gain in health or reduction in disease burden resulting from a health intervention in relation to the cost. Cost-effectiveness analysis helps identify interventions that are likely to produce the greatest improvements in health status for the available resources and is measured in dollars per disability-adjusted life-year.
Disability-adjusted life-year (DALY).	An indicator developed for the calculation of disease burden that quantifies, in a single indicator, time lost due to premature death with time lived with a disability. It is calculated as the present value of the future years of disability-free life that are lost as the result of the premature deaths or cases of disability occurring in a particular year.
Elimination.	Reduction of the number of new infections to zero in a defined geographic area, with continued interventions required to prevent reestablishment of transmission.
Eradication.	The permanent reduction to zero of new infections worldwide.
Global burden of disease.	An indicator that quantifies the loss of healthy life from disease, measured in disability-adjusted life-years.
Intervention (in health care).	A specific activity meant to reduce disease risks, treat illness, or palliate the consequences of disease and disability.
Life expectancy.	The age to which a newborn baby survives.
Maternal mortality.	The death of a woman while pregnant or within two months after pregnancy.
Outreach.	Disease prevention and health promotion activities that are aimed at segments of the general population, outside of hospitals, clinics, and other service delivery sites. Often, outreach refers to activities in which health workers conduct home visits to provide information and basic health commodities, and to refer patients or clients to services.

Surveillance.   The ongoing systematic collection and analysis of data about an infectious disease, which can lead to action being taken to control or prevent the disease. Effective surveillance systems detect health events; collect epidemiological, clinical, and/or laboratory information; and investigate and confirm cases and outbreaks.

Total fertility rate.   The average number of children borne by each woman; a synthetic measure based on current levels of age-specific fertility.

Vertical program.   Such health programs deliver health services, often through a disease-specific intervention, that are not fully integrated in the services of the health systems. Traditionally, vertical programs have had a centralized management structure and reporting and accounting systems that are separate from the government systems. In many but not all cases, external donors largely finance vertical programs.

Index

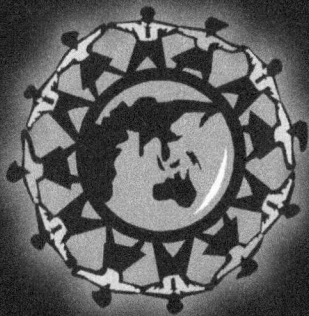

The
ESSENTIAL PUBLIC HEALTH SERIES
from Jones and Bartlett Publishers

Essential Public Health is an introductory series that captures the full range of issues that affect the public's health from the impact of AIDS to the cost of health care. Edited by Richard Riegelman, the series takes the big picture "population health" perspective by introducing concepts and content that are fundamental to the study and practice of public health. The series will be closely tied to the new public health core competencies, which will serve as the basis for the certifying examination by the National Board of Public Health Examiners.

CURRENT AND FORTHCOMING TITLES IN THE SERIES:

Public Health 101: Healthy People–Healthy Populations
Richard Riegelman, MD, MPH, PhD

Essentials of Public Health
Bernard J. Turnock, MD, MPH

Essential Case Studies in Public Health: Putting Public Health into Practice
Katherine Hunting, PhD, MPH & Brenda L. Gleason, MA, MPH

Essentials of Evidence-Based Public Health
Richard Riegelman, MD, MPH, PhD

Epidemiology 101
Robert H. Friis, PhD

Essentials of Infectious Disease Epidemiology
Manya Magnus, PhD, MPH

Essential Readings in Infectious Disease Epidemiology
Manya Magnus, PhD, MPH

Essentials of Biostatistics in Public Health
Lisa M. Sullivan, PhD (with Workbook: *Statistical Computations Using Excel*)

Essentials of Public Health Biology: A Guide for the Study of Pathophysiology
Constance Urciolo Battle, MD

Essentials of Environmental Health
Robert H. Friis, PhD

Essentials of Global Health
Richard Skolnik, MPA

Case Studies in Global Health: Millions Saved
Ruth Levine, PhD & the What Works Working Group

Essentials of Health, Culture, and Diversity
Mark Edberg, PhD

Essentials of Health Behavior: Social and Behavioral Theory in Public Health
Mark Edberg, PhD

Essential Readings in Health Behavior: Theory and Practice
Mark Edberg, PhD

Essentials of Health Policy and Law
Joel B. Teitelbaum, JD, LLM & Sara E. Wilensky, JD, MPP

Essential Readings in Health Policy and Law
Joel B. Teitelbaum, JD, LLM & Sara E. Wilensky, JD, MPP

Essentials of Health Economics
Diane M. Dewar, PhD

Essentials of Community Health
Jaime Gofin, MD, MPH & Rosa Gofin, MD, MPH

Essentials of Program Planning and Evaluation
Karen McDonnell, PhD

Essentials of Public Health Communication and Informatics
Claudia Parvanta, PhD; Patrick Remington, MD, MPH; Ross Brownson, PhD; & David E. Nelson, MD, MPH

Essentials of Public Health Ethics
Ruth Gaare Bernheim, JD, MPH & James F. Childress, PhD

Essentials of Management and Leadership in Public Health
Robert Burke, PhD & Leonard Friedman, PhD, MPH

Essentials of Public Health Preparednes
Rebecca Katz, PhD, MPH

ABOUT THE EDITOR:
Richard Riegelman, MD, MPH, PhD is professor of Epidemiology-Biostatistics, Medicine, and Health Policy and founding dean at George Washington University School of Public Health and Health Services in Washington, DC.